ADVANCES IN CANCER RESEARCH

VOLUME 21

Contributors to This Volume

A. J. Bedford

Baruj Benacerraf

Ernest H. Y. Chu

G. B. Clements

E. H. Cooper

M. Essex

David H. Katz

T. E. Kenny

Keen A. Rafferty, Jr.

Michael B. Shimkin

Gary D. Stoner

James E. Trosko

ADVANCES IN CANCER RESEARCH

Edited by

GEORGE KLEIN
Department of Tumor Biology
Karolinska Institutet
Stockholm, Sweden

SIDNEY WEINHOUSE
Fels Research Institute
Temple University Medical School
Philadelphia, Pennsylvania

Consulting Editor

ALEXANDER HADDOW
Chester Beatty Research Institute
Institute of Cancer Research
Royal Cancer Hospital
London, England

Volume 21 — 1975

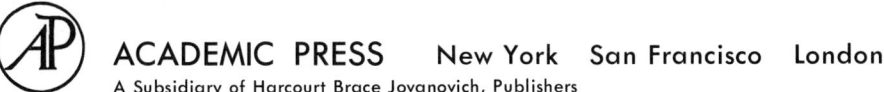

ACADEMIC PRESS   New York   San Francisco   London
A Subsidiary of Harcourt Brace Jovanovich, Publishers

COPYRIGHT © 1975, BY ACADEMIC PRESS, INC.
ALL RIGHTS RESERVED.
NO PART OF THIS PUBLICATION MAY BE REPRODUCED OR
TRANSMITTED IN ANY FORM OR BY ANY MEANS, ELECTRONIC
OR MECHANICAL, INCLUDING PHOTOCOPY, RECORDING, OR ANY
INFORMATION STORAGE AND RETRIEVAL SYSTEM, WITHOUT
PERMISSION IN WRITING FROM THE PUBLISHER.

ACADEMIC PRESS, INC.
111 Fifth Avenue, New York, New York 10003

United Kingdom Edition published by
ACADEMIC PRESS, INC. (LONDON) LTD.
24/28 Oval Road, London NW1

LIBRARY OF CONGRESS CATALOG CARD NUMBER: 52-13360

ISBN 0-12-006621-1

PRINTED IN THE UNITED STATES OF AMERICA

CONTENTS

CONTRIBUTORS TO VOLUME 21 ix

Lung Tumors in Mice: Application to Carcinogenesis Bioassay

MICHAEL B. SHIMKIN AND GARY D. STONER

I.	Introduction	2
II.	Frequency and Distribution	3
III.	Morphology	5
IV.	Histogenesis	7
V.	Growth and Transplantation	11
VI.	Biochemical Characteristics	13
VII.	Host Factors	15
VIII.	Environmental Influences	20
IX.	Virus Aspects	23
X.	Lung Tumor Induction with Chemicals	25
XI.	Lung Tumor Induction with Other Agents	35
XII.	Lung Tumor Bioassay	38
XIII.	Explants and Embryos	44
XIV.	Conclusions	46
	References	48

Cell Death in Normal and Malignant Tissues

E. H. COOPER, A. J. BEDFORD, AND T. E. KENNY

I.	Introduction	59
II.	Cell Loss in Embryogenesis	61
III.	Transmission Electron Microscopy	65
IV.	Microcinematography	68
V.	Scanning Electron Microscopy	71
VI.	Chromosome Aberrations as a Cause of Cell Loss . . .	74
VII.	Identification of Dead Cells *in Vitro*	77
VIII.	Assessment of Tumor Cell Death *in Vivo*	78
IX.	The Blood Supply of Tumors and Tumor Cell Necrosis . .	80
X.	Immune Elimination of Cancer Cells	82
XI.	Phagocytosis and Autolysis	90
XII.	Tumor Cell Loss by Differentiation	93
XIII.	Cell Loss in Experimental Tumors	96
XIV.	Cell Loss in Human Tumors	100
XV.	Cell Loss and the Treatment of Tumors	106
	Addendum: Mathematical Treatment of Cell Loss in Tumors .	108
	References	114

The Histocompatibility-Linked Immune Response Genes

BARUJ BENACERRAF AND DAVID H. KATZ

I.	Immune Responses Controlled by Histocompatibility-Linked Ir Genes. Species Distribution	121
II.	The Mapping of Mouse H-Linked Ir Genes	130
III.	Relationship of H-Linked Ir Genes to Immunoglobulin Structural Genes	133
IV.	The Cell Type Where Histocompatibility-Linked Ir Genes are Expressed	135
V.	The Demonstration of Suppressor T Cells Specific for GAT^{10} in Genetic Nonresponder Mice	140
VI.	The Role of Histocompatibility Gene Products in T–B Cell Interactions	143
VII.	Identification of I Region Gene Products	159
VIII.	Relationship of Histocompatibility Gene Products to Each Other in Nature and Function	162
IX.	Function of Products of H-Linked Ir Genes and of Other I Region Gene Products: Relationship of These Products to Activation of Immunocompetent Cells	165
X.	The Histocompatibility-Linked Ir Genes and Disease	168
	References	171

Horizontally and Vertically Transmitted Oncornaviruses of Cats

M. ESSEX

I.	Introduction	175
II.	Characteristics of Feline Oncornaviruses	178
III.	Antigenic Structure and Serologic Detection	181
IV.	Virus–Host Cell Relationships	186
V.	Cell Surface Antigens Induced by Feline Oncornaviruses	191
VI.	Experimental Induction of Tumors with Feline Oncornaviruses	194
VII.	Immune Response to Experimental Infections	199
VIII.	Virus Transmission and Natural History of Feline Leukemia	205
IX.	Comparison of Feline Oncornavirus Infectivity Patterns to Those of Other Oncogenic or Potentially Oncogenic Viruses	230
X.	Public Health Significance of Feline Oncornaviruses	233
XI.	Summary and Conclusions	235
	References	237

Epithelial Cells: Growth in Culture of Normal and Neoplastic Forms

KEEN A. RAFFERTY, JR.

I.	Introduction	249
II.	Aging Revisited	251

III. Senescence and Cell Type	. . . .	253
IV. Epithelial Cells *in Vivo* and Limits on Division Potential	. . .	261
V. Summary and Conclusions	. . . .	268
References	. . . .	270

Selection of Biochemically Variant, in Some Cases Mutant, Mammalian Cells in Culture

G. B. CLEMENTS

I. Introduction	. . . .	274
II. Selection and Characterization of Variant Cells	. . . .	282
III. Drug-Resistant Variants	. . . .	289
IV. Variants with Altered Expression of Antigenic Surface Components or Immunoglobulin Production (Table XVIII)	. . . . . .	358
V. Variants with Altered Nutritional Requirements	. . . .	364
VI. Temperature-Sensitive Conditionally Lethal Cells	. . . .	370
VII. Variants Resistant to Physical Agents	. . . . . .	376
VIII. Spontaneous Variants	. . . .	379
IX. Conclusions	. . . .	379
References	. . . .	380

The Role of DNA Repair and Somatic Mutation in Carcinogenesis

JAMES E. TROSKO AND ERNEST H. Y. CHU

I. Introduction	. . . .	391
II. Mutagenicity of Chemical Carcinogens	. . . . . .	393
III. Molecular Basis for Mutagenesis and Carcinogenesis	. . .	395
IV. DNA Damage and Its Repair	. . . .	400
V. Factors Influencing DNA Repair	. . . .	407
VI. Evolutionary Perspectives of Somatic Mutagenesis	. . . .	417
VII. Summary and Conclusion	. . . .	419
References	. . . .	420

SUBJECT INDEX	. . . .	427
CONTENTS OF PREVIOUS VOLUMES	. . . .	432

CONTRIBUTORS TO VOLUME 21

Numbers in parentheses refer to the pages on which the authors' contributions begin.

A. J. BEDFORD, *Department of Experimental Pathology and Cancer Research, School of Medicine, University of Leeds, Leeds, England* (59)

BARUJ BENACERRAF, *Department of Pathology, Harvard Medical School, Boston, Massachusetts* (121)

ERNEST H. Y. CHU, *Department of Human Genetics, University of Michigan Medical School, Ann Arbor, Michigan* (391)

G. B. CLEMENTS,[1] *Department of Tumor Biology, Karolinska Institute, Stockholm, Sweden* (273)

E. H. COOPER, *Department of Experimental Pathology and Cancer Research, School of Medicine, University of Leeds, Leeds, England* (59)

M. ESSEX, *Department of Microbiology, School of Public Health, Harvard University, Boston, Massachusetts* (175)

DAVID H. KATZ, *Department of Pathology, Harvard Medical School, Boston, Massachusetts* (121)

T. E. KENNY, *Department of Experimental Pathology and Cancer Research, School of Medicine, University of Leeds, Leeds, England* (59)

KEEN A. RAFFERTY, JR., *Department of Anatomy, The University of Illinois at the Medical Center, Chicago, Illinois* (249)

MICHAEL B. SHIMKIN, *Department of Community Medicine, University of California at San Diego, La Jolla, California* (1)

GARY D. STONER, *Department of Community Medicine, University of California at San Diego, La Jolla, California* (1)

JAMES E. TROSKO, *Department of Human Development, Michigan State University, East Lansing, Michigan* (391)

---

[1] Present address: Pathology Department, Western Infirmary, Glasgow, G11 6NT Scotland.

LUNG TUMORS IN MICE:
APPLICATION TO CARCINOGENESIS BIOASSAY[*]

Michael B. Shimkin and Gary D. Stoner

Department of Community Medicine
University of California at San Diego, La Jolla, California

I. Introduction	2
II. Frequency and Distribution.	3
III. Morphology	5
IV. Histogenesis	7
V. Growth and Transplantation	11
VI. Biochemical Characteristics	13
VII. Host Factors	15
A. Influence of Heredity	15
B. Effect of Age	17
C. Immunologic Factors	18
VIII. Environmental Influences	20
A. Effect of Germ-Free State	20
B. Effect of Atmospheric Oxygen	21
C. Metabolic Inhibitors and Other Chemicals	22
IX. Virus Aspects	23
X. Lung Tumor Induction with Chemicals	25
A. Polycyclic Hydrocarbons	26
B. Carbamates and Aziridines	27
C. Alkylating Agents	28
D. Nitrosamines	28
E. Hydrazine Derivatives	32
F. Aminoazo and Other Compounds	33
G. Food Additives, Drugs, etc.	34
XI. Lung Tumor Induction with Other Agents	35
A. Ionizing Radiation	35
B. Tobacco	36
C. Air Pollutants	37
D. Metals and Miscellaneous	38
XII. Lung Tumor Bioassay	38
A. Selection of Animals	39
B. Administration of Chemicals	40
C. Interpretation	42
XIII. Explants and Embryos	44
XIV. Conclusions	46
References	48

[*] Prepared with support of Contract NIH-NO1-CP3-3232 from the National Cancer Institute.

I. Introduction

A young adult mouse of the inbred strain A is given a single injection of a carcinogenic chemical, such as 3-methylcholanthrene or urethane. The mouse is killed 13 weeks later. Its lungs will be studded with pearly-white nodules.

An untreated strain A mouse sacrificed at the same time should be free of lung nodules. At one year of age, however, the majority of strain A mice will have solitary lung nodules. A "spontaneous" nodule, and multiple nodules induced by a carcinogenic chemical, are illustrated in Fig. 1, reproduced from a publication of 1940 (*301*).

The nodules are the primary adenomatous alveologenic lung tumors of the mouse, one of the commoner neoplasms in the species *Mus musculus*. The first description of the tumor is usually attributed to Livingood (*207*) in 1896. Slye, Holmes, and Wells (*310*) in 1914 reported on 160 mice with lung tumors found among 6000 mice of their colony. Murphy and Sturm (*245*) in 1925 first induced lung tumors by cutaneous paintings of tar. Clara Lynch (*209*) in 1926 began genetic studies using spontaneous and induced lung tumors in inbred strains of mice. Heston (*136*) in 1940 extended genetic studies to the relationship of specific genes. Grady and Stewart (*120*) in 1940 clarified the histogenesis of the neoplasm as arising from alveolar lining cells. Shimkin (*301*) in 1940 and Andervont and Shimkin (*9*) in

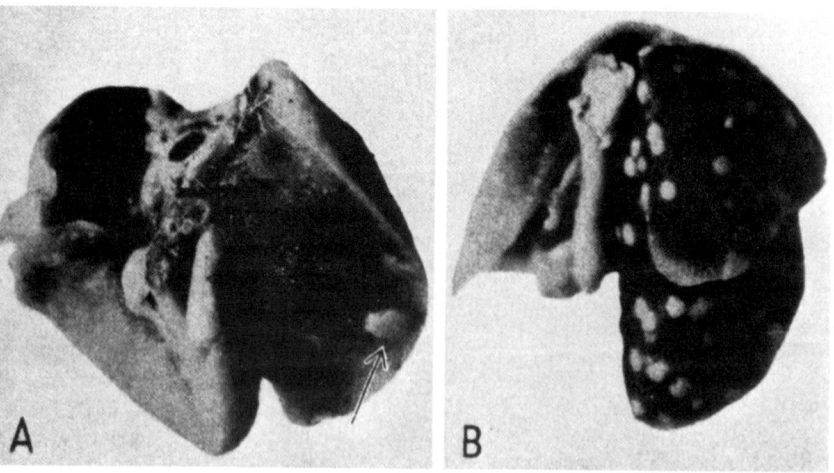

FIG. 1. (A) Spontaneous lung tumor in strain A male mouse 8 months old. ×3.5. (B) Induced multiple lung tumors in strain A male mouse 13 weeks after intravenous injection of 1.5 mg of 3-methylcholanthrene. ×3.5. From Shimkin (*301*). Copyright 1940, American Medical Association.

1941 applied lung tumors in mice to quantitative bioassays of chemicals for carcinogenic activity.

A review on the subject (303) appeared in the 1955 volume of *Advances in Cancer Research*. In 1965 an international conference on lung tumors in animals was held in Perugia. The proceedings, edited by Severi (295), include some 70 papers and discussions by over 100 participants.

This review updates the information on lung tumors in mice, with emphasis on the use of the mouse lung for quantitative investigations in carcinogenesis, especially bioassay of chemicals for carcinogenic activity. Comparative oncology of the lung, included in the first review (303) and well represented at the Perugia conference (295), was excluded from this presentation.

References cited in this review were selected primarily from papers published since 1955. The expansion of interest in lung tumors in mice is indicated by the number of papers during the decade after 1964 being almost double that of the previous decade. There is also wider geographic distribution of the research than was evident in 1955, with increased participation of investigators from Japan, Italy, and France.

II. Frequency and Distribution

The 1972 listing of inbred strains and substrains of mice includes 244 entries (315). Specific data on the incidence of spontaneous lung tumors is given for some 24 strains.

There is general agreement that the A strain, originated by Strong (323), has the highest incidence of lung tumors. Strain SWR (the inbred "Swiss") is next in susceptibility. Strains BALB/c, CR, O20, and DD are of intermediate susceptibility. Among the relatively resistant strains are the CBA and C3H. The most resistant strains are the DBA, C57BL, and C57L. A wide spectrum of susceptibility to spontaneous lung tumors extends, therefore, from strain A mice, in which lung nodules begin to appear in a few animals as young as 3–4 months and rise steadily to almost 100% by 24 months, to C57BL mice, in which lung tumors are seen only rarely in old animals. Multiplicity of lung tumors, as well as frequency, is another indicator of susceptibility. In the more susceptible strains, two or more nodules per animal are encountered in older mice, whereas only single nodules are seen in the more resistant strains.

Inbreeding of mouse strains was conducted without reference to the occurrence of lung tumors, so that the segregation of this characteristic was unpremeditated. Inbreeding itself does not cause lung tumors. Andervont and Dunn (8) found pulmonary tumors in 21% of 225 wild house mice raised in captivity and surviving to an average age of 18 months.

The characteristic of lung tumor frequency is more constant for the strain and is less influenced by the usual environmental conditions of geography and diet than is the frequency of mammary, hepatic, or lymphogenous neoplasms. Pulmonary tumors are not related to the sex of the animal, although males of strain A usually have slightly more tumors than females (307). There is no relationship between susceptibility of mouse strains to lung tumors and the susceptibility to other spontaneous or induced neoplasms. The major determinants for the appearance of lung tumors in mice are the genetic constitution and the age of the animal.

The lungs of mice susceptible to the development of spontaneous lung tumors are also exquisitely sensitive to the induction of tumors by exogenous carcinogenic stimuli. Many investigations (24, 80, 171, 212, 285, 331, 352) on lung tumors in mice reiterate that the susceptibility to carcinogens is in direct relation to the spontaneous occurrence of the tumors. Thus, strain A mice are the most susceptible to a wide variety of carcinogens, in terms of earlier appearance and greater multiplicity of tumors. Strain C57BL is among the most resistant to all chemical classes of carcinogens.

TABLE I
SUSCEPTIBILITY TO LUNG TUMORS (LT) IN 7 STRAINS
OF MICE AND THEIR F_1 HYBRIDS[a]

Strains	Spontaneous LT		Urethane-induced LT	
	Incidence (%)	Age (months)	Incidence (%)	Mean No.
A	71	23	100	17.1
GR	42	14	100	15.3
O20	58	21	100	12.1
CBA	18	27	38	0.5
C3H	14	21	21	0.3
DBA	9	21	17	0.2
C57BL	7	22	7	0.1
F_1 hybrids				
O20 × GR	—	—	100	13.7
C57 × GR	—	—	100	5.7
O20 × DBA	32	12	100	3.7
C57 × CBA	—	—	63	0.9
C3H × C57BL	—	—	30	0.3

[a] Data of Bentvelzen and Szalay (24).

Table I summarizes results of Bentvelzen and Szalay (24) of Holland, reiterating the parallelism between induced and spontaneous lung tumors. This parallelism is maintained in newborn (52, 212, 285) and in fetal (24, 249) mice.

The parallelism between induced and spontaneous tumors has been used as an argument for the view that the induction of lung tumors is an accleration of a process already inherent in the animal. This is applicable in some degree to any neoplastic reaction that an animal can manifest.

III. Morphology

Small primary pulmonary tumors have a uniform gross and microscopic appearance. In the gross, or after fixation, the tumors are pearly-white, glistening, discrete round nodules, often situated just below the visceral pleura (Fig. 1). There is no predilection for side or lobe. The tumors are sharply contrasted against the normal tissue of the lung and have a rubbery consistency. With practice, the tumors can be correctly identified with the naked eye or under a dissecting microscope when they are a millimeter or less in diameter. The presence of a superimposed pneumonic consolidation may obscure small tumors, and the presence of an obvious tumor elsewhere may make distinction difficult between primary pulmonary tumor and metastasis.

Under the microscope (Fig. 2), the tumor is devoid of a capsule and infiltrates and compresses the surrounding pulmonary tissue,

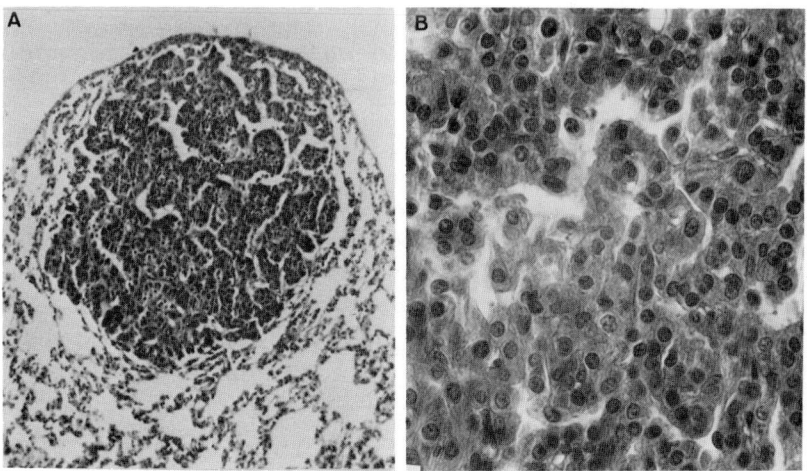

FIG. 2. Lung tumor in strain A mouse 84 days after intraperitoneal injection of 20 mg of urethane. (A) ×80; (B) ×600. From Shimkin and Polissar (304).

with the intact somewhat thickened pleura over the mass. The tumor is usually of a uniform adenomatous pattern, consisting of closely packed columns of cuboidal or columnar cells. The cells are uniform in size and shape, with a homogeneous, acidophilic cytoplasm and round, hyperchromatic nucleus of moderate size. Cilia are not encountered. Mitotic figures are rare. The sparse stroma is composed of adult-appearing fibroblasts, and there are few blood vessels. The margins of the tumor are usually devoid of inflammatory reaction, lymphocytic infiltration, or increase in fibrous elements. Small areas of necrosis and small cysts may be encountered in the larger masses (*83–85*).

Well over 95% of all pulmonary tumors in mice present this appearance. There seems to be no morphological difference between the neoplasms seen in noninbred mice and in mice of various homozygous strains. The tumors are the same whether they are spontaneous or induced by carcinogenic agents, except that the latter are multiple, whereas spontaneous tumors usually are single.

A proportion of larger tumors have histologic features of malignancy, such as structural and cellular anaplasia, increased number of mitotic figures, and invasion of surrounding tissue. The tumors are then classified as adenocarcinomas (*148*). Hemorrhage, necrosis, and fibrosis are encountered in the less differentiated tumors. Areas of histologic malignancy may be found in only a portion of a tumor that otherwise would be designated as an adenoma (*235*). Admixtures of sarcomatous-appearing elements also are seen.

The proportion of lung tumors that are diagnosed as adenocarcinomas rather than adenomas depends upon the age of the animals or the time after the induction of the tumors. Small nodules visible at, say, 16 weeks after urethane, will be monotonously uniform adenomas. In mice over 1 year old, one-third of the tumors may be designated as adenocarcinomas. Classification by histologic patterns such as papillary or columnar (*6*) is no longer fashionable.

Metastases are a feature of larger, older tumors. Wells *et al.* (*366*) in 1941 reported that among 2865 mice with spontaneous lung tumors, 104, or 3.6%, had distant metastases. BALB/c mice receiving daily urethane at 17–19 months had multiple lung tumors, of which 45% were classified as carcinomas and one-third of these had metastases (*270*). Turusov *et al.* (*353*) in 1974 published that among 2439 mice with induced and spontaneous lung tumors, there were distant metastases in 87, or 3.6%. The most frequent sites were mediastinal lymph nodes, 57; chest wall, 31; heart, 29; kidney, 24; and liver, 12; in 49 mice there were multiple metastatic deposits. The proportion of metastases also depends upon the age and survival of mice, as well as upon the care with which metastases are sought at autopsy.

Chromosome patterns of spontaneous pulmonary adenomas of strain A mice and of pulmonary adenomas from strain A animals treated with urethane were analyzed by Di Paolo (75). Stemlines of the primary pulmonary adenomas were diploid, pseudodiploid, and aneuploid, with a preponderance of aneuploid. Tumors having a diploid mode also had cells with abnormal karyotypes. Serially transplanted adenomas underwent further alteration of stemlines. It is not known whether the abnormal chromosome patterns have oncogenic significance.

IV. Histogenesis

Grady and Stewart (120) in 1940 established that lung tumors induced with polycyclic hydrocarbons in mice originate from the alveolar lining cells. Alveolar cell origin of these tumors has been accepted by practically all investigators (13, 86, 135, 251). Mori (232) examining 96 lung tumors induced by 4-nitroquinoline 1-oxide, concluded that 9 arose from bronchial epithelium. Biancifiori et al. (27), in a study of hydrazine-induced lung tumors in BALB/c mice, stated that, although most of the tumors arise from the alveoli, "the possibility of bronchial origin cannot be excluded for some." Although the great majority of the tumors are undoubtedly alveologenic, generalization to all lung tumors in all strains and all carcinogens requires caution.

Electron microscopy (294) and quantitative morphometry (365) during the past decade have added new dimensions to knowledge about the cellular components of the lung.

The normal pulmonary alveolar tissue of the mouse, and other species, contains 7 types of cells: (a) type 1 alveolar epithelial cells, (b) type 2 alveolar epithelial cells (c) alveolar macrophages, (d) capillary endothelial cells and blood elements within the capillaries, (e) connective tissue cells, (f) septal macrophages or histiocytes, and (g) leukocytes in connecting tissue spaces. Septal macrophages and leukocytes are seen rarely in normal lung (38). A schematic representation is furnished in Fig. 3. The two types of alveolar cells are photographed in Fig. 4.

The two types of epithelial cells lie on the alveolar basement membrane and are connected by tight junctions, as in other epithelia. They completely cover the alveolar surface. Type 1 alveolar cells (also called type A alveolar cells) have a greatly extended cytoplasm that spreads out and covers almost the entire alveolar sur-

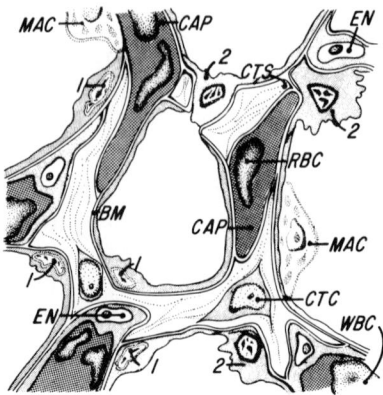

FIG. 3. Schematic representation of the components of a murine lung alveolus. Redrawn from Brooks (38). Type 1 and type 2 cells lie on basement membrane (BM). MAC, macrophage; CTS, connective tissue space, CTC, connective tissue cell; EN, endothelial cell; CAP, blood capillary; RBC, red, and WBC, white blood cell.

face. Type 2 alveolar cells are cuboidal to irregular in shape, with short cytoplasmic projections. They generally occur in niches of the alveolar wall and may extend across the alveolar septum to border on adjacent alveoli.

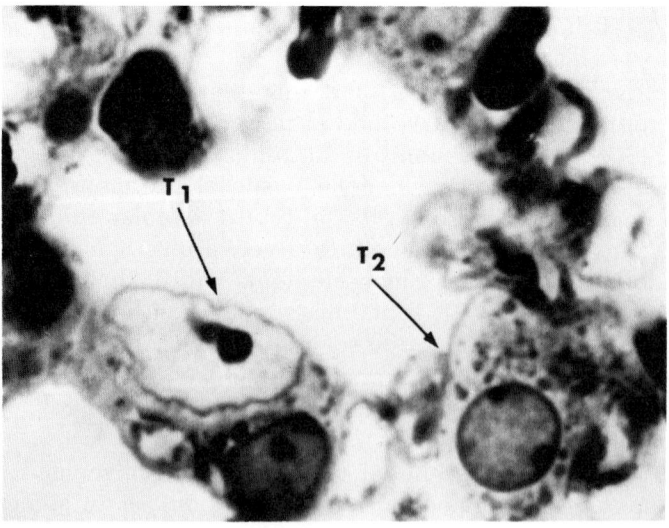

FIG. 4. Type 1 (T_1) and type 2 (T_2) alveolar cells of the lung of mouse receiving urethane. ×1000. From Kauffman (161).

Type 2 cells (also called granular pneumocytes, great alveolar cells, type B alveolar cells, and septal cells) have numerous, structurally unique cytoplasmic organelles, called lamellar inclusion bodies. They also contain numerous mitochondria, a few granular endoplasmic reticula, and zones of Golgi lamellae and vesicles. Lamellar bodies appear to be the source of pulmonary surfactant that is discharged into the alveoli (177). Surfactant is composed principally of dipalmitoyllecithin (41, 60). Many type 2 alveolar cells are high in glycogen content (38).

Alveolar macrophages are separated from the basement membrane by type 1 or 2 cells. They contain phagocytized material, and have broad cytoplasmic pseudopods. It seems clear that these macrophages are of hematopoietic origin.

Type 2 cells are found singly and well separated from each other by the intervening cytoplasmic layer of the type 1 cells. Brooks (38) stated that the two epithelial cells occur in approximately one-to-one proportion. Kauffman (161) gave the numbers found in mouse lung as 0.88×10^7 for type 2 cells and 0.29×10^7 for type 1 cells, or approximately 3 to 1 preponderance for type 2 cells.

Evans et al. (97–99) studied the renewal of alveolar epithelium in rats exposed to nitrous oxide and established that type 2 cells are progenitors of type 1 cells. In young adult Swiss-Webster mice, the estimated life-span of type 2 cells was 20–25 days, for type 1, greater than 30 days, and for alveolar macrophages, 5–10 days. After type 2 cells divide, one or both may transform into type 1 cells.

Electron microscopic studies on the induction of lung tumors in mice receiving urethane (18, 19, 39, 150, 157, 172, 327), polycyclic hydrocarbons (14), hydrazine sulfate (42), nitroso compounds (263), as well as spontaneous tumors (39) and tumors induced in vitro (107) uniformly conclude that these tumors arise from type 2 cells of the alveolar epithelium. The conclusion is based upon structural similarity between type 2 cells and the cells of the tumors, and the presence of lamellar inclusion bodies in the tumor cells. Brooks and Adkinson (40) made quantitative comparisons of type 2 cells and cells of lung tumors, and found that the nucleus-cytoplasm ratio in tumor cells was increased (0.59 in tumors vs 0.36 for type 2 cells). There were more mitochondria, cytosomes, and heterochromatin in the cytoplasm of type 2 cells than in tumor cells, and more nucleoli, granular endoplastic reticulum and euchromatin in the cytoplasm of tumor cells than in type 2 cells.

Quantitative measurements (198, 199, 306) of cell numbers, cell cycles, and DNA synthesis, as measured by tritiated thymidine uptake, have been applied to mouse lungs following exposure to carcinogens, usually urethane. These studies have sought to elucidate the events preceding carcinogenesis and the mechanism of carcinogenesis. Intriguing findings have been recorded, but it remains to be elucidated which findings are part of the carcinogenic process and which are "nonspecific" effects of the chemical.

Shimkin and Polissar (304) in 1957 reported that after a single intraperitoneal dose of urethane to A strain mice, the lungs show focal areas of increased cellularity. Neyman and Scott (247) used this information in developing a two-stage hypothesis of carcinogenesis, although there was no evidence that the focal cellularity was a precursor or related to the eventual appearance of lung tumors. White et al. (367), in fact, could not replicate the finding of focal cellularity, and attributed Shimkin and Polissar's observations to enhancement of inflammatory reactions by urethane. Kauffman (158–161), however, also observed general increase in pulmonary cellularity, and then extended her studies in mice maintained on urethane in drinking water by specifying the changes to cell types. During the first 2 weeks, there was a depression in the number of type 1 and 2 alveolar cells, and in the alveolar macrophages, but by 3 weeks the number of the cells doubled or tripled above the numbers seen in normal lungs. The greatest proportional increase was in type 2 cells, and doublets of such cells were often encountered whereas in normal lungs type 2 cells usually occur singly between type 1 cells.

Thus, following continual exposure to urethane, there is at least a doubling of the alveolar lining cells, which may be called a general hyperplasia. From this doubling of 1×10^7 type 2 cells arise some 100 discrete tumors. Carcinogenesis, therefore, is an event that transpires once in approximately 100,000 cells, a rare clonal occurrence. The initial stimulus of urethane seemingly affects not only type 2 cells, but type 1 cells and macrophages, but the continued alteration toward neoplasia involves a small subpopulation of type 2 cells. This involvement seems to be distributed at random throughout the lung. Whether these events are best typified as one- or two-stage process (143, 247), or the first stages of a much greater continuum of progressive steps, remains conjectural.

Calafat et al. (47) compared electron-microscopic changes in the lungs of the susceptible GR strain and the resistant C3H strain following exposure to dimethylnitrosamine (DMN). Nuclear alterations, characterized first by the formation of plaques of dark-staining material in the nucleolus, and subsequent segregation of the nucleolar components, appeared in the bronchial epithelium within 1 hour, and later in the alveolar epithelium. The changes were similar in the two strains of mice. The same group (70) also studied the methylation of lung DNA following ^{14}C-labeled DMN. Radioactivity in the guanine and adenine fractions was appreciably higher in the DNA of the susceptible GR strain than in the resistant C3H strain. Divertie et al. (79) also reported that cell DNA synthesis, as measured by tritiated thymidine, was prolonged in lungs of mice predisposed to the development of lung tumors.

Further quantitative studies targeted at type 2 cells should be informative.

V. Growth and Transplantation

The development of pulmonary tumors in strain A mice following a single exposure to urethane appears to proceed through a rapid phase of initiation and a slower phase of subsequent tumor growth (304). A collection of some 70 cells at the largest circumference of a mass could be convincingly designated as a tumor under an optical microscope. The growth rate was rapid during the first 2–3 weeks, and then decelerated. At the maximum, a doubling time of 4.4 days was calculated, and the deceleration was attributed to mitotic activity being restricted to the outer surfaces of the organoid masses. Backward extrapolation of the curve led to the time of urethane injection and a single-cell mass, suggesting that the initiation of the process began very quickly after the pulse stimulus.

During the initial stage there is a continual increase in the number of recognizable tumor nodules, until a plateau is reached by approximately 16 weeks. If serial sections are examined under the microscope, however, the plateau is reached by 7 weeks, indicating the effect of recognition rather than of induction.

Yuhas (375) measured the volume of tumors in RFM mice at 6–12 months after a single dose of intraperitoneal urethane, and found a doubling time of 1.6 months. Comparison of the growth of lung tumors in strain A and C3H mice showed that the growth rate in the more resistant C3H strain was 0.6 that of the rate for A mice (305).

These observations cover the adenoma stage of lung tumor evolution. Later, the growth rate of some of the tumors probably accelerates again in concert with the acquisition of more malignant morphologic and biologic characteristics. No numerical data are available for this stage of tumor growth in the lungs. The accelerated growth and the acquisition of aggressive behavior are best supported by studies on transplantation of the tumors.

Transplantation of lung tumors was initially studied by Andervont (7), at the time when a major question was the histogenesis of the alveolar lining cells, especially as to whether they were derived from mesenchymal or ectodermal elements. On transplantation, some of the tumors retained their adenomatous pattern, and others became spindle-celled in appearance. The latter could be interpreted either as spindle-celled epithelial elements or as sarcomatous, and the issue remained unresolved (127, 128). Klein (178) related the size of the tumors to their ability to grow subcutaneously; the larger the primary lung tumor, the more takes there were, and the shorter was the latent period before growth commenced.

Kimura (168) performed meticulous experiments that repeated and extended Andervont's observations. He showed that transplanted tumors upon serial transplantation progressively grew more rapidly, became less differentiated, and yielded metastases. Eventually the transplants became anaplastic, the cells spindle in appearance, and finally able to grow as ascitic tumors. On the basis of his studies of primary tumors and their transplants, the author concluded that the pulmonary tumor of the mouse was a "progressive tumor" with an easily defined continuum from the benign-appearing adenoma to the anaplastic, metastasizing ascitic neoplasm. His scheme is presented in Fig. 5.

Thus, a single dose of a carcinogen not only induces changes in type 2 alveolar pneumocytes that eventuate in an adenomatous tumor, but the changes continue through many generations of cells toward an increasingly malignant neoplasm. In this continuum, in which discrete events remain to be defined, selection as well as possible further mutational changes must be involved. Such selection, natural and experimental, is accentuated by serial transplantation. Peacock (259), using an ingenious *in vivo* "plating technique," obtained 4 separate tumor clones from a lung carcinoma, as a demonstration of the presence of subpopulations in such tumors.

It should be emphasized that the scheme proposed by Kimura (168) must be truncated. Lung adenomas are elicited in a rare proportion of type 2 alveolar cells exposed to a carcinogen. Morphological adenocarcinomas are observed later, in but a small percentage of the adenomas. On transplantation, the more rapidly dividing cells would predominate in the subsequent growths.

That some of the intermediary cellular changes are terminal rather than progressive is also shown by the successful *in vitro* culture of adenoma cells (319). After 42 passages in culture, epithelial cells derived from urethane-induced pulmonary adenoma did not ex-

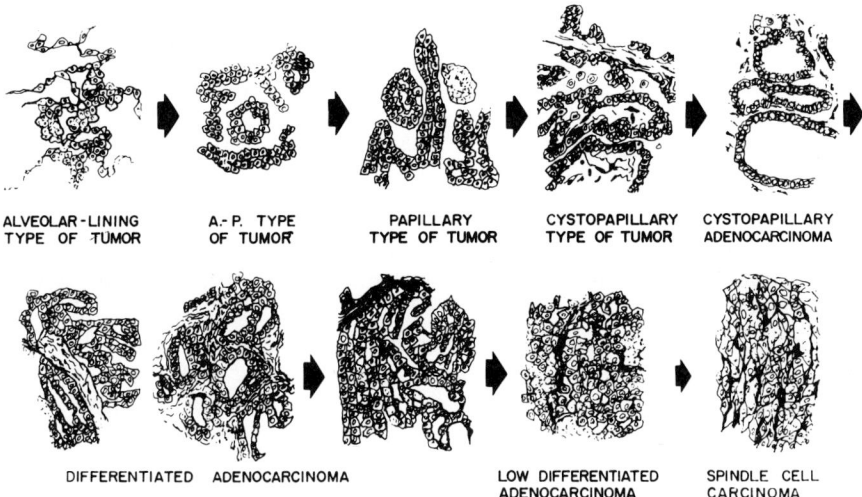

FIG. 5. Schematic representation of progression in the lung tumor complex in mice. A.-P. = alveolar-papillary. As discussed in the text, such progression is truncated. From Kimura (168).

hibit many of the characteristics of transformed cells *in vitro*, such as the ability to grow in soft agar, loss of contact inhibition, and tumorigenicity in appropriate hosts. However, they were aneuploid with an average number of 110 chromosomes per cell. Their origin from type 2 alveolar cell was indicated by the appearance on electron microscopy of numerous lamellar inclusion bodies in the cytoplasm.

The question of whether carcinogenesis of the mouse lung is a one-step mutation or a multistep reaction is complicated by the progressive changes in the cell population, with selection for the more rapidly dividing and better-surviving cells. It remains unanswered as to whether the whole progressive process is triggered by one event or requires additional stimuli for the later stages to occur. Tissue culture of clonal derivatives should be a useful approach to this problem.

VI. Biochemical Characteristics

The rat liver and hepatomas remain the favorite material for the biochemist–oncologist, for a number of excellent theoretical and practical reasons. The mouse lung and its tumors are sparsely represented in the biochemical oncologic literature.

Greenstein (126) in 1947 showed by quantitative chemical analyses that lung tumors in mice contained less alkaline phosphatase than the normal lung tissue. Burt et al. (46) found no alkaline phosphatase by histochemical study of lung tumors induced in strain A mice with methylcholanthrene. Griciute and Rudali (131) used the Gomori histochemical reaction for alkaline phosphatase, and found it to be high in the lungs of mice of strains AKR, C3H, and XVII G, but absent in strain C57BL. Lung tumors induced in XVII G strain were devoid of the enzyme. Urethane and methylcholanthrene failed to induce the enzyme in the resistant C57BL mice.

Nebert and Gelboin (245a) examined the levels of methylcholanthrene-inducible aryl hydrocarbon hydroxylase (AHH) activity in the lungs of six strains of mice (A, "Swiss," C3H, AKR, DBA, and C57GK) of differing susceptibilities to chemical carcinogens. There was no correlation between the levels of inducible AHH activity and lung tumor susceptibility.

Usunov (356) and Ganter and Maral (115) conducted histochemical studies on urethane-induced lung tumors, and found increased activity of the oxidoreductive enzymes, succinic dehydrogenase, and cytochrome oxidase in the adenomas. Tumor cells resembled bronchial rather than alveolar cells in these characteristics. Although Usunov (356) suggested that this may indicate bronchogenic origin of the tumors, it more likely represents dedifferentiation.

Suzuki (326) examined 23 enzymes histochemically in mouse and rat lung tumors induced by 4-nitroquinoline 1-oxide and reported the following: (a) β-glucuronidase, DPN-diaphorase, TPN-diaphorase, lactic dehydrogenase, and glucose-6-phosphate dehydrogenase activities were consistently higher in lung tumors of mice (dd strain males) and rats than in normal lung tissues. (b) Leucine aminopeptidase activity was seen only in the adenomas and adenocarcinomas of both species, but not in normal lung. (c) In mice, monoamine oxidase, glutamic dehydrogenase, and ethanol dehydrogenase activities were higher in tumors considered to be originating in the bronchioles than in tumors originating in the alveoli. They were also higher in the bronchioles than in the alveoli of normal lungs. (d) In mice, alkaline phosphatase was not found in alveolar epithelial cells of normal lung or in adenomas, but was observed in adenocarcinomas. Acid phosphatase activity was low in adenoma and normal lung of both species.

Yamane et al. (373) studied lactic dehydrogenase in mouse lung and tumors produced by 4-nitroquinoline 1-oxide. The enzyme was increased in the tumor by 2.5–3.5 times over normal lung, and the isoenzymes shifted toward the embryonic pattern of decreases in fractions I and II and increases in fractions IV and V.

Azzopardi and Thurlbeck (*15, 16*) reported that the principal enzymes of the three major pathways for carbohydrate metabolism; viz., the Embden–Meyerhof, the Krebs cycle, and the hexose monophosphate shunt function at all stages of adenoma development following urethane, as do the enzymes of the terminal hydrogen transport chain. The enzymic pattern of the tumor cells, although qualitatively similar to that of the type 2 alveolar cells, was one of greater activity throughout. The oxidative enzyme, succinic dehydrogenase, was of particular interest because the adenoma cells showed a reversal to the fetal pattern of activity of the alveolar septa, i.e., both adenoma cells and alveolar cells derived from the fetus exhibit strong succinic dehydrogenase activity whereas its activity in the adult alveolar cell is very low.

Urethane-induced adenomas have been used for the study of pulmonary surfactant biosynthesis by Snyder *et al.* (*313*). Adenoma cells contained significant quantities of disaturated phosphatidylcholine, the main constituent of lung surfactant. In addition, the adenoma homogenate was capable of synthesizing surfactant as demonstrated by the incorporation of palmitic acid-1-^{14}C into phosphatidylcholine with palmitate at positions 1 and 2 of the glycerol moiety. Normal lung and squamous cell carcinoma also incorporated palmitic acid into phosphatidylcholine, but at a much slower rate than adenoma cells. The major incorporation of palmitic acid-1-^{14}C into phosphatidylcholine in the adenoma homogenate did not take place via the cytidine diphosphate choline pathway or by methylation of phosphatidylethanolamine, the two major pathways for surfactant biosynthesis in the human fetus (*119*).

Mizushima (*228*) published an interesting account of hyperestrogenism produced by transplantable pulmonary tumors of mice, as a manifestation of inappropriate hormone secretion.

Lung tumors in mice, as other neoplasms, biochemically appear to revert toward embryonic patterns. They demonstrate the specific biochemical property of producing surfactant. This marker makes possible and desirable more systematic studies on the relationship of the marker to the induction and subsequent evolution of this neoplasm.

VII. Host Factors

A. INFLUENCE OF HEREDITY

The characteristic of different frequencies of pulmonary tumors in different strains of mice was applied to genetic studies by Clara

Lynch in 1926. By 1955 the investigations were extended to many strains and carcinogens (*139, 303*). In these and more recent investigations (*24, 101, 214, 223*) crosses between the high-tumor strains and low-tumor strains resulted in F_1 generations that resembled the high-tumor strain. The back-cross generations resembled the strain to which the F_1 mice were mated. The general conclusion was that susceptibility was inherited in a dominant manner, but that multiple genetic factors or modifying factors had to be involved. Reciprocal crossing had no effect on lung tumor susceptibility (*223*).

Heston et al. (*137–145*) examined the relation of pulmonary tumor susceptibility to 13 known mouse genes. An association was elicited between susceptibility and the yellow (AY) gene, 4 genes were associated with a decrease in susceptibility, and no association was found for 8 genes. These studies also concluded that the susceptibility to pulmonary tumors in mice was determined by genetic factors to a major degree. Deringer and Heston (*72*) added information that the dominant spotting (W), caracul (Ca), and fused (Fu) genes had no significant association with lung tumors. The effect of the AY genes was eliminated as an indirect result of increased normal growth (*357*). Bloom (*33*) also related lung tumor susceptibility to body size.

Falconer and Bloom (*100*) in 1961 proposed that a single gene, which they named *ptr*, was responsible for up to three-fourths of the difference in susceptibility to lung tumors between strains A and C57BL. They random-bred 4 strains of mice and selected the subsequent breeding lines by examining the susceptibility of the parents to tumor induction with urethane. Within 9 generations they were able to restitute 2 lines, one resembling the susceptible A strain and the other the resistant C57BL strain (*34, 101*). They concluded that 54.5% of pulmonary-tumor resistance was heritable by a single gene. Bentvelzen and Szalay (*24*) also concluded that resistance to pulmonary tumors in C57BL mice is mediated primarily by a single gene. Heston (*140*) in a review, presented at the Perugia conference, stated that in the C57BL strain one predominant gene may be involved, but that for other strains there are multiple genetic factors.

There is no doubt that the genetic background of the mouse is an important determinant in its susceptibility or resistance to pulmonary tumors. However, the degrees of susceptibility or resistance are relative, and are modified by a variety of environmental factors. The most resistant strains, such as C57BL, will develop lung tumors after exposure to polycyclic hydrocarbons, urethane, or 4-nitroquinoline

N-oxide (*171*). The tumors merely appear later and in smaller numbers than in the more susceptible strains.

B. Effect of Age

Fetal (*41, 44, 80, 249*) and newborn (*68, 102, 103, 250, 262, 279, 318, 352, 358*) mice develop more pulmonary tumors following exposure to urethane and other carcinogens than adult mice. In a typical experiment reported by Kaye and Trainin (*163*) 12 weeks after a single dose of 1 mg per gram body weight of urethane yielded a mean of 4.9 adenomas in young adult SWR mice, and a mean of 18.2 in neonatal animals.

Kaye (*162*) and Mirvish *et al.* (*224, 225*) established that catabolism of urethane was much slower in young animals than in adults. In adult SWR mice, there was practically total excretion of a single dose of urethane within 7 hours, whereas in newborn animals, only 20% was eliminated during the first 24 hours, a rate calculated at one-tenth that of the adult.

Domsky *et al.* (*82*) recorded that 7,12-dimethylbenzanthracene (DMBA) also was eliminated more slowly in newborn than in adult Swiss mice; the rate in newborns was approximately half that of the adult.

The effects of host metabolism on the elimination of carcinogens are relevant to all investigations concerned with factors modifying carcinogenesis. An increased number of tumors following some procedure should raise the question of whether the procedure might not decrease the rate of catabolism of the carcinogen. It is reasonable to postulate that the greater response of newborn mice to many carcinogens, as reviewed by Toth (*337*) is related to incompletely developed hepatic detoxification pathways, and to incomplete immunologic competence. Cell proliferation in the lung is also at a higher level in fetal and newborn animals (*64*), and it may be related to greater risk to carcinogenesis.

Fetal and newborn lung tissues are more susceptible to carcinogenesis at the tissue level. Heston and Steffee (*144*) showed that subcutaneous transplants of lungs from A strain fetuses, 12–18 days of age, into adult hosts of A strain or ALF_1 and LAF_1 crosses produced tumors following intravenous injection of dibenzanthracene in 28 or 29 transplants, for an average of 3.7 lung tumors per transplant. Transplants of adult lung tissue produced tumors in 23 of 57 transplants, for an average of 0.5 lung tumor per transplant. The authors noted that fetal lung tissue grew in mass following transplantation subcutaneously, whereas adult tissue merely survived.

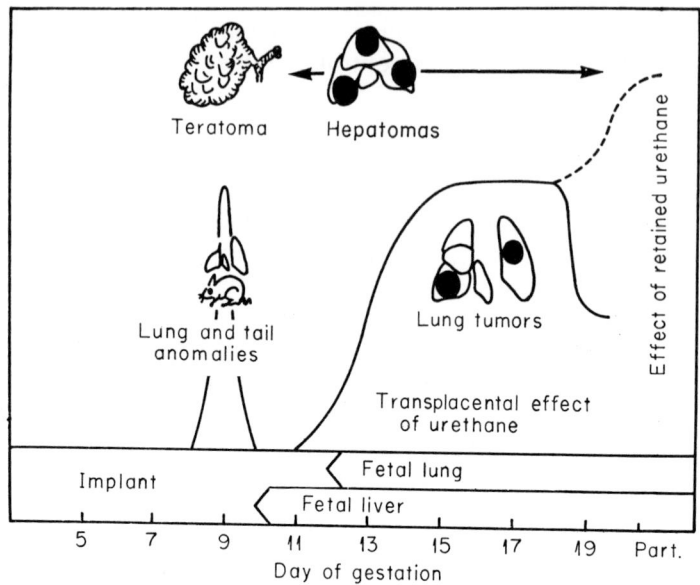

FIG. 6. Time relations of teratogenesis, carcinogenesis, and organogenesis. From Nomura and Okamoto (249). Implant, implantation of ovum; Part, parturition. Reprinted from GANN by permission of the copyright owner, the Japanese Cancer Association.

Kimura et al. (170) also reported that there was greater tissue susceptibility to carcinogenesis of newborn mouse lungs as compared with adult lungs. The authors transplanted newborn and adult lung subcutaneously into A strain hosts, and exposed the hosts to intraperitoneal 3-methylcholanthrene. Fifteen weeks later 16 of 19 newborn lung transplants bore lung tumors, whereas 9 of 19 adult lung transplants had tumors, a significant difference.

Nomura and Okamoto (249) have related carcinogenesis and teratogenesis to fetal development. Malformations of the fetus can be initiated by day 9 of gestation. Hepatic carcinogenesis can occur by day 11, and pulmonary carcinogenesis by day 13, or a day following the appearance of lung buds. Carcinogenesis, therefore, is related to organogenesis, as shown in Fig. 6.

C. IMMUNOLOGIC FACTORS

Transplantation tests have shown that lung adenomas are weakly antigenic. Prehn (268) observed transplantation immunity against only 1 of 8 urethane-induced lung adenomas. Pasternak et al. (254) found that none of six diethylnitrosamine-induced lung tumors could elicit a transplantation resistance. However, there is evidence of an immunological control over the development of adenomas, and particularly that of thymus-dependent immune functions.

Duhig (88, 89) in 1965 noted that thymectomy of mice at 4 or 5 weeks was associated with an increase in lung tumors that was significant at the 5% level, but the author did not quite believe the observation and called for further study. Ribacchi and Giraldo (271, 272) reported that neonatal thymectomy of BALB/c mice led to earlier and greater number of lung tumors following exposure to urethane. The observation was repeated by others (1, 69, 191). Splenectomy or cortisone had no effect (69). Sanford et al. (290) did not observe a higher frequency of spontaneous lung tumors in thymectomized BALB/c mice as compared with sham-operated controls (20/40 vs 23/37). They do note, however, that *multiple* lung tumors occurred in 10 of the thymectomized mice and in only 1 of the sham-operated.

The effect of neonatal thymectomy upon lung tumor induction was also studied by Trainin and Linker-Israeli (347–350). Enhancement of lung tumor formation by thymectomy was demonstrated with 7,12-dimethylbenzanthracene (DMBA) (350), urethane (347), and for spontaneous tumors (349). In a typical experiment in Swiss mice receiving urethane, 31 thymectomized mice had a mean of 14.1 lung tumors, and the controls, 7.5 lung tumors per mouse. Antilymphocyte serum also increased the response to urethane, and a thymic implant in thymectomized mice brought the response back to the response level in intact mice, of 6.6 tumors per mouse (348). Antilymphocyte serum also increased the lung tumor response to DMBA (19).

Stutman (324) observed different results on the role of thymus-dependent immune functions in the development of lung tumors. He found that athymic nude mice and normal nude mice showed no significant differences in either latent period or incidence of sarcomas or lung adenomas within 120 days after administration of 3-methylcholanthrene at birth.

Other data, however, further indicate the influence of cell-mediated immunity on lung adenoma development. Pretreatment of mice with BCG (living bacillus Calmette-Guerin) and trehalose-6,6-dimycolate (cord factor) reduced the number of urethane-induced lung tumors, according to Bekierkunst et al. (23); the effect was attributed to the host cellular reaction. Colnaghi et al. (61) demonstrated that sensitized lymphoid cells taken from SWR mice previously injected with extracts from lung adenomas reacted *in vitro* against target cells from adenomas. The same group (216) observed that treatment of 10-day-old BALB/c mice with urethane and cortisone suppressed their immune response and the number of lung tumors was directly related to the degree of immunological impairment.

Lappé and Prehn (*191*) reported that treatment of 4-day-old BALB/c mice with 1 mg of urethane depressed their immune response as measured by skin allograft survival, and these mice had more lung tumors than untreated animals (1.62 per mouse for urethane vs 0.62 for controls). In a similar study, Lappé and Steinmuller (*192*) found that urethane at doses of 120–150 mg was not immunosuppressive in adult BALB/c mice, although the 150-mg dose depressed the response of C57BL and DBA/2 mice. These data suggest that the pronounced susceptibility of newborn and weanling mice to the carcinogenic effect of urethane, and probably other chemicals, is related, at least in part, to age-dependent factors in immune responses.

The role of humoral immunity on the development of lung adenomas has not been thoroughly investigated. In one study with SWR mice (*350*) depression of humoral immunity was unrelated to the production of lung tumors by urethane.

VIII. Environmental Influences

A. Effect of Germ-Free State

Pollard et al. (*265, 266*) found that germ-free SWR mice developed more lung tumors following subcutaneous methylcholanthrene than did conventional mice. Kelly et al. (*164*) recorded that their germ-free mice had "about the same susceptibility" to pulmonary tumors as the conventional colony.

In 1970, however, two laboratories reported that germ-free mice developed fewer lung tumors than conventional mice.

Burstein et al. (*45*) studied germ-free and conventional mice exposed to a single intraperitoneal injection of 20 mg of urethane. Germ-free BALB/c mice showed a lower frequency (9 of 17) and mean number (1.7) of lung tumors per animal than the conventional mice (17 of 20, and a mean of 3.2 lung tumors per animal).

Grant and Roe (*121, 276*) compared C3H mice raised under germ-free and "minimal disease" conditions that were injected with a single subcutaneous dose of dimethylbenzanthracene. Germ-free mice displayed lung tumors in 6 of 109 mice between 28 and 42 weeks, as compared with 33 of 122 among conventional animals, but this difference disappeared by 80 weeks. There was no significant difference in the untreated mice. The authors reported similar effects for primary liver tumors as well: significantly greater frequency was found up to 40 weeks in the conventional mice, but the difference disappeared by 80 weeks and was not significant in the mice not receiving DMBA. The authors (276) interpreted their results as showing that the induction of pulmonary and of hepatic tumors was a cocarcinogenic rather than a carcinogenic effect.

Burstein et al. (45) discussed their results in terms of possible differences of urethane metabolism in the germ-free state as compared with conventional mice. They pointed out the requirement of bacterial conversion of cycasin to the proximal carcinogen, but this is not required for urethane. Their conclusion is cautiously correct: "The reason for a lower susceptibility to lung tumorigenesis by urethane in germ-free mice remains to be determined." It may also be considered that the conventional mice in the experiments of Roe and Grant (276) and of Burstein et al. (45) may have been exposed to unidentified environmental carcinogens from which the germ-free mice were protected. In any case, it is clear that germ-free mice do develop spontaneous and induced lung tumors, and that the influence of the germ-free state is not striking.

B. Effect of Atmospheric Oxygen

Mori-Chavez (240–242) in a series of reports from Peru compared strain A mice maintained at high altitudes and at sea level. He found at high altitudes a somewhat higher frequency of spontaneous lung tumors as well as urethane-induced tumors. The tumors were reported to be larger in mice living at high altitudes. His conclusion was that lower atmospheric pressures increased susceptibility to lung tumors.

Laboratory studies, however, seem to reach the opposite conclusions. Altschul and Whitehead (5) indicated that oxygen deficiency during days 6 and 15 of pregnancy led to a decrease in lung tumors in the progeny. Heston and Pratt (142) exposed mice to 100% and 8% oxygen for 48 hours after dibenzanthracene. Lung tumors were increased by high-oxygen and decreased by low-oxygen conditions. Exposure of newborn strain A mice to these conditions did not alter their spontaneous lung tumor incidence. Di Paolo (73, 74) kept strain A mice injected with urethane in a hyperoxic environment of 70% oxygen and compressed air, and found that these conditions significantly increased the number of lung tumors. Ellis et al. (91), simulating atmospheric pressures of high altitudes, found *fewer* lung tumors induced by urethane in strain A and 3 other strains of mice kept under reduced pressures than in mice at ambient pressures.

C. Metabolic Inhibitors and Other Chemicals

In 1957 Rogers (282) published that the lung tumor response to urethane was potentiated by treating the mice with aminopterin, adenine, and oxaloacetic acid, and inhibited by thymine, asparagine, and orotic, dihydroorotic, ureidosuccinic, and cytidylic acid and was not influenced by thymidylic acid. He constructed a scheme suggesting that urethane acted in the pathway of nucleic acid synthesis below orotic acid. Unfortunately, the observations could not be confirmed by Kaye and Trainin (163), who found no effect on lung-tumor production by urethane in SWR mice treated with thymidine, thymine, orotic acid, or aminopterin. Strain A mice maintained on thymine in drinking water did have some reduction in the spontaneous lung tumor frequency (0.21 vs 0.81 tumors per mouse).

Actinomycin D, 5-fluorouracil, puromycin, and cycloheximide, chemicals that inhibit nucleic acid or protein synthesis at various metabolic steps, did not affect the induction of lung tumors by urethane in strain A mice (306).

Lespagnol et al. (200, 201) and Adenis et al. (2) noted that phenobarbital, which induces microsomal hepatic enzymes, inhibited lung tumor induction with urethane in Swiss mice. In groups of 35 mice each, urethane alone induced a mean of 21.6 ± 3.1 tumors; urethane plus phenobarbital yielded only 9.1 ± 2.0 tumors. Sulfanilamide also had an inhibitory effect: 6.3 lung tumors per mouse were produced in 52 of 63 mice when it was given as well as urethane, versus a mean of 19 lung tumors in all of 18 mice on urethane alone. p-Aminobenzoic acid and butyl and isoamyl carbamate had no significant effects. Enzyme induction could be expected to enhance the excretion of urethane, but no excretion-rate studies are available.

The phenobarbital effect was confirmed by others (67, 372). Yamamoto et al. (372) also found that pretreatment by microsomal enzyme inducers, chlordane, phenobarbital, and β-naphthoflavone reduced the yield of lung tumors in strain A mice receiving urethane. The authors reported also that the number of lung tumors following 3-methylcholanthrene plus urethane was the same as following urethane alone. The possible blocking of methylcholanthrene carcinogenesis by urethane deserves confirmation and extension. Urethane carcinogenesis was not influenced by administration of homologous esters or N-substituted derivatives of carbamic acid (267).

Wattenberg and Leong (363, 364) showed that β-naphthoflavone in the diet increased the activity of benzpyrene hydroxylase in the lung, which resulted in a marked reduction in lung tumors in strain

A exposed to dimethylbenzanthracene (DMBA) or benzpyrene (BP). The inhibitory effect of flavones was related to their activity of inducing BP-hydroxylase.

The effect of the antioxidant, butylated hydroxyanisole (BHA) on carcinogen-induced lung adenomas has been studied by Wattenberg (362). Intraperitoneal administration of BHA caused a decreased number of pulmonary adenomas resulting from subcutaneous administration of diethylnitrosamine and 4-nitroquinoline-N-oxide. BHA also protected against DMBA, BP, uracil mustard, and urethane-induced pulmonary tumor formation when given initially in the diet followed by exposure of the mice to the carcinogens, and against lung tumors induced by DMBA, DBA, and 7-OH-DMBA when given simultaneously in the diet with the carcinogen.

Adenine derivatives were reported to reduce lung tumor induction by urethane (11). Arginine glutamate failed to inhibit lung tumor formation in strain A mice receiving isoniazid and hydrazine (371). Vitamin E hypo- and hypervitaminosis had no effect on lung tumor induction by dibenzanthracene in strain A mice (312). More lung tumors were observed in mice on a high-casein diet than on a low-casein diet following injection with DMBA (359) or urethane (176). Phorbol promoted lung and liver tumor induction by dimethylnitrosamine in newborn AKR mice, but not when the mice were 10 days old (10).

Steroid hormones and the sex of the animals do not have a significant influence on lung tumors. However, Rudali et al. (284–286) claimed that estrogens inhibited lung tumor induction with 3-methylcholanthrene, whereas testosterone had no effect. Somatotropin was reported to promote urethane-induced lung tumors (173). Meisels and Auger (215) found lung tumors following intravaginal dimethylbenzanthracene were increased by treatment of the animal with cortisone and decreased by estrogen due to the effect on absorption of the carcinogen through the altered vaginal epithelium. Decreases in lung tumor induction by cortisone (118) and by estrogen in oil (167) also seem related to the effects of solvents and absorption.

IX. Virus Aspects

The presence of virus particles in pulmonary tumors in mice was established in two reports (43, 169) published in 1972. Previously several authors (175, 269) described dense elementary particles in pulmonary tumor cells examined by electron microscopy. These particles were probably lamellar structures characteristic of type 2 alveolar cells rather than virus particles (135).

Kimura et al. (169) found typical A-type and C-type particles intracisternally in transplanted lung tumors that grew in ascitic form, or in vitro. Bucciarelli and Ribacchi (43) also recorded C-type particles in 6 of 17 primary lung tumors in BALB/c mice, and in 10 of 16 transplanted lung tumors. A-type particles were detected in 15 of 17 neoplasms and in 7 of 11 normal lungs. Immunofluorescent studies showed the presence of group-specific (gs) antigens of type-C RNA viruses.

The role of these virus particles in the induction of pulmonary tumors is not clear. They are seen in many other mouse tumors and in embryonic tissues grown in vitro (31, 51). Klarner and Albrecht (174) in 1966 claimed that cell-free filtrates from urethane-induced lung tumors, when injected into newborn A strain mice, significantly increased the number of lung tumors. Kimura et al. (169), however, elicited no increase in lung tumors with cell-free extracts known to contain viruslike particles, and the filtrates produced no leukemias or sarcomas.

Thus, oncornavirus particles have been observed in lung tumors in mice. Their role, if any, in the development of pulmonary tumors, is not established. Kimura et al. (169) postulated that the particles may represent incomplete or inactive viral genome, and concluded that this "still remains a problem to be solved in the future."

Several investigations have explored the effect of induced virus infection on lung tumor production in mice. Steiner and Loosli (317) in 1950 observed no effect of human influenza type A on the frequency of lung tumors in mice of strains A and C57BL. Casazza et al. (49) infected mice intranasally with influenza A_2 virus and then treated them with urethane. The number of tumors was not significantly affected. The authors suggested that this could have been anticipated since the chemical affects alveoli while the virus affects bronchial epithelium.

Kotin et al. (185–188) infected C57BL mice with 3 myxoviruses (PR-8, Lee strain of influenza B, and Sendai), and exposed the mice to an artificial smog of ozonized gasoline. Among 330 controls, 28, or 8.5%, had lung tumors; 231 exposed to smog had 45, or 19%, and 270 influenza-infected mice had 17 lung tumors, or 7%. The outstanding finding, however, was that among 328 mice infected with influenza and exposed to smog, 33 had bronchogenic squamous carcinomas as well as 16 with adenomatous tumors.

Staemmler et al. (316) in 1970 reported that albino mice infected with PR8 strain of influenza virus A developed pulmonary squamous cell carcinomas and adenocarcinomas. The microphotographs appear convincing. This work deserves attempt at confirmation and extension.

Frolov (*113*) also infected mice with influenza B and A_2 and found an increase in alveologenic tumors in the infected mice as compared with the untreated controls. Mice infected with influenza and injected with urethane, however, had the same number of lung tumors as mice that received urethane alone. Leuchtenberger and Leuchtenberger (*202, 203*) studied the effect of cigarette smoke and influenza virus *in vivo* and *in vitro*, and found only the atypical bronchial proliferations to be anticipated with influenza.

Squartini, Olivi, and Severi (*314*), in a reanalysis of data on foster-nursed and non-foster-nursed BALB/c mice, concluded that the introduction of mammary tumor virus and lymphatic leukemia virus by foster nursing significantly reduced the spontaneous lung tumor incidence. Stoner *et al.* (*320*) found that lung tumor induction by methylcholanthrene and by urethane was suppressed by pretreating the mice with the Moloney strain of murine sarcoma virus. The virus itself did not induce lung tumors. Stromskaya (*322*) reported that the incidence of pulmonary tumors in mice that received a myeloid chloroleukemia virus and urethane was the same as in mice injected with urethane only.

Corbett and Nettesheim (*63*) contribute an interesting observation that influenza virus reduced the enzyme benzpyrene hydroxylase in lungs of BALB/c mice 10 days after infection. This indicates that respiratory infections may affect the metabolism of chemical carcinogens. The possible interplay between viruses and chemicals is also suggested in a preliminary report (*289*) that interferon inhibited the induction of fibrosarcomas and lung tumors in mice injected with methylcholanthrene. The thoughtful review of the induction of cancer by combinations of viruses and other agents, by Roe and Rowson (*278*), is a resource for future studies.

X. Lung Tumor Induction with Chemicals

The lung tumor test has been applied to most major groups of chemical carcinogens. The lung tumor reaction, indeed, was the first evidence of the carcinogenic properties of urethane (*224*) and of isonicotinic hydrazide (*153, 154*). In this and the following section are presented summary data on the major groups of chemical and other carcinogens that have been applied to the lung tumor reaction. The summaries are meant as examples of the use of the lung tumor response for carcinogenesis bioassay, rather than as complete data on such tests.

A. POLYCYCLIC HYDROCARBONS

Table II summarizes findings on 10 polycyclic hydrocarbons and related compounds, following single intravenous injection of approximately 0.25 mg of aqueous dispersions with sodium sulfosuccinate as a wetting agent. On the basis of micromoles per kilogram dose that induced a mean of 1 lung tumor per adult mouse of strain A approximately 6 months after a single exposure, polycyclic hydrocarbons include some of the more potent carcinogenic agents that have been identified. The compounds include two on which the data are indicative of a marginal response, and two that demonstrated no activity. Conclusions regarding these compounds should be limited to the actual dose of the chemical to which the animals were exposed. The conditions of the experiment, such as the route of administration and the vehicle also modify the response. The pulmonary tumor response, moreover, does not necessarily parallel carcinogenic activity as measured by the induction of sarcomas at the site of injection (9).

Walters and Roe (358, 359, 361) have contributed studies on 7,12-dimethylbenz[a]anthracene (DMBA), a carcinogenic polycyclic hy-

TABLE II
COMPARATIVE CARCINOGENICITY OF POLYCYCLIC HYDROCARBONS AND RELATED COMPOUNDS, MEASURED BY INDUCTION OF LUNG TUMORS (LT)[a,b]

Compound	Dose (μmoles/kg)	Mice with LT/ No. of mice	Mean No. LT/mouse	μMoles/kg for 1 LT response
3-Methylcholanthrene, 0.1 mg	15	15/15	11	0.9
3-Methylcholanthrene, 0.5 mg	74	6/6	47	
Dibenz[ah]anthracene	36	10/10	31	1.0
7H-Dibenzo[cg]carbazole	38	12/12	5.7	6.0
Benzo[a]pyrene	40	10/10	3.7	9.5
Dibenz[aj]aceanthrylene	33	9/10	2.7	14
Dibenz[ah]acridine	36	11/12	2.0	18
8-Methylbenzo[c]phenanthrene	42	6/11	0.7	—
7-Methylbenzo[a]pyrene	38	5/10	0.6	—
5-Methoxy-7-propylbenz[a]anthracene	33	1/10	0.1	—
Benz[a]anthracene	44	2/11	0.2	—
Untreated controls	—	4/19	0.2	—

[a] Strain A mice, 8–12 weeks old, received single intravenous injection of 0.25 mg of methylcholanthrene in aqueous dispersion and were killed 20 weeks later.
[b] Data from Andervont and Shimkin (9) and Shimkin (301).

drocarbon frequently used in cancer research, relating the dose to the lung tumor response in adult and newborn BALB/c mice. Klein (180) produced lung tumors in infant BAF_1 mice by intragastric methylcholanthrene and benzpyrene, but not with deoxycholic acid.

B. Carbamates and Aziridines

Table III summarizes data on eight esters of carbamic acid and 14 N-alkylated urethanes examined by Larsen (193–195). Only three carbamates other than urethane produced significantly more lung tumors than the controls, and all were much weaker than the ethyl

TABLE III
Comparative Carcinogenicity of Some Esters of Carbamic Acid and N-Alkylated Carbamates Measured by Induction of Lung Tumors (LT)[a,b]

Compound	Dose per injection (mg/gm)	Mice with LT/ No. of mice	Mean No. LT per mouse
Untreated controls	—	24/141	0.18
Esters of carbamic acid			
Ethyl (urethane)	0.5	102/102	76.9
Isopropyl	0.5	46/51	3.7
n-Propyl	0.5	49/78	0.95
Trichloroethyl	0.25	22/53	0.54
Methyl	0.5	7/46	0.19
n-Butyl	0.25	4/33	0.12
Isoamyl	0.5	3/23	0.13
Chloroethyl	0.5	7/46	0.15
N-Alkylated carbamates			
Methyl	0.5	31/34	6.9
Dimethyl	0.5	43/53	2.7
Ethyl	0.5	19/22	4.0
Diethyl	0.375	27/29	2.5
n-Propyl	0.5	37/37	3.7
Di-n-propyl	0.5	37/39	2.3
Isopropyl	0.5	35/35	26.6
Disopropyl	0.5	38/48	1.6
n-Butyl	0.5	12/38	0.5
Di-n-butyl	0.5	10/49	0.2
Diphenyl	0.5	7/44	0.2
Methylene diurethane	0.5	37/37	28.6
Ethylene diurethane	0.5	44/45	8.2
Ethylidene diurethane	0.5	48/48	45.5

[a] Data from Larsen (193–195).
[b] Strain A mice, male and female, 10–12 weeks old, were injected intraperitoneally weekly for 13 doses and killed at 6 months of age.

compound. The methyl ester was entirely negative. Eight alkylated urethanes were active, but all less than urethane itself.

Larsen (*193–195*) also tested 12 barbiturates, including Nembutal, Luminal, and Seconal, and 9 hypnotics, including chloral hydrate and paraldehyde; all were clearly negative. Also, no increase in lung tumors was elicited with some possible metabolic derivatives of urethane such as urea, thiourea, and ethanol.

Twenty years later, the carbamates were reexamined (*309*). Table IV includes 6 compounds also tested by Larsen (*194, 195*). The results were in good agreement.

On the basis of molar dose, the polycyclic hydrocarbons include chemicals that are over 1000-fold more potent as inducers of lung tumors than are the carbamates. Carbamoyls include chemicals that are more active than the carbamates, but still less than the more active polycyclic hydrocarbons.

C. ALKYLATING AGENTS

Table V presents some of the data of a survey (*307*) of 29 alkylating agents, including many that are used as chemotherapeutic agents in disseminated neoplasms of man. Uracil mustard was found to be the most active, with nitrogen mustard and melphalan in the same order of activity as the more active polycyclic hydrocarbons. The aziridines of Table V also are alkylating agents.

In this study, 3–8 dose levels were used for each agent, so that dose-response relationships could be studied in more detail. Plotting log-dose against the mean number of lung tumors produced a series of parallel lines (*376*). Thus, the more active carcinogens, such as nitrogen mustard, could be compared directly with weaker agents such as epodyl, using the dose that induced 1 lung tumor per adult strain A mouse.

D. NITROSAMINES

Table VI is a summary on 8 nitrosamine compounds tested on SWR mice. The experiment of Mirvish and Kaufman (*227*) included urethane and allows a comparison of the susceptibility of SWR and A strain mice. To the same dose of urethane, A strain mice yielded approximately 4 times more lung tumors than SWR mice. Dimethylnitrosamine (DMN) is the most active compound of the series, in the range of the more active polycyclic hydrocarbons, and the ethyl compound (DEN) is approximately one-tenth as active in the induction of lung tumors.

The induction of lung tumors and other neoplasms in mice with DMN and DEN has been studied by Clapp *et al.* (*56–58*), Toth *et al.*

TABLE IV
COMPARATIVE CARCINOGENIC ACTIVITY OF CARBAMATES AND AZIRIDINES
MEASURED BY INDUCTION OF LUNG TUMORS (LT)[a,b]

Compound	Total dose (μmoles/kg)	Mice with LT/ total mice	LT Mean No.	Dose for 1 LT response (μmoles/kg)
Carbamates				
Ethyl (urethane)	26,933	12/12	24.5	1,963
N-Hydroxyethyl	22,834	15/15	18.6	1,995
Allyl	2,755	10/14	1.3	2,123
N-Cyanoacetylethyl	15,374	13/13	4.0	2,265
N-Acetylethyl	18,302	15/16	3.2	2,371
Isopropyl	23,275	8/10	1.5	26,300
N-Methylnaphthyl	1,190	6/15	0.7	—
n-Propyl	23,275	9/12	0.8	—
N,N-Dimethylolmethoxyethyl	1,339	5/16	0.4	—
Diethyl bicarbamate	1,358	3/13	0.3	—
sec-Butyl	10,238	4/14	0.3	—
n-Hexyl	18,014	4/16	0.3	—
N-Phenylisopropyl	13,392	1/10	0.1	—
Benzyl	15,869	3/15	0.2	—
Phenyl	17,501	2/8	0.5	—
β-Chloroethyl	19,416	2/12	0.4	—
β-Hydroxypropyl	20,150	3/14	0.2	—
n-Butyl	20,477	2/14	0.3	—
Methallyl	20,851	3/12	0.3	—
β-Hydroxyethyl	22,834	8/16	0.5	—
Methyl	31,954	10/16	0.1	—
Aziridines				
3,4-Dichlorophenyl-N-carbamoyl	101	12/15	1.3	85
m-Chlorophenyl-N-carbamoyl	1,219	10/10	5.0	173
Phenyl-N-carbamoyl	1,478	12/12	2.0	194
Cyclohexyl-N-carbamoyl	1,426	11/15	1.0	1,426
p-Methoxyphenyl-N-carbamoyl	1,248	10/16	0.7	—
p-Tolyl-N-carbamoyl	1,358	10/16	0.8	—
o-Ethoxyphenyl-N-carbamoyl	1,167	5/15	0.5	—
p-Fluorophenyl-N-carbamoyl	1,330	4/12	0.5	—
Water-vehicle control	—	6/31	0.2	
Tricaprylin-vehicle control	—	7/28	0.3	
Untreated control	—	2/31	0.1	

[a] Data from Shimkin *et al.* (*309*).
[b] A-strain mice 20 weeks after 12 thrice-weekly intraperitoneal injections.

TABLE V
COMPARATIVE CARCINOGENIC ACTIVITY OF ALKYLATING COMPOUNDS MEASURED
BY INDUCTION OF LUNG TUMORS (LT)[a,b]

Compound	Total dose (μmoles/kg)	Mice with LT/ total mice	Mean LT	Dose for 1 LT response (μmoles/kg)
Uracil mustard (M)	38.0	30/30	20.3	1
Nitrogen M	17.5	36/38	2.8	3
Melphalan	56.2	40/41	4.0	4
Aziridylbenzoquinone	88.7	24/28	2.9	12
Chloroquine M	38.9	12/15	1.4	18
Quinacrine ethyl M	60.0	8/12	1.3	30
Benzimidazole M	357	17/17	3.6	36
Mannitol M	381	20/22	2.4	60
TESPA	111	20/24	1.7	60
Chlorambucil	493	45/47	5.1	60
Hydroquinone M	42.7	16/25	1.4	66
Aniline M	863.3	26/26	5.5	96
OPSPA	515	20/24	2.0	120
Cytoxan	516	20/27	1.3	360
Naphthylamine M	4,477	25/29	2.0	1,200
Diepoxybutane	2,232	21/27	1.5	1,320
Mannitol Myleran	14,196	25/27	3.2	3,000
Epodyl	27,480	12/17	1.2	14,400
Chloroethylmesulfan	3,800	16/27	0.9	—
Quinacrine ethyl M/2	1,284	18/27	0.9	—
Quinacrine propyl M	2.93	8/27	0.4	—
Quinacrine M	16.6	13/15	0.5	—
Quinacrine propyl M/2	17.5	7/19	0.4	—
5-Chloroquine M	24.6	6/19	0.4	—
Benzalpurine M	35.9	7/28	0.5	—
Chloroquine M pamoate	92.4	13/30	0.7	—
Epoxypropidine	204	10/21	0.6	—
5-Chloroquine M pamoate	696	12/24	0.8	—
Diepoxypiperazine	1,212	17/28	0.6	—
Controls	—	272/777	0.4	—

[a] Data from Shimkin et al. (307).

[b] A-strain mice 39 weeks after 12 thrice-weekly intraperitoneal injections.

[c] TESPA, Phosphine sulfide, tris (1-aziridinyl-); OPSPA, Phosphine sulfide, bis (1-aziridinyl) morpholino-.

(341, 346), and others (4, 146, 229). Takayama and Oota (330, 331) recorded positive lung tumor responses to DMN in ddN, ICR, and C3H mice. Active related compounds include N-nitrosomorpholine (244), N,N'-dinitrosopiperazine (291), N-nitrosomethylurea (112, 165, 336), and N-nitrosohexamethyleneimine (4). Nitrosonornicotine, a

TABLE VI
COMPARATIVE CARCINOGENICITY OF SOME NITROSAMINES MEASURED BY INDUCTION OF LUNG TUMORS (LT)[a,b]

Compound	MW	Total dose Mg/kg	Total dose Mmoles/kg	No. mice +/ mice	Mean No. LT/mouse
Urethane	89	2,000	22.4	29/32	6.0 ± 3.6
Dimethylnitrosamine (DMN)	74	20	0.27	33/33	7.8 ± 3.2
Diethylnitrosamine (DEN)	102	200	1.96	28/29	5.3 ± 3.2
Dibutylnitrosamine	158	250	1.58	14/20	1.3 ± 1.0
Nitrosopiperidine[c]	114	107	0.94	16/30	0.7 ± 0.8
N-Acetyl-S-carbethoxycysteine	235	300	1.28	2/18	0.1 ± 0.3
S-Carbamylcysteine	164	800	4.88	11/40	0.4 ± 0.8
S-Carbobenzyloxycysteine	255	400	1.56	8/29	0.3 ± 0.5
Dimethylsulfoxide (DMSO)	78	11,000	141.0	9/20	0.7 ± 0.9
Untreated	–	–	–	10/36	0.3 ± 0.5

[a] Data from Mirvish and Kaufman (227).

[b] SWR males and females, 9–13 weeks old, receiving 2 intraperitoneal injections at 1–2 week intervals, in water or DMSO, sacrificed at 6 months.

[c] One injection only.

compound that could occur in tobacco smoke, induced lung tumors in mice (35, 36).

The lung tumor bioassay procedure was applied effectively by Greenblatt et al. (123–125) and Mirvish et al. (226, 227) to the problem of possible in vivo conversion of nitrites and amines to carcinogenic nitrosamines. Table VII summarizes one investigation. It demonstrates the induction of lung tumors in mice that received sodium nitrite in drinking water and some secondary amines in food. Subsequent work (124), quantitating the optimum doses for the combination, showed that 6.25 gm/kg of piperazine in food and 2.0 gm/l of $NaNO_2$ in water produced a mean of 31 lung tumors per animal. However, the amino acids proline, hydroxyproline, or arginine, secondary amines occurring naturally in food, plus $NaNO_2$ in water, did not increase the number of lung tumors in Swiss mice (123). Nitrosation in vivo was demonstrated for methyl and ethylurea, by formation of nitrosoureas and an increase in lung tumors (226).

The N-nitroso compounds are systemic carcinogens with a great variety of organotropism, and they produce a galaxy of neoplasms in many species of animals. The lung tumor response in mice is but one such carcinogenic effect, which does not parallel carcinogenic activity in other species and in other sites. The reviews of Magee and Barnes (211) Montesano (230), and Druckrey (87) are useful references.

TABLE VII
LUNG TUMORS (LT) FOLLOWING CONCURRENT SODIUM NITRITE
IN DRINKING WATER AND SECONDARY AMINES IN FOOD[a,b]

Compound	Dose (mmoles/kg)	Mice with LT/ total mice	Mean No. LT/mouse
None	–	20/144	0.18
NaNO$_2$	14.5	14/74	0.22
Piperazine (P)	72.5		
Morpholine (M)	72.5	21/142	0.19
Methylalanine (MA)	18.1		
P + NaNO$_2$			
M + NaNO$_2$		91/148	1.57
MA + NaNO$_2$			
Dinitrosopiperazine	0.28		
Nitrosomorpholine	0.69	87/133	3.7
Nitrosomethylalanine	0.52		

[a] Data of Greenblatt et al. (125).
[b] Swiss mice, male and female, 6–11 weeks old, treated for 28 weeks and killed at 40 weeks.

E. HYDRAZINE DERIVATIVES

In 1957 Juhász et al. (153) reported the appearance of lung tumors in 7 of 14 mice receiving isonicotinic acid hydrazide (INH) intraperitoneally, whereas 50 untreated mice were free of lung tumors. The observation was repeated and extended by Biancifiori et al. (26–30) and others (152, 166, 237, 261, 342, 344). A comparative study of 8

TABLE VIII
COMPARATIVE CARCINOGENICITY OF SOME HYDRAZINES MEASURED
BY LUNG TUMOR (LT) INDUCTION[a,b]

Compound	Total dose (mg)	Mice with LT/ total mice	Mean No. LT/mouse
Isoniazid	502	38/38	3.79
Hydrazine	283	22/22	17.86
Isonicotinic acid	326	4/21	0.24
Iproniazid	260	14/40	0.55
Phenylhydrazine	200	16/30	0.80
Benzoylhydrazine	330	36/40	4.05
2-Methoxybenzoylhydrazine	150	19/20	2.15
4-Methoxybenzoylhydrazine	300	38/40	3.50
Untreated	–	17/150	0.1

[a] Data of Biancifiori and Ribacchi (28) and Clayson et al. (59).
[b] BALB/c mice receiving compounds daily via stomach tube; survival 43–59 weeks.

hydrazine derivatives is given in Table VIII. Hydrazine sulfate was a more active inducer of lung tumors than isoniazid, and isonicotinic acid was negative (59).

Hydrazine sulfate induced lung tumors in newborn mice, by oral, intraperitoneal, and percutaneous routes (218–221, 339, 340). Among active related compounds were 4-(isonicotinylhydrazone)pimelic acid (222), pyrazinamide, and semicarbazide (239), 1,1-dimethylhydrazine (277), procarbazine HCL and some of its degradation products (165), benzoylhydrazine (338), and 1-carbamoyl-2-phenylhydrazine (343). INH produced lung tumors but inhibited the appearance of mammary tumors in C3H mice (345).

F. AMINOAZO AND OTHER COMPOUNDS

Table IX presents lung tumor induction by four carcinogenic chemicals with the predominant biological effect of hepatotoxicity and hepatomagenicity in the rat. Mice are considerably more resistant to the hepatic effects of these chemicals than are rats.

Aflatoxin B_1, a carcinogen elaborated by *Aspergillus flavus*, is the most active of the four in producing lung tumors, and on a molar dose basis is about 10 times as active as urethane (370). Aminoazotoluene is intermediate in activity, and the aminofluorene compounds the least active. The N-hydroxy derivative of 2-acetylaminofluorene is of the same order of activity for lung tumor induction as the parent

TABLE IX
LUNG TUMORS (LT) FOLLOWING INJECTIONS OF AMINOAZO DYE, AMINOFLUORENES, AND AFLATOXIN[a,b]

Compound	MW	Dose Mg/mouse	Dose μMoles/kg	Mice with LT/ total mice	Mean No. LT/ mouse	Dose to produce one LT/mouse (μmoles/kg)
2-Amino-5-azotoluene	225	105	18,700	15/15	4.1	4,560
2-Acetylaminofluorene	223	120	27,000	20/21	2.3	11,739
N-Hydroxy-2-acetylaminofluorene	240	120	25,000	16/19	1.9	13,158
Aflatoxin B_1	312	5.6	700	14/14	5.6	121

[a] Data of Andervont and Shimkin (9), Stoner et al. (unpublished), and Wieder et al. (370).

[b] Strain A mice injected intraperitoneally in 12 thrice-weekly doses and killed at 24 weeks.

compound. Red Prontosil, containing a diazo compound, produced lung tumors in 8 of 32 mice at 12 months, whereas no lung tumors were evident in 28 controls (3).

Two naturally occurring carcinogens of plant origin, cycasin and bracken fern, also induce lung tumors in mice. Cycasin induced lung tumors in newborn mice of the DD strain (147). Bracken fern, on feeding to Swiss mice evoked leukemia in all of 33 animals and multiple lung tumors in 5; 38 controls were free of tumors (253).

Mori et al. (231–236, 238) and other investigators in Japan (148, 248), have contributed extensive studies on the induction of lung tumors with 4-nitroquinoline-1-oxide (NQO). A related compound, 4-hydroxyaminoquinoline-1-oxide was much less active (236).

In a study over five generations of strain A mice, Shabad et al. (298) found lung tumors in 56 of 164 mice (34%) exposed to DDT, as compared with 15 of 138 controls (11%), and concluded that DDT is a weak carcinogen.

G. Food Additives, Drugs, etc.

The lung tumor induction bioassay has been applied to chemicals grouped by their use rather than by their structural relationships. The activity of urethane, an anesthetic once popular in veterinary practice, led Larsen (193) to survey other hypnotics. Alkylating agents are used widely in cancer chemotherapy, and include many with carcinogenic activity (307). Metronidazole, a nitroimidazole derivative used in the treatment of *Trichomonas vaginalis*, produced a significant increase in lung tumors in mice (287). Phenprobamate was reported as negative following administration to newborn Swiss mice (151). Table X presents lung-tumor-induction data on 18 selected drugs, used primarily in cancer chemotherapy. It seems reasonable to repeat the suggestion (302) that the carcinogenic potentiality in animals be considered in the choice of drugs for prolonged, reversible diseases.

Epstein et al. (93) tested six food additives by parenteral administration to infant Swiss mice. Safrole was found to yield a positive response, increasing lung tumors in both sexes and hepatomas in males. The total single dose administered was 6.6 mg. Sodium cyclamate in doses of 20–25 mg, increased hepatomas and lung tumors in three strains of mice (283).

Stoner et al. (321) tested 41 food additives by repeated intraperitoneal injections into adult strain A mice. Cinnamyl anthranilate produced a significant increase in lung tumors, an observation reproduced by a second series of test. Safrole and saccharin were negative under the conditions employed.

TABLE X
LUNG TUMOR RESPONSE TO SOME SELECTED CHEMOTHERAPEUTIC AGENTS[a,b]

Compound	Total dose (μmoles/kg)	Mice with LT/ total mice	Mean No. LT/mouse	Dose for + response
Triethylene melamine	25	24/28	26	8
Thio-TEPA	499	16/20	1.5	143
Estradiol mustard	2,028	19/19	4.9	179
β-Deoxythioguanosine	581	10/14	1.0	653
Isophosphamide	5,000	10/12	1.8	1428
1-Propanol-3,3'-imino dimethanesulfonate	3,374	8/12	1.0	3427
Phenesterin	18,605	19/19	3.9	3588
Imidazole mustard	5,340	11/13	1.0	5187
Aminopterin	4	7/23	0.3	—
Adriamycin	66	4/16	0.4	—
Potassium arsenite	300	9/24	0.4	—
Emetine	385	6/16	0.5	—
Stilbamidine	2,200	4/17	0.2	—
Cortisone	3,450	7/24	0.3	—
Phenazopyridine	6,200	6/18	0.5	—
Phenformin	7,317	5/19	0.3	—
Acronycine	8,099	5/17	0.3	—
Tolbutamide	177,580	8/20	0.4	—
Control	—	18/94	0.2	—

[a] Strain A mice receiving 12 thrice-weekly intraperitoneal injections and killed at 6 months.
[b] Data from Stoner et al. (321) and Shimkin (302).

XI. Lung Tumor Induction with Other Agents

A. IONIZING RADIATION

The frequency of lung tumors was increased slightly but significantly in mice exposed daily to 8.8 R (208). A single total body exposure of C57BL mice to 100 R X-rays markedly increased the frequency of lung tumors (63, 246).

Exposure of mice to total body radiation at doses that inhibit cellular division in the lung, however, also inhibits the appearance of urethane-induced lung tumors (53, 54, 62, 88, 90, 108–111, 129). In adult LAF_1 mice, such inhibition occurs with 500–900 R (110). The effect is observed whether urethane precedes X-rays or is given after X-ray exposure. The persistence of effect is indicated as being as long as 8 weeks by Foley and Cole (108), and less than 2 weeks by Bartlett (21). There is no X-ray inhibition of urethane lung tumor induction if the thorax is shielded (109), and inhibition when only the thorax is exposed. Induction of lung tumors by nitrogen mustard was not inhibited by total body radiation at lower doses (89, *141*).

Inhalation of radon, 3×10^3 ME for 4–8 months, by white mice was reported to increase lung tumors (355), but the controls leave something to be desired and emphasis was upon whether the tumors were benign or malignant. Intratracheal administration of plutonium 239 (37) and ruthenium 106 increased lung tumors in BAF_1 mice (*334, 335*). At high doses, however, the number of lung tumors was decreased. Inhalation of plutonium 239 prior to urethane also inhibited lung tumor induction (37). Thorotrast did not yield clearly positive results (*132*).

The mechanism of inhibition of urethane-induced lung tumors by ionizing radiation appears to be through direct action on cellular replication. Foley *et al.* (*111*) showed that a 800 R dose of X-rays sharply reduced the proportion of thymidine-^{3}H-labeled nuclei, an effect that was enhanced by urethane. Cividalli *et al.* (55) found that the rate of catabolism of urethane was not affected by 400 R whole-body X-rays exposure in newborn mice of several strains. Radiation at this dose level inhibits lung tumor induction by urethane, but leukemogenesis is enhanced. The thymus seems not to be involved in the inhibitory effect of X-rays on urethane-induced lung tumors (*20, 21*).

B. Tobacco

The lung tumor reaction has been applied to studies on tobacco smoke and its condensates. Positive but rather unimpressive results were obtained by several investigators. Mühlbock (*243*) exposed 020 × $DBAF_1$ to intermittent cigarette smoke for 2 years and found lung tumors in 23 of 29; untreated controls had tumors in 10 of 32 animals. Essenberg *et al.* (94–96) exposed strain A mice to daily intermittent cigarette smoke for 1 year; 18 of 28 mice had tumors as compared with 12 of 30 controls. He also found a marginal increase of lung tumors when high-nicotine cigarettes were used, and could not relate the effect to the arsenic content. Harris and Negroni (*133, 134*) exposed the resistant C57BL mice to cigarette smoke every other day, and found lung tumors in 4%, as compared with none in the controls.

Tobacco "tars" were applied intraorally in Swiss mice by Di Paolo *et al.* (76, 77), doubling the frequency of lung tumors. Tobacco smoke condensates also increased the number of lung tumors in strain A mice receiving low doses of urethane (78). Mori (*234*) reported a similar enhancement by cigarette smoke of NQO-induced lung tumors. Modest increases in lung tumors followed parenteral injection of tobacco "tar" in several strains of mice (*104, 189, 329*).

Leuchtenberger *et al.*'s (*204–206*) studies of tobacco smoke were equivocal. No increase in lung tumors was seen in 231 CF_1 mice exposed to cigarette smoke. Bronchitis and atypical epithelial changes resembling carcinoma *in situ* were described (*206, 213*). Shabad (*297*) mentioned that cigarette smoke failed to increase lung tumors in albino mice in his experiments.

Tobacco smoke and its condensates seem to be of only weak activity insofar as induction of lung tumors in mice is concerned.

C. Air Pollutants

Air pollutants represent variable mixtures of undefined materials, and may include carcinogens. Investigations on the carcinogenic effects, including the induction of lung tumors, can be divided into exposure of mice to the environments being studied, the reproduction of such environments under laboratory conditions, and the testing of fractions of materials collected in the field.

Lifetime exposure of mice to ambient air in Los Angeles and filtered air, as reported by Gardner *et al.* (*116*) and Emik *et al.* (*92*), did not increase the frequency of lung tumors in A or C57BL mice, although pulmonary infections were definitely increased. In respiratory chambers, in which the concentration of atmospheric pollutants can be raised above ambient conditions, ozonized gasoline did yield an increase in lung tumors in C57BL mice (*186, 187*).

Extracts of particulate atmospheric pollutants gathered in New York City were made by Asahina *et al.* (*12*) and injected into infant Swiss mice. High frequencies of single and multiple lung tumors were found in mice given injections of basic, neutral, and aromatic fractions and oxyneutral subfractions.

The mouse lung tumor reponse has been applied to a variety of industrial inhalation hazards. Lynch *et al.* (*210*) exposed mice to air with asbestos. Lung tumors were found in 46% of 127 dusted mice, and 18% of the tumors were multiple, whereas 36% of 222 controls had lung tumors, of which 8% were multiple. Baetjer *et al.* (*17*) exposed mice and rats to chromate dust. Lung tumors appeared at an earlier age among the dust-exposed mice and among mice injected intravenously with zinc chromate, but the effects were not significant. Inhalation of aluminum oxide by ddN mice produced proliferative changes in the lungs and 1 squamous cell carcinoma in 19 animals (*181*). Peacock and Spence (*260*) reported that inhalation of SO_2 doubled the lung tumor frequency of mice over that of the controls. Gaseous formaldehyde produced atypical metaplastic changes in the bronchi of C3H mice, but no increase in lung tumors (149). Aerosols of phenols from coal tar were used thrice weekly for 55 weeks on C3H mice; there were 23 lung tumors, including 4 adenocarcinomas in 32 mice, but 11 adenomas and no adenocarcinomas in 20 controls (354). Exposure of A and C3H mice to "tar vapors" under industrial conditions increased the lung tumor response only when benzopyrene was added (217). Inhalation of bis(chloroethyl) ether by strain A mice produced a significant response of multiple lung tumors (197). A positive response was elicited also to urethane aerosols (252).

D. Metals and Miscellaneous

Data on the lung tumor response to metals are limited and are based usually on low levels of lifetime exposure. Furst and Haro (114) and Sunderman (325) have furnished recent reviews on metal carcinogenesis.

Schroeder and his associates (292, 293) studied the effect of chromium, lead, cadmium, nickel, and titanium in Swiss mice, the metal salts being added to drinking water at 5 ppm. No carcinogenic effects were detected. Further lifetime observations on mice receiving 5 μg/ml in drinking water of arsenite, germanate, stannous or vanadyl ions also were negative. In fact, mice on arsenite had significantly fewer tumors of all types, including of the lung, compared with mice receiving tin, vanadium, or the controls. Zirconium, antimony, niobium, and fluoride in trace amounts also failed to influence the frequency of tumors (155, 156). Selenium and tellurium produced liver tumors in rats, but no lung or other tumors in Swiss mice (293). Tin or zinc salts in drinking water or food did not increase the lung tumor frequency in stock mice (360).

A group of 29 fatty acids and esters, lactones, and epoxy and peroxy compounds were examined by Swern et al. (328). All were negative for lung tumor induction, although some sarcomas at the site of injection were elicited. In a series of extracts of fungi, *Candida parapsilosis* yielded increased frequency of leukemias and lung tumors (32); the work requires confirmation and extension.

XII. Lung Tumor Bioassay

The lungs of mice provide a biological material for quantitative bioassay of carcinogenic chemicals and other carcinogenic agents. Experiences with practically every type of carcinogen elicited by this and other determinations during the past 35 years allow the suggestion of standardized bioassay procedures.

A. SELECTION OF ANIMALS

Mice of strain A, males and females, 6–8 weeks old and weighing 15–20 gm, are preferred. This is the most susceptible strain. Its spontaneous lung tumor occurrence from 2 to 18 months of age is given in Table XI. Its lung tumor frequency and its response to carcinogens has been stable and reproducible over 30 years.

Inbred strains of mice yield more reproducible data with smaller deviations of the means than noninbred mice (264, 308) or the F_1 crosses of inbred strains. SWR strain is next in susceptibility to strain A, and BALB/c is another susceptible strain (71). The F_1 crosses reflect the more susceptible strain, but there is greater variation in lung tumor counts than in the parent strains (139).

There does not appear to be much gained by using more resistant strains, such as C3H, for pulmonary-induction studies. The response is delayed and the number of tumors is reduced, and the *relative* background occurrence of spontaneous lung tumors requires the same meticulous consideration as in the more susceptible strains.

TABLE XI
Lung Tumors in Untreated Strain A Mice as a Function of Age[a]

Age (months)	Mice (No.)	Mice with lung tumors No.	Mice with lung tumors %	Tumors per mouse (mean No.)
2	20	0	0	0
3	60	1	1.7	0.02
4	66	2	3.0	0.04
5	69	2	2.9	0.04
6	83	6	7.3	0.06
7	115	13	11.3	0.11
8	127	16	12.6	0.15
9	121	30	24.7	0.28
10	212	68	32.1	0.36
11	106	41	38.7	0.47
12	178	71	40.0	0.58
13	104	50	48.0	0.63
14	132	57	42.5	0.57
15	192	129	67.1	1.06
16	43	29	67.5	1.09
17	50	31	62.0	1.06
18	136	105	77.1	1.43

[a] Data from Heston (137) and Shimkin (301).

C57BL, one of the more resistant strains, is useful for investigations in which *avoidance* of alveologenic carcinoma may be desirable, such as induction of bronchogenic carcinoma with inhalants.

Inbred strains are essential for quantitative, exact biological work. Strict brother-to-sister breeding must be maintained for the stock. Pen breeding is adequate for the derivation of experimental animals, as in most bioassays.

It is established that fetal mice are most susceptible, and newborn mice more susceptible to lung tumor carcinogenesis than adult mice. We do not use fetal or newborn mice for practical reasons of logistics that are particularly compelling when the animals are obtained from outside sources. Pregnant mice do not stand travel well and abort following exposure to many toxic compounds. Newborn mice are harder to obtain, handle, and inject than adults. The advantages of using newborn mice seem to be less than the difficulties and inconveniences (*117*). They may be useful in some special situations, such as when only a small amount of chemical is available (275).

Sex does not have an important effect on lung tumors in mice. Strain A males have a consistently slightly higher frequency of lung tumors than females after injections with various vehicles (*307*), but this can be disregarded in the usual bioassay investigation. Truhaut *et al.* (*351*) indicate that, with benzopyrene, females were more sensitive. Since the metabolism of some chemicals is distinctly different in the two sexes, initial bioassays with chemicals should include groups of both sexes. This becomes mandatory with agents which on preliminary toxicology studies indicate a sex difference.

The mice are weighed and assigned randomly to the treatment groups, the vehicle-injected and untreated controls, and to the positive controls to be injected with urethane. Standard environmental and dietary (*332*) conditions are assumed. The absence of infectious diseases and parasites is also assumed, but requires constant vigilance.

B. ADMINISTRATION OF CHEMICALS

The chemicals are tested after preliminary toxicology determinations of the maximum tolerated doses.

The plan is to have 3 groups of 20 to 30 mice each at 3 dose levels. The first dose level is at the maximum-tolerated of a series of 24 intraperitoneal injections given 3 times per week for 8 weeks. The second dose level is one-half of the first. The strain A mouse lung regularly distinguishes a 2-fold difference in doses of carcinogens, so that the second group provides data toward a dose-response relationship; moreover, this group helps assure data on maximum exposure in case the first group suffers unanticipated delayed mortality. Also, general toxicity with loss of weight can inhibit tumor formation, and there are examples of better tumor induction with doses less than the maximum tolerated. The third group is set at one-fifth of the top dose. The three groups provide the essential information on dose-response, upon which much of the interpretation depends.

This dose-response consideration is seldom evident in the literature. It should be emphasized that response at different levels is one of the primary needs of a pharmacologic investigation, and for comparisons of different chemicals or conditions under which they are tested.

The intraperitoneal route is selected for convenience, and because the dose exposure of the animals is best assured. The question asked of this system is whether a chemical is carcinogenic for the lung of strain A mice. It is not intended to mimic exposure conditions in man (127). Thus, the more "natural" routes such as by ingestion or by inhalation, are reserved for later extensions. Of course, compounds that are soluble and stable in water may be given conveniently in the drinking water. Intragastric instillations (179) or intravenous injections are more difficult technically than intraperitoneal injections, and at the primary bioassay stage do not seem to be justified.

The route of the exposure (48, 190, 215) and the physical form in which the chemical is administered affect the tumor response. The chemical must reach the lung, and the subsequent dose and time over which the dose is effective will modify the extent of the reaction. For polycyclic hydrocarbons, the intravenous route is the most effective, producing the maximum contact of the lung with the chemical. The size of the particles of the chemicals is important; the particles must be small enough to be tolerated and large enough to remain impinged in the lung. Intravenous injection is impractical for insoluble carcinogens requiring large doses for effect, such as the aminoazo chemicals.

The response to subcutaneous and intraperitoneal injections is affected by the vehicle used for the compound. The chemical must be released and absorbed in order to reach the lung. Such release must not be too rapid, so that the chemical is active over a maximum period.

Since studies on the absorption and excretion of every chemical to be tested are impractical, the pulmonary-tumor response must be considered relative to the conditions of the experiment. Excretion is also affected by the dose and schedule of administration (368, 369). The relative carcinogenic potency of a series of compounds given by the intravenous route, using aqueous dispersions, may not be the same as the relative potency by subcutaneous injection in a triglyceride.

With all these considerations in mind, however, experience has shown that the chief determinant of the tumor response is the total dose of the chemical to which the mouse is exposed (308, 369).

It is taken for granted that the animals are carefully observed for toxic and other pharmacologic reactions. Body weights, obtained weekly or more frequently during the course of injections, and monthly thereafter, are the best single determinations of the general condition of the animals.

Induced lung tumors have been applied to therapeutic experiments (81, 130), in which the number and size of the tumors in the treated group was compared with appropriate controls. An outstanding example of the use of this system was contributed by Yuhas (375), who investigated the effect of radiotherapy plus a radioprotective drug on urethane-induced lung tumors in RFM mice. Using lungs cleared to render them semitransparent (333), the volume of the nodules could be estimated. The study showed that the tumor volume could be reduced by treatment to one-fourth that of the controls.

C. INTERPRETATION

In the pulmonary-tumor system, a definite time of sacrifice allows the easiest and most definitive interpretation of the data. In strain A mice, 24 weeks are satisfactory, and for most tests, 12 or 16 weeks are sufficient. The animals are sacrificed by any convenient method, the lungs with the mediastinum placed in a fixative (Tellyesniczky's is useful because its acetic acid shrinks the normal lung, making the nodules more evident). The typical pearly-white nodules on the surfaces of the lung are counted at leisure under a dissecting microscope, by two independent observers. Representative sections are then taken for histologic preparations. A "complete autopsy" is desirable on all animals, and tissues that appear grossly abnormal are also preserved for histologic examination.

The analysis and presentation of the data involve comparison with the control groups, after assurance that the pulmonary tumor response among the untreated animals is in the anticipated spontaneous range, and that the response to mice that have received a single intraperitoneal dose of urethane (1 mg per gram body weight) is also in the anticipated range (usually 1 tumor per 1 mg of urethane).

The statistically tested difference between the number of lung tumors in the vehicle-injected controls and the treated mice determines whether a positive carcinogenic response has been elicited. Occurrence of lung tumors deviates to some degree from Poisson's distribution (264). For groups of 20–30 mice, levels of statistical significance ($P < 0.05$) may be reached when a mean of 0.7–0.8 tumor per mouse is observed and compared with a mean of 0.2–0.3 lung tumors among the controls at the age of 8–9 months (Table XI). Most tests are considered positive if several conditions are met: (a) the mean number of lung tumors in the test animals is significantly increased, preferably to 1 or more per mouse, (b) there is a dose-response relationship, (c) the mean number of lung tumors in the vehicle-injected and untreated controls is approximately the anticipated number for untreated mice of the same age. Occasionally, statistical significance is obtained because control animals demonstrate fewer than the anticipated number, and is obviously not acceptable data on which to conclude a positive effect.

Zweifel (376) has published the statistical probability concepts that guide the interpretation of the data. For practical purposes, this involves the plotting of the mean number of tumors versus the log of the molar dose of the chemical (Fig. 7). With several dose levels, a linear dose-response is obtained, and the "carcinogenic index" for the compound is the dose at which the response line transects the 1 tumor-per-mouse level. Lung tumor data limited to single doses can be assumed to follow the same dose-response slope in strain A mice.

The dose-response for adult strain A mice for a wide variety of chemicals is therefore, a series of parallel lines. This slope should be steeper for newborn mice of strain A, demonstrating their greater responsiveness, and flatter for more resistant strains of mice. Appropriate nomograms for conversion are feasible and would be useful, but have not been developed.

As with any bioassay procedure, a proportion of tests will be indeterminate for a variety of reasons. These must be repeated, preferably at higher doses. There is little question when all of the test animals have the lungs studded with lung nodules. A test that depends entirely on statistical analysis is much less convincing. For "negative" compounds, it must be emphasized that the conclusion has to be limited to the dose to which the animal was exposed, and to other conditions of the experiment.

And, finally, positive data obtained on lung tumor bioassay identifies chemicals for further testing in other animal systems such as life-term studies on rats.

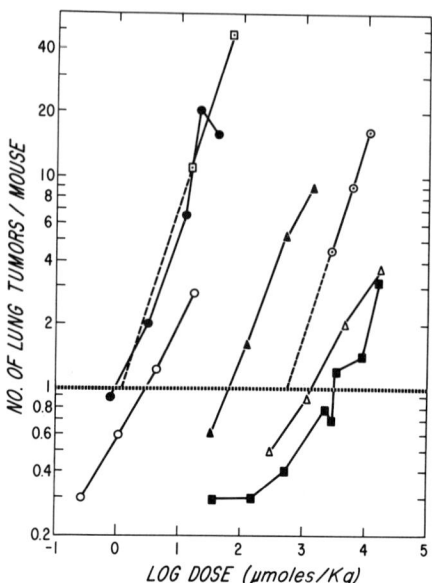

FIG. 7. Logarithmic plot of number of lung tumors per mouse as a function of log dose with selected compounds. ▫, 3-methylcholanthrene; ●, uracil M; ○, HN$_2$; ▲, chlorambucil; ⊙, urethane; △, naphthylamine; ■, mannitol myleran. From Shimkin et al. (307).

XIII. Explants and Embryos

It was known by 1955 that (a) primary pulmonary tumors could be induced in embryo lungs by transplacental exposures, (b) pulmonary tissue implanted intramuscularly or subcutaneously would give rise to tumors following either exposure of the host or of the transplant to a carcinogen, and (c) embryo or newborn mice were more susceptible to the induction of pulmonary tumors than adult mice, in that such tumors appeared earlier and in greater number.

These findings have intrigued a number of investigators to apply them for the purpose of developing what they hoped would be short-term tests for carcinogenic activity of chemicals. In one permutation, Peacock et al. (255–259) minced embryos of BALB/c strain mice, exposed the mince to polycyclic hydrocarbons or other carcinogens, and implanted the mince into thigh muscle of adult BALB/c mice. The tissue was removed after 16 weeks and examined for the histologic evidence of malignant changes. *In vitro* exposure of lung tissue to nitrogen mustard led to development of lung tumors (280), but not to urethane (25, 281). Peacock (256) in 1965 also injected pregnant

BALB/c mice within 3 days of term with isoniazid or urethane, killed the animals 48 hours later, and implanted the fetal tissues into adult mice. The dose of the compounds had to be restricted because of abortion. Sixteen weeks later 8 of 78 implants of tissue exposed to isoniazid had adenomas, but none appeared in 31 urethane-treated implants.

Flaks and Laws (*105–107, 196*) varied the experiments by explanting lungs of BALB/c mice and exposing them to 3-methylcholanthrene in organ culture for 1–6 days, and then implanting the tissue into homologous animals. Recovery of the tissue showed lung tumors 3–12 months later. Tumors occurred more frequently in embryonic lungs than in lungs taken from weanling mice. Davies *et al.* (65, 66) repeated the work and obtained essentially identical results; however, higher doses of methylcholanthrene were necessary to obtain tumors.

Kolesnichenko (*182–184*) and Shabad *et al.* (*296, 299*) reported another scheme, in which strain A mice were injected with 3 doses of urethane during the second half of pregnancy, the animals were killed, and the embryo lungs were maintained in organ culture. The author describes the histologic appearance of adenomas within 4 to 14 days of cultivation. Unfortunately, the reports do not contain data on the abortion rate among pregnant females exposed to the doses of up to 100 mg of urethane. Since the initial reports, their scheme has been extended to nitrosamines (*311*).

The use of mouse lungs for quantitative carcinogenesis investigations resembles some of the contemporary *in vitro* studies in which cells are plated and observed for the appearance of foci of transformed cells. Carcinogen-treated cells often require several passages *in vitro* before they can produce tumors on transplantation into appropriate animals.

The lungs of mice of susceptible strains can be visualized as lattices with the target type 2 alveolar cells being progenitors of the adenomas. The adenomas require time or passage in order to demonstrate progression of morphologic and biologic properties to the overt malignant stage.

The advantages of the mouse lung over even theoretical *in vitro* systems of the future include (a) the participation of the host in the carcinogenic reaction, thus facilitating demonstration of carcinogens that require metabolic conversion, (b) the homeostatic mechanisms of the tissue and host that are lost *in vitro*, (c) easier maintenance of mice and lesser probabilities of extraneous complications. It is premature to consider cost (including time) of the two procedures for carcinogenesis testing, but if several transfers of *in vitro* cells, and at least partial confirmation of *in vitro* transformation are necessary, lung tumor observations in 12–16 weeks may not be significantly longer than *in vitro* techniques.

Transplacental *in vivo–in vitro* techniques become particularly complicated and expensive if there is requirement for embryonic tissues or the use of pregnant mice, which tend to abort when exposed to toxic chemicals. Truly rapid, uncomplicated *in vitro* assays of carcinogenesis would be a great boon. One requirement is for stable yet reactive cell lines, the equivalent of homozygous mouse strains that are irreplaceable for biologic investigations. It also requires the demonstration that certain morphologic criteria *in vitro* represent the equivalent of neoplastic change *in vivo*. Tests requiring production of tumors *in vivo* by cells maintained *in vitro* defeat the rapid bioassay purposes of the *in vitro* system.

One of the advantages of the *in vitro* systems is the ability to observe morphological changes under a microscope. This is not possible for mouse lungs *in situ*, but perhaps explants to the ears or to the anterior chamber of the eye (22) might provide such accessibility. It may also be rewarding to sacrifice strain A mice following exposure to carcinogens *in vivo*, and then to observe the lung tissue *in vitro* (50). Perhaps islands of type-2 derived cells, identifiable *in vivo* as early as 21 days following urethane as adenomas, may be visualized even earlier under *in vitro* conditions.

XIV. Conclusions

Pulmonary tumors in mice have now attracted cancer investigators in many laboratories throughout the world, but the system has failed to gain acceptance as a bioassay screening procedure for carcinogenic activity of chemicals. The criticisms of the system are that the adenoma has no counterpart in human neoplastic pathology, and that the numerical increase and earlier appearance of the tumors merely accelerates a process already present in the animal rather than being a true inductive process. Thus it could be considered as more in the nature of cocarcinogenesis than that of carcinogenesis (273). These criticisms are valid, of course, but apply to some degree to most, if not all, bioassay systems.

Complete one-to-one relationship of one animal model to the human situation (122) is probably in the realm of searches for the philosopher's stone. The value of any experimental model lies in the questions proposed to it.

The lung-tumor response in strain A mice is easily and clearly positive to all major types of chemical carcinogens. Estrogenic and other steroid hormones, with the targets of endocrine-regulated tissues, are an exception.

The lung tumor of the mouse has demonstrated its ability to pick up undetected, unpredicted neoplastic responses, such as to urethane and to isoniazid. The carcinogens picked up by the lung tumor system, without exceptions known to us, have been shown to be carcinogenic for other tissues and in other species of animals. Although lung tumors are the earliest neoplasms induced by urethane, for example, further work showed the compound to be an intriguing multipotential carcinogen (224). Its possible carcinogenic potential in man of course remains unestablished.

An instructive example of the use of the lung tumor response in mice was published by Roe *et al.* (274). Mice delivered by a commercial source had a higher-than-anticipated frequency of lung tumors, and the offspring of these mice had a lower frequency. It was learned that the commercial dealer used creosote on his wooden cages. Creosote was tested by skin painting, and it evoked skin and pulmonary tumors. Pulmonary tumors were also evoked by a concentration of creosote that yielded no skin tumors. Thus, an environmental carcinogen was detected by an increase in lung tumors in mice.

Pulmonary tumors in mice are not a suitable "model" for studies directed at bronchogenic carcinoma. Inhalation experiments are probably better carried out on larger animals. The small dose exposure possible on intratracheal injection in mice, as well as the high mortality with the procedure, makes this route of limited use. Access to the alveolar cell lining is probably better achieved by the intravenous route. The important role of impingement of carcinogens in the lung as a necessary factor in bronchogenic carcinogenesis was shown by Shabad *et al.* (300) with India ink powder in rats and by Saffioti and Borg (288) with hematite in hamsters. The technique has been extended with Freund's adjuvant to mice (374), and it should be useful to explore it further.

What, then, is the value of the lung tumor test? We believe that its value lies especially in two areas. The first is that it is one of the fastest *in vivo* systems for the evocation of a neoplastic reaction. Large numbers of compounds can be screened within a 6-month period for this one end-point. Positive compounds require extension to other systems, such as lifetime exposure of rats. Proof of the negative, i.e., safety in the sense of absence of carcinogenic activity, is much more difficult. Any bioassay approach to this standard is hazardous. We anticipate that in the future, *in vitro* tests, such as mutagenicity tests in bacteria and mammalian cell transformation, will replace many of the longer *in vivo* procedures. Yet we remain convinced that carcinogenesis is a complex for which any single screening procedure is probably intellectually simplistic.

The second value of the mouse lung tumor is that it is a reproducible, stable, rapid, biological model for a wide variety of quantitative investigations in carcinogenesis. It provides a three-dimensional lattice of the lung in which a known, identifiable subpopulation of cells, the type 2 alveolar pneumocytes, can be accelerated into conversion into neoplasms. A limitation of the model is that the animal has to be sacrificed in order to make the necessary observations. Perhaps the addition of *in vitro* culture techniques will obviate this limitation.

REFERENCES

1. Adenis, L., Vlaeminck, M. N., and Driessens, J. (1969). *C. R. Soc. Biol.* **163**, 2147–2150.
2. Adenis, L., Vlaeminck, M. N., and Driessens, J. (1970). *C. R. Soc. Biol.* **164**, 560–562.
3. Albert, Z. (1955). *Patol. Pol.* **6**, 77–81.
4. Althoff, J., Pour, P., Cardesa, A., and Mohr, U. (1972). *Z. Krebsforsch.* **78**, 78–81.
5. Altschul, R., and Whitehead, W. F. (1957). *Beitr. Pathol. Anat. Allg. Pathol.* **117**, 331–336.
6. Amaral-Mendes, J. J. (1969). *J. Pathol.* **97**, 415–427.
7. Andervont, H. B. (1939). *Pub. Health Rep.* **54**, 1519–1524.
8. Andervont, H. B., and Dunn, T. B. (1962). *J. Nat. Cancer Inst.* **28**, 1153–1163.
9. Andervont, H. B., and Shimkin, M. B. (1941). *J. Nat. Cancer Inst.* **1**, 225–239.
10. Armuth, V., and Berenblum, I. (1972). *Cancer Res.* **32**, 2259–2262.
11. Asadov, D. A. (1968). *Vop. Onkol.* **14** (1), 82.
12. Asahina, S., Andrea, J., Carmel A., Arnold, E., Bishop, Y., Jodei, S., Coffin, D., and Epstein, S. S. (1972). *Cancer Res.* **32**, 2263–2268.
13. Asari, S. (1958). *Acta Pathol. Jap.* **8**, 27–43.
14. Auger, C., and Meisels, A. (1967). *Laval Med.* **38**, 680–685.
15. Azzopardi, A., and Thurlbeck, W. M. (1967). *Lab. Invest.* **16**, 706–716.
16. Azzopardi, A., and Thurlbeck, W. M. (1969). *Amer. Rev. Resp. Dis.* **100**, 801–812.
17. Baetjer, A. M., Lowney, J. F., Steffee, H., and Budacz, V. (1959). *AMA Arch. Ind. Health* **20**, 124–135.
18. Balo, J., Kendrey, G., and Veres, J. (1968). *Magy. Onkol.* **12**, 83–89.
19. Baroni, C. D., Mingazzini, P., Pesando, P., Cavallero, A., Uccini, S., and Scelsi, R. (1972). *Tumori* **58**, 397–408.
20. Bartlett, G. L. (1970). *Int. J. Cancer* **5**, 384–388.
21. Bartlett, G. L. (1970). *Int. J. Cancer* **6**, 56–62.
22. Baudot, S., and May, R. M. (1964). *Bull. Ass. Fr. Etude Cancer* **51**, 541–561.
23. Bekierkunst, A., Levij, I. S., Yarkoni, E., Vilkas, E., and Lederer, E. (1971). *Science* **174**, 1240–1242.
24. Bentvelzen, P. A. J., and Szalay, G. (1966). Cited in ref. 295, pp. 835–844.
25. Berenblum, I., Kaye, A. M., and Trainin, N. (1960). *Cancer Res.* **20**, 38–43.

26. Biancifiori, C., Bucciavelli, E., Clayson, D. B., and Santilli, F. E. (1964). *Brit. J. Cancer* **18**, 543–550.
27. Biancifiori, C., Giornelli Santilli, F. E., Milia, U., and Bucciarelli, E. (1966). Cited in ref. 295, pp. 881–895.
28. Biancifiori, C., and Ribacchi, R. (1962). *Nature (London)* **194**, 488–489.
29. Biancifiori, C., Santilli, F. E., Bucciarelli, E., and Ribacchi, R. (1963). *Lav. Ist. Anat. Istol. Patol. Univ. Studi Perugia* **23**, 209–220.
30. Biancifiori, C., and Severi, L. (1966). *Brit. J. Cancer* **20**, 528–538.
31. Biczysko, W., Pienkowski, M., Solter, D., and Koprowski, H. (1973). *J. Nat. Cancer Inst.* **51**, 1041–1050.
32. Blank, F., Chin, O., Just, G., Meranze, D. R., Shimkin, M. B., and Wieder, R. (1968). *Cancer Res.* **28**, 2276–2281.
33. Bloom, J. L. (1964). *J. Nat. Cancer Inst.* **33**, 599–606.
34. Bloom, J. L., and Falconer, D. S. (1964). *J. Nat. Cancer Inst.* **33**, 607–618.
35. Boyland, E., and Roe, F. J. C. (1966). Cited in ref. 295, pp. 667–676.
36. Boyland, E., Roe, F. J. C., Gorrod, J. W., and Mitchley, B. C. V. (1964). *Brit. J. Cancer* **18**, 265–270.
37. Brightwell, J., and Heppleston, A. G. (1973). *Brit. J. Radiol.* **46**, 180–182.
38. Brooks, R. E. (1966). *Amer. Rev. Resp. Dis.* **94**, 112–113.
39. Brooks, R. E. (1968). *J. Nat. Cancer Inst.* **41**, 719–742.
40. Brooks, R. E., and Adkinson, B. (1971). *J. Nat. Cancer Inst.* **47**, 639–644.
41. Brown, E. S. (1964). *Amer. J. Physiol.* **207**, 402–406.
42. Bucciarelli, E., Biancifiori, C., and Rosi, F. (1968). *Lav. Ist. Anat. Istol. Patol. Univ. Studi Perugia* **28**, 41–55.
43. Bucciarelli, E., and Ribacchi, R. (1972). *J. Nat. Cancer Inst.* **49**, 673–684.
44. Bulay, O. M., and Wattenberg, L. W. (1971). *J. Nat. Cancer Inst.* **46**, 397–402.
45. Burstein, N. A., McIntire, K. R., and Allison, A. C. (1970). *J. Nat. Cancer Inst.* **44**, 211–214.
46. Burt, R. C., Killmeyer, L. A., and Grauer, R. C. (1959). *J. Histochem. Cytochem.* **7**, 182–188.
47. Calafat, J., Den Engelse, L., and Emmelot, P. (1970). *Chem. Biol. Interactions* **2**, 309–320.
48. Campbell, J. S., Yang, Y. H., and Bolton, J. D. (1965). *Arch. Pathol.* **79**, 588–594.
49. Casazza, A. M., Gaetani, M., Ghione, M., and Turolla, E. (1965). *Tumori* **51**, 401–418.
50. Chan, P. C., Sanders, F. K., and Wynder, E. L. (1969). *Nature (London)* **223**, 847–848.
51. Chase, D. G., and Piko, L. (1973). *J. Nat. Cancer Inst.* **51**, 1971–1975.
52. Chieco-Bianchi, L., Fiore-Donati, L., Tridente, G., and De Benedictis, G. (1965). *Tumori* **51**, 53–68.
53. Chouroulinkov, I., Riviere, M. R., Arnold, J., and Guerin, M. (1966). *C. R. Soc. Biol.* **160**, 234–237.
54. Chouroulinkov, I., Riviere, M. R., and Guerin, M. (1965). *Bull. Ass. Fr. Etude Cancer* **52**, 331–348.
55. Cividalli, G., Mirvish, S. S., and Berenblum, I. (1965). *Cancer Res.* **25**, 855–858.
56. Clapp, N. K. (1973). *Int. J. Cancer* **12**, 728–833.
57. Clapp, N. K., and Craig, A. W. (1967). *J. Nat. Cancer Inst.* **39**, 903–916.
58. Clapp, N. K., Craig, A. W., and Toya, R. E. (1968). *J. Nat. Cancer Inst.* **41**, 1213–1228.
59. Clayson, D. B., Biancifiori, C., Milia, U., and Giornelli-Santilli, F. E. (1966). Cited in ref. 295, pp. 869–877.

60. Clements, J. A., Nellenbogen, J., and Trahan, H. J. (1970). *Science* **169**, 603–604.
61. Colnaghi, M. I., Ménard, S., and Della Porta, G. (1971). *J. Nat. Cancer Inst.* **47**, 1325–1331.
62. Conklin, J. W., Upton, A. C., and Christenberry, K. W. (1965). *Cancer Res.* **25**, 20–28.
63. Corbett, H., and Nettesheim, P. (1973). *J. Nat. Cancer Inst.* **50**, 779–782.
64. Crocker, T. T., Teeter, A., and Nielsen, B. (1970). *Cancer Res.* **30**, 357–361.
65. Davies, R. F., Major, I. R., and Aberdeen, E. R. (1970). *Brit. J. Cancer* **24**, 785–787.
66. Davies, R. F., Major, I. R., and Aberdeen, E. R. (1971). *Brit. J. Cancer* **25**, 565–567.
67. De Azevedo, E., and Silva, E. (1967). *Hospital (Rio de Janeiro)* **72**, 205–219.
68. De Benedictis, G., and Mariorano, G. (1962). *Brit. J. Cancer* **16**, 686–689.
69. Della Porta, G., Colnaghi, M. I., and Parmi, L. (1970). *Tumori* **56**, 121–135.
70. Den Engelse, L., Bentvelzen, P. A. J., and Emmelot, P. (1970). *Chem. Biol. Interactions* **1**, 395–406.
71. Deringer, M. K. (1965). *J. Nat. Cancer Inst.* **35**, 1047–1052.
72. Deringer, M. K., and Heston, W. E. (1955). *J. Nat. Cancer Inst.* **16**, 763–768.
73. Di Paolo, J. A. (1959). *J. Nat. Cancer Inst.* **23**, 535–540.
74. Di Paolo, J. A. (1962). *Cancer Res.* **22**, 299–403.
75. Di Paolo, J. A. (1965). *J. Nat. Cancer Inst.* **34**, 337–343.
76. Di Paolo, J. A., and Levin, M. L. (1965). *J. Nat. Cancer Inst.* **34**, 595–600.
77. Di Paolo, J. A., and Moore, G. E. (1959). *J. Nat. Cancer Inst.* **23**, 529–534.
78. Di Paolo, J. A., and Sheehe, P. A. (1962). *Cancer Res.* **22**, 1058–1060.
79. Divertie, M. B., Shorter, R. G., and Titus, J. L. (1968). *Thorax* **23**, 83–86.
80. Diwan, B. A., and Meier, H. (1974). *Cancer Res.* **34**, 764–770.
81. Djioev, F. K. (1965). *Vop. Onkol.* **11**(9), 51–54.
82. Domsky, I. I., Lijinsky, W., Spencer, K., and Shubik, P. (1963). *Proc. Soc. Exp. Biol. Med.* **113**, 110–112.
83. Driessens, J., Clay, A., Vanlerenberghe, J., and Adenis, L. (1962). *C. R. Soc. Biol.* **156**, 655–657.
84. Driessens, J., Clay, A., Vanlerenberghe, J., Adenis, L., and Quandale, P. (1963). *C. R. Soc. Biol.* **157**, 1448–1449.
85. Driessens, J., Clay, A., Vanlerenberghe, J., Dupont, A., Demaille, A., and Adenis, L. (1963). *Bull. Cancer* **50**, 171–182.
86. Driessens, J., Dupont, A., and Demaille, A. (1963). *C. R. Soc. Biol.* **157**, 560–563.
87. Druckrey, H. (1973). *Xenobiotika* **3**, 271–303.
88. Duhig, J. T. (1965). *Arch. Pathol.* **79**, 177–179.
89. Duhig, J. T. (1965). *Arch. Pathol.* **79**, 180–184.
90. Duplan, J. F. (1962). *Bull. Ass. Fr. Etude Cancer* **49**, 260–269.
91. Ellis, H. A., Styles, J. A., and Heppleston, A. G. (1966). *Brit. J. Cancer* **20**, 375–384.
92. Emik, L. O., Plata, R. L., Campbell, K. I., and Clarke, G. L. (1971). *Arch. Environ. Health* **23**, 335–342.
93. Epstein, S. S., Fujii, K., Andrea, J., and Mantel, N. (1970). *Toxicol. Appl. Pharmacol.* **16**, 321–334.
94. Essenberg, J. M. (1957). *West. J. Surg., Obstet. Gynecol.* **65**, 161–163.
95. Essenberg, J. M., Horowitz, M., and Gaffney, E. (1955). *West. J. Surg., Obstet. Gynecol.* **63**, 265–267.
96. Essenberg, J. M., Leavitt, A. M., and Gaffney, E. (1956). *West. J. Surg., Obstet. Gynecol.* **64**, 35–36.

97. Evans, M. J., Cabral, L. J., Stephens, R. J., and Freeman, G. (1973). *Amer. J. Pathol.* **70**, 175-198.
98. Evans, M. J., Cabral, L. J., Stephens, R. J., and Freeman, G. (1973). *Amer. J. Pathol.* **70**, 199-208.
99. Evans, M. J., Stephens, R. J., Cabral, L. J., and Freeman, G. (1972). *Arch. Environ. Health* **24**, 180-188.
100. Falconer, D. S., and Bloom, J. L. (1961). *Nature (London)* **191**, 1070-1071.
101. Falconer, D. S., and Bloom, J. L. (1964). *Brit. J. Cancer* **18**, 322-332.
102. Fiore-Donati, L., De Benedictis, G., Malorano, G., and Chieco-Bianchi, L. (1961). *Naturwissenschaften* **48**, 409-410.
103. Flaks, A. (1965). *Brit. J. Cancer* **19**, 547-550.
104. Flaks, A. (1966). *Brit. J. Cancer* **20**, 145-147.
105. Flaks, A. (1967). *Brit. J. Cancer* **21**, 390-392.
106. Flaks, A., and Laws, J. O. (1968). *Brit. J. Cancer* **22**, 839-842.
107. Flaks, B., and Flaks, A. (1972). *J. Pathol.* **108**, 211-217.
108. Foley, W. A., and Cole, L. J. (1963). *Cancer Res.* **23**, 1176-1180.
109. Foley, W. A., and Cole, L. J. (1964). *Cancer Res.* **24**, 1910-1917.
110. Foley, W. A., and Cole, L. J. (1966). *Radiat. Res.* **27**, 87-91.
111. Foley, W. A., Cole, L. J., Ingram, B. J., and Crocker, T. T. (1963). *Nature (London)* **199**, 1267-1268.
112. Frei, J. V. (1970). *Cancer Res.* **30**, 11-17.
113. Frolov, A. F. (1970). *Vop. Onkol.* **16**(5), 72-76.
114. Furst, A., and Haro, R. T. (1969). *Progr. Exp. Tumor Res.* **12**, 102-133.
115. Ganter, P., and Maral, R. (1966). *C. R. Soc. Biol.* **160**, 46-49.
116. Gardner, M. B., Loosli, G. G., Hanes, B., Blackmore, W., and Teebken, D. (1970). *Arch. Environ. Health* **20**, 310-317.
117. Gargus, J. L., Paynter, O. E., and Reese, W. H., Jr. (1969). *Toxicol. Appl. Pharmacol.* **15**, 552-559.
118. Gillman, T., Hathorn, M., and Penn, J. (1956). *Brit. J. Cancer* **10**, 394-400.
119. Gluck, L., Kulovich, M. V., Eidelman, A. I., Cardero, L., and Khazin, A. F. (1972). *Pediat. Res.* **6**, 81-99.
120. Grady, H. G., and Stewart, H. L. (1940). *Amer. J. Pathol.* **16**, 417-432.
121. Grant, G. A., and Roe, F. J. C. (1969). *Nature (London)* **223**, 1060.
122. Grasso, P., and Crompton, R. F. (1972). *Food Cosmet. Toxicol.* **10**, 418-426.
123. Greenblatt, M., and Lijinsky, W. (1972). *J. Nat. Cancer Inst.* **48**, 1389-1392.
124. Greenblatt, M., and Mirvish, S. S. (1973). *J. Nat. Cancer Inst.* **50**, 119-124.
125. Greenblatt, M., Mirvish, S. S., and So, B. T. (1971). *J. Nat. Cancer Inst.* **46**, 1029-1034.
126. Greenstein, J. P. (1947). "Biochemistry of Cancer," pp. 224-225. Academic Press, New York.
127. Griciute, L. A. (1957). *Arkh. Patol.* **19**(4), 22-31, 88.
128. Griciute, L. A. (1958). *Vop. Onkol.* **4**(1), 39-48.
129. Griciute, L. A. (1961). *Vop. Onkol.* **7**(3), 64-68.
130. Griciute, L. A. (1964). *Vop. Onkol.* **10**(12), 59-63.
131. Griciute, L. A., and Rudali, G. (1969). *Rev. Fr. Etud. Clin. Biol.* **14**, 75-80.
132. Guimaraes, J. P., and Lamerton, L. F. (1956). *Brit. J. Cancer* **10**, 527-532.
133. Harris, R. J. C., and Negroni, G. (1966). Cited in ref. 295, pp. 497-512.
134. Harris, R. J. C., and Negroni, G. (1967). *Brit. Med. J.* **iv**, 637-641.
135. Hattori, S., Matsuda, M., and Wada, A. (1965). *Gann* **56**, 275-280.
136. Heston, W. E. (1940). *J. Nat. Cancer Inst.* **1**, 105-111.
137. Heston, W. E. (1942). *J. Nat. Cancer Inst.* **3**, 79-82.

138. Heston, W. E. (1954). *J. Nat. Cancer Inst.* **15**, 755–789.
139. Heston, W. E. (1957). *Proc. Int. Genet. Symp., Tokyo, 1956*, pp. 219–224.
140. Heston, W. E. (1966). Cited in ref. 295, pp. 43–56.
141. Heston, W. E., Lorenz, E., and Deringer, M. K. (1963). *Cancer Res.* **13**, 573–577.
142. Heston, W. E., and Pratt, A. W. (1959). *J. Nat. Cancer Inst.* **22**, 707–717.
143. Heston, W. E., and Schneiderman, M. A. (1953). *Science* **117**, 109–111.
144. Heston, W. E., and Steffee, C. H. (1957). *J. Nat. Cancer Inst.* **18**, 779–793.
145. Heston, W. E., and Vlahakis, G. (1961). *J. Nat. Cancer Inst.* **27**, 1189–1196.
146. Hilfrich, J., Althoff, J., and Mohr, U. (1970). *Z. Krebsforsch.* **75**, 240–242.
147. Hirono, I., and Shibuya, C. (1970). *Gann* **61**, 403–407.
148. Hisamatsu, T., Mori, K., and Okamoto, K. (1965). *Gann* **56**, 77–79.
149. Horton, A. W., Tye, R., and Stemmer, K. L. (1963). *J. Nat. Cancer Inst.* **30**, 31–43.
150. Itagi, K. (1956). *Acta Tuberc. Jap.* **6**, 75–90.
151. Jahn, U., Adrian, R. W. (1966). *Arzneim. Forsch.* **16**, 1539–1543.
152. Jones, C. D., Fairchild, D. G., and Morse, W. C. (1971). *Amer. Rev. Resp. Dis.* **103**, 612–617.
153. Juhász, J., Baló, J., and Kendrey, G. (1957). *Z. Krebsforsch.* **62**, 188–196.
154. Juhász, J., Baló, J., and Szende, B. (1963). *Z. Krebsforsch.* **65**, 434–438.
155. Kanisawa, M., and Schroeder, H. A. (1967). *Cancer Res.* **27**, 1192–1195.
156. Kanisawa, M., and Schroeder, H. A. (1969). *Cancer Res.* **29**, 892–895.
157. Karrer, H. E. (1956). *J. Biophys. Biochem. Cytol.* **2**, 241–252.
158. Kauffman, S. L. (1969). *Amer. J. Pathol.* **54**, 83–93.
159. Kauffman, S. L. (1971). *Amer. J. Pathol.* **64**, 531–540.
160. Kauffman, S. L. (1972). *Amer. J. Pathol.* **68**, 317–326.
161. Kauffman, S. L. (1974). *Lab. Invest.* **30**, 170–175.
162. Kaye, A. M. (1960). *Cancer Res.* **20**, 237–241.
163. Kaye, A. M., and Trainin, N. (1966). *Cancer Res.* **26**, 2206–2212.
164. Kelly, M G., Newton, W. L., and O'Gara, R. W. (1963). *Cancer Res.* **23**, 978–982.
165. Kelly, M. G., O'Gara, R. W., Yancey, S. T., and Botkin, C. (1968). *J. Nat. Cancer Inst.* **41**, 619–626.
166. Kelly, M. G., O'Gara, R. W., Yancey, S. T., Gadekar, K., Botkin, C., and Oliverio, V. T. (1969). *J. Nat. Cancer Inst.* **42**, 337–344.
167. Kendrey, G., Baló, J., and Juhász, J. (1958). *Acta Morphol.* **8**, 95–104.
168. Kimura, I. (1971). *Acta Pathol. Jap.* **21**, 13–56.
169. Kimura, I., Miyake, T., Ishimoto, A., and Ito, Y. (1972). *Gann* **63**, 563–574.
170. Kimura, I., Miyake, T., and Ito, Y. (1970). *Proc. Soc. Exp. Biol. Med.* **134**, 504–506.
171. Kinosita, R., and Tanaka, T. (1966). Cited in ref. 295, pp. 717–728.
172. Kitamura, H. (1964). *Acta Pathol. Jap.* **14**, 147–166.
173. Klarner, P. (1956). *Z. Krebsforsch.* **61**, 276–279.
174. Klarner, P., and Albrecht, B. (1966). *Naturwissenschaften* **53**, 44.
175. Klarner, P., and Gieseking, R. (1960). *Z. Krebsforsch.* **64**, 7–21.
176. Klarner, P., and Klarner, R. (1957). *Z. Krebsforsch.* **62**, 85–89.
177. Klaus, M., Reiss, O. K., Tooley, W. H., Piel, C., and Clements, J. A. (1962). *Science* **137**, 750–751.
178. Klein, M. (1957). *Cancer Res.* **17**, 655–658.
179. Klein, M. (1962). *J. Nat. Cancer Inst.* **29**, 1035–1046.
180. Klein, M. (1963). *Cancer Res.* **23**, 1701–1707.
181. Kobayoshi, N., Ide, G., Katsuki, H., and Yamane, Y. (1968). *Gann* **59**, 433–436.
182. Kolesnichenko, T. S. (1966). *Vop. Onkol.* **12**(12), 39–47.
183. Kolesnichenko, T. S. (1968). *Vop. Onkol.* **14**(6), 83–88.

184. Kolesnichenko, T. S. (1971). *Vop. Onkol.* **17**(7), 59–62.
185. Kotin, P. (1964). *Proc. Can. Cancer Res. Conf.* **6**, 475–498.
186. Kotin, P., and Falk, H. L. (1956). *Cancer (Philadelphia)* **9**, 910–917.
187. Kotin, P., Falk, H. L., and McCammon, C. J. (1958). *Cancer (Philadelphia)* **11**, 473–481.
188. Kotin, P., and Wisely, D. V. (1963). *Progr. Exp. Tumor Res.* **3**, 186–215.
189. Kourilsky, R., and Happert, J. L. (1964). *Bull. Ass. Fr. Etude Cancer* **51**, 243–267.
190. Kuwahara, A., Otsuka, H., and Nagamatsu, A. (1972). *Gann* **63**, 499–502.
191. Lappé, M. A., and Prehn, R. T. (1970). *Cancer Res.* **30**, 1357–1361.
192. Lappé, M. A., and Steinmuller, D. S. (1970). *Cancer Res.* **30**, 674–678.
193. Larsen, C. D. (1946). *J. Nat. Cancer Inst.* **7**, 5–8.
194. Larsen, C. D. (1947). *J. Nat. Cancer Inst.* **8**, 99–101.
195. Larsen, C. D. (1948). *J. Nat. Cancer Inst.* **9**, 35–37.
196. Laws, J. O., and Flaks, A. (1966). *Brit. J. Cancer* **20**, 550–554.
197. Leong, B. K. J., MacFarland, H. M., and Reese, W. H., Jr. (1971). *Arch. Environ. Health* **22**, 663–666.
198. Lesca, P., Toutain, D., and Truhaut, R. (1968). *C. R. Acad. Sci., Ser. D* **266**, 174–177.
199. Lesca, P., Toutain, D., and Truhaut, R. (1969). *C. R. Acad. Sci., Ser. D* **268**, 1238–1240.
200. Lespagnol, A., Adenis, L., and Driessens, J. (1967). *C. R. Soc. Biol.* **161**, 612–614.
201. Lespagnol, A., Adenis, L., Cazin, J. C., and Driessens, J. (1969). *C. R. Soc. Biol.* **163**, 2145.
202. Leuchtenberger, C., and Leuchtenberger, R. (1965). *Oncologia (Basel)* **19**, 81–104.
203. Leuchtenberger, C., and Leuchtenberger, R. (1966). Cited in ref. 295, pp. 445–463.
204. Leuchtenberger, C., and Leuchtenberger, R. (1971). *Schweiz. Med. Wochenschr.* **101**, 1374–1381.
205. Leuchtenberger, C., Leuchtenberger, R., and Doolin, P. F. (1958). *Cancer (Philadelphia)* **11**, 490–506.
206. Leuchtenberger, R., Leuchtenberger, C., Zebrun, W., and Shaffer, P. (1960). *Cancer (Philadelphia)* **13**, 956–958.
207. Livingood, L. E. (1896). *Bull. Johns Hopkins Hosp.* **7**, 177–178.
208. Lorenz, E., Heston, W. E., Deringer, M. K., and Eschenbrenner, A. B. (1946). *J. Nat. Cancer Inst.* **6**, 349–353.
209. Lynch, C. (1926). *J. Exp. Med.* **43**, 339–355.
210. Lynch, K. M., McIver, F. A., and Cain, J. R. (1957). *AMA Arch. Ind. Health* **15**, 207–214.
211. Magee, P. N., and Barnes, J. M. (1967). *Advan. Cancer Res.* **10**, 163–246.
212. Matsuyama, M., and Suzuki, H. (1968). *Brit. J. Cancer* **22**, 527–532.
213. May, R. M., and Bonchard, J. (1960). *C. R. Acad. Sci.* **250**, 1569–1571.
214. Medvedev, N. N. (1958). *Dokl. Akad. Nauk SSR* **119**, 594–597.
215. Meisels, A., and Auger, C. (1968). *Acta Cytol.* **12**, 237–242.
216. Ménard, S., Colnaghi, M. I., and Cornalba, G. (1973). *Brit. J. Cancer* **27**, 345–350.
217. Mestitzova, M., and Kossey, P. (1961). *Neoplasma* **8**, 27–39.
218. Milia, U. (1965). *Lav. Ist. Anat. Istol. Patol. Univ. Studi Perugia* **25**, 73–81.
219. Milia, U. (1966). Cited in ref. 295, pp. 863–868.
220. Milia, U., Biancifiori, C., and Giornelli-Santilli, F. E. (1965). *Lav. Ist. Anat. Istol. Patol. Univ. Studi Perugia* **25**, 165–171.

221. Milia, U., and DiLeo, F. P. (1965). *Lav. Ist. Anat. Istol. Patol. Univ. Studi Perugia* **25**, 149–154.
222. Milia, U., Gaetani, M., and Biancifiori, C. (1964). *Lav. Ist. Anat. Istol. Patol. Univ. Studi Perugia* **24**, 39–47.
223. Miller, E. W., and Pybus, F. C. (1954). *Brit. J. Cancer* **8**, 466–484.
224. Mirvish, S. S. (1968). *Advan. Cancer Res.* **11**, 1–42.
225. Mirvish, S. S., Cividalli, G., and Berenblum, I. (1964). *Proc. Soc. Exp. Biol. Med.* **116**, 265–268.
226. Mirvish, S. S., Greenblatt, M., and Choudari Kommineni, V. R. (1972). *J. Nat. Cancer Inst.* **48**, 1311–1315.
227. Mirvish, S. S., and Kaufman, L. (1970). *Int. J. Cancer* **6**, 69–73.
228. Mizushima, M. (1972). *Acta Pathol. Jap.* **22**, 53–75.
229. Mohr, U., and Althoff, J. (1965). *Z. Krebsforsch.* **67**, 152–155.
230. Montesano, R. (1970). *Tumori* **56**, 335–344.
231. Mori, K. (1961). *Gann* **52**, 265–270.
232. Mori, K. (1964). *Gann* **55**, 315–323.
233. Mori, K. (1965). *Gann* **56**, 513–518.
234. Mori, K. (1966). *Gann* **57**, 537–541.
235. Mori, K., and Hirafuku, I. (1964). *Gann* **55**, 205–209.
236. Mori, K., Kondo, M., Koibuchi, E., and Hashimoto, A. (1967). *Gann* **58**, 105–106.
237. Mori, K., and Yasuno, A. (1959). *Gann* **50**, 107–110.
238. Mori, K., and Yasuno, A. (1961). *Gann* **52**, 149–154.
239. Mori, K., Yasuno, A., and Matsumoto, K. (1960). *Gann* **51**, 83–89.
240. Mori-Chavez, P. (1962). *J. Nat. Cancer Inst.* **28**, 55–73.
241. Mori-Chavez, P. (1962). *J. Nat. Cancer Inst.* **29**, 945–961.
242. Mori-Chavez, P. (1966). Cited in ref. 295, pp. 845–861.
243. Mühlbock, O. (1955). *Ned. Tijdschr Geneesk.* **99**, 2276–2278.
244. Müller, H. A. (1964). *Z. Krebsforsch.* **66**, 303–309.
245. Murphy, J. B., and Sturm, E. (1925). *J. Exp. Med.* **42**, 693–700.
245a. Nebert, D. W., and Gelboin, H. V. (1969). *Arch. Biochem. Biophys.* **134**, 76–89.
246. Nettesheim, P., Hanna, M. G., Jr., and Doherty, D. (1970). *In* "Inhalation Carcinogenesis" (M. G. Hanna, Jr., P. Nettesheim, and J. R. Gilbert, eds.), AEC Symposium Series No. 21, pp. 437–448. USAEC, Oak Ridge, Tennessee.
247. Neyman, J., and Scott, E. L. (1967). *Proc. 5th Berkeley Symp. Math. Statist. Probabil.*, pp. 745–776.
248. Nishizuka, Y., Nakakuki, K., and Sakakura, T. (1964). *Gann* **55**, 495–508.
249. Nomura, T., and Okamoto, E. (1972). *Gann* **63**, 731–742.
250. O'Gara, R. W., Kelly, M. G., Brown, J., and Mantel, N. (1965). *J. Nat. Cancer Inst.* **35**, 1027–1042.
251. Okada, Y., Daido, S., and Ishiko, S. (1962). *Acta Tuberc. Jap.* **11**, 73–82.
252. Otto, H., and Plötz, D. (1966). *Z. Krebsforsch.* **68**, 284–292.
253. Pamukcu, A. M., Erturk, E., Price, J. M., and Bryan, G. T. (1972). *Cancer Res.* **32**, 1442–1445.
254. Pasternak, G., Hoffman, F., and Graffi, A. (1966). *Folia Biol. (Prague)* **12**, 299–304.
255. Peacock, P. M. (1962). *Brit. J. Cancer* **16**, 701–706.
256. Peacock, P. M. (1965). *Brit. J. Cancer* **19**, 812–815.
257. Peacock, P. M., and Dick, E. (1963). *Brit. J. Cancer* **17**, 59–61.
258. Peacock, P. M., and Peacock, P. R. (1966). *Brit. J. Cancer* **20**, 127–133.
259. Peacock, P. R. (1965). *J. Pathol. Bacteriol.* **89**, 285–293.
260. Peacock, P. R., and Spence, J. B. (1967). *Brit. J. Cancer* **21**, 606–618.

261. Pershin, G. N., Makeeva, O. O., Grushina, A. A., and Chernov, V. A. (1972). *Vop. Onkol.* 18(6), 50–53.
262. Pietra, G., Spencer, K., and Shubik, P. (1959). *Nature (London)* 183, 1689.
263. Pluot, M., Hopfner, C., Adnet, J. J., and Caulet, T. (1972). *Z. Krebsforsch.* 77, 279–291.
264. Polissar, M. J., and Shimkin, M. B. (1954). *J. Nat. Cancer Inst.* 15, 377–403.
265. Pollard, M., Matsuzawa, T., and Salomon, J. C. (1964). *J. Nat. Cancer Inst.* 33, 93–99.
266. Pollard, M., and Salomon, J. C. (1963). *Proc. Soc. Exp. Biol. Med.* 112, 256–259.
267. Pound, A. W. (1972). *Brit. J. Cancer,* 26, 216–225.
268. Prehn, R. T. (1963). *Ann. N. Y. Acad. Sci.* 101, 107–113.
269. Raine, C. S., Field, E. J., and Joyce, G. (1967). *Beitr. Pathol. Anat. Allg. Pathol.* 135, 117–123.
270. Ribacchi, R., Biancifiori, C., Milia, U., DiLeo, F. P., and Bucciarelli, E. (1963). *Lav. Ist. Anat. Istol. Patol. Univ. Studi Perugia* 23, 103–114.
271. Ribacchi, R., and Giraldo, G. (1966). *Lav. Ist. Anat. Istol. Patol. Univ. Studi Perugia* 26, 127–136.
272. Ribacchi, R., and Giraldo, G. (1966). Cited in ref. 295, pp. 823–834.
273. Roe, F. J. C. (1966). Cited in ref. 295, pp. 101–126.
274. Roe, F. J. C., Bosch, D., and Boutwell, R. K. (1958). *Cancer Res.* 18, 1176–1178.
275. Roe, F. J. C., Dipple, A., and Mitchley, B. C. (1972). *Brit. J. Cancer* 26, 461–465.
276. Roe, F. J. C., and Grant, G. A. (1970). *Int. J. Cancer* 6, 133–144.
277. Roe, F. J. C., Grant, G. A., and Millican, D. M. (1967). *Nature (London)* 216, 375–376.
278. Roe, F. J. C., and Rowson, K. E. K. (1968). *Int. Rev. Exp. Pathol.* 6, 181–227.
279. Roe, F. J. C., Rowson, K. E. K., and Salaman, M. H. (1961). *Brit. J. Cancer* 15, 515–530.
280. Rogers, S. (1955). *J. Nat. Cancer Inst.* 15, 1379–1390.
281. Rogers, S. (1955). *J. Nat. Cancer Inst.* 15, 1675–1683.
282. Rogers, S. (1957). *J. Exp. Med.* 105, 279–306.
283. Rudali, G., Coezy, E., and Muranyi-Kovacs, I. (1969). *C. R. Acad. Sci., Ser. D* 269, 1910–1912.
284. Rudali, G., Juliard, L., and Desormeaux, B. (1957). *C. R. Soc. Biol.* 150, 1853–1855.
285. Rudali, G., Yourkovski, N., and Juliard, L. (1962). *Bull. Ass. Fr. Etude Cancer* 49, 270–277.
286. Radali, G., Yourkovski, N., Juliard, L., and Desormeaux, B. (1957). *C. R. Soc. Biol.* 151, 246–247.
287. Rustia, M., and Shubik, P. (1972). *J. Nat. Cancer Inst.* 48, 721–729.
288. Saffiotti, U., and Borg, S. A. (1964). *Chicago Med. Sch. Quart.* 24, 10–17.
289. Salerno, R. A., Whitmire, C. E., and Garcia, I. M. (1972). *Nature (London)* 239, 31–32.
290. Sanford, B. H., Kohn, H. I., Daly, J. J., and Soo, S. F. (1973). *J. Immunol.* 110, 1437–1439.
291. Schmähl, D., and Thomas, C. (1965). *Z. Krebsforsch.* 67, 11–15.
292. Schroeder, H. A., Balassa, J. J., and Vinton, W. H., Jr. (1964). *J. Nutr.* 83, 239–250.
293. Schroeder, H. A., and Mitchener, M. (1972). *Arch. Environ. Health* 24, 66–71.
294. Schulz, H. (1959). "Die Submikroscopische Anatomie und Pathologie der Lunge." Springer-Verlag, Berlin and New York.
295. Severi, L., ed. (1966). "Lung Tumors in Animals," *Proc. 3rd Quadrennial Conf. Cancer, Univ. Perugia, 1965.*

296. Shabad, L. M. (1968). Z. Krebsforsch. **70**, 198-203.
297. Shabad, L. M. (1971). Cancer (Philadelphia) **27**, 51-55.
298. Shabad, L. M., Kolesnichenko, T. S., and Nikonova, T. V. (1973). Int. J. Cancer **11**, 688-693.
299. Shabad, L. M., Kolesnichenko, T. S., and Smetanin, E. Y. (1971). J. Nat. Cancer Inst. **47**, 987-1005.
300. Shabad, L. M., Pylev, L. N., and Kolesnichenko, T. S. (1964). J. Nat. Cancer Inst. **33**, 135-142.
301. Shimkin, M. B. (1940). Arch. Pathol. **29**, 239-255.
302. Shimkin, M. B. (1954). Cancer (Philadelphia) **7**, 410-413.
303. Shimkin, M. B. (1955). Advan. Cancer Res. **3**, 223-267.
304. Shimkin, M. B., and Polissar, M. J. (1955). J. Nat. Cancer Inst. **16**, 75-97.
305. Shimkin, M. B., and Polissar, M. J. (1958). J. Nat. Cancer Inst. **21**, 595-610.
306. Shimkin, M. B., Sasaki, T., McDonough, M., Baserga, R., Thatcher, D., and Wieder, R. (1969). Cancer Res. **29**, 994-998.
307. Shimkin, M. B., Weisburger, J. H., Weisburger, E. K., Gubareff, N., and Suntzeff, V. (1966). J. Nat. Cancer Inst. **36**, 915-935.
308. Shimkin, M. B., Wieder, R., Marzi, D., Gubareff, N., and Suntzeff, V. (1967). Proc. 5th Berkeley Symp. Math. Statist. Probabil., pp. 707-719.
309. Shimkin, M. B., Wieder, R., McDonough, M., Fishbein, L., and Swern, D. (1969). Cancer Res. **29**, 2184-2190.
310. Slye, M., Holmes, H. F., and Wells, H. G. (1914). J. Med. Res. **30**, 417-442.
311. Smetanin, E. Y. (1970). Vop. Onkol. **16**(11), 124-125.
312. Smith, W. E., Yazdi, E., and Miller, L. (1972). Environ. Res. **5**, 152-163.
313. Snyder, C., Malone, B., Nettesheim, P., and Snyder, F. (1973). Cancer Res. **33**, 2437-2443.
314. Squartini, F., Olivi, M., and Severi, L. (1966). Cited in ref. 295, pp. 273-283.
315. Staats, J. (1972). Cancer Res. **32**, 1609-1646.
316. Staemmler, M., Foitzik, E., and Heidenreich, M. (1970). Z. Krebsforsch. **74**, 283-294.
317. Steiner, P. E., and Loosli, C. G. (1950). Cancer Res. **10**, 385-392.
318. Stich, H. F. (1960). J. Nat. Cancer Inst. **25**, 649.
319. Stoner, G. D., Kikkawa, Y., and Kniazeff, A. J. (1975). Cancer Res. (in press).
320. Stoner, G. D., Kniazeff, A. J., Shimkin, M. B., and Hoppenstand, R. D. (1974). J. Nat. Cancer Inst. **53**, 493-498.
321. Stoner, G. D., Shimkin, M. B., Kniazeff, A. J., Weisburger, J. H., Weisburger, E. K., and Gori, G. B. (1973). Cancer Res. **33**, 3069-3085.
322. Stromskaya, T. P. (1970). Vop. Onkol. **16**(2), 63-65.
323. Strong, L. C. (1936). J. Hered. **27**, 21-24.
324. Stutman, O. (1974). Science **183**, 534-536.
325. Sunderman, F. W., Jr. (1971). Food Cosmet. Toxicol. **9**, 105-120.
326. Suzuki, T. (1966). Gann **57**, 169-184.
327. Svoboda, D. J. (1962). Cancer Res. **22**, 1197-1201.
328. Swern, D., Wieder, R., McDonough, M., Meranze, D. R., and Shimkin, M. B. (1970). Cancer Res. **30**, 1037-1046.
329. Takayama, S. (1970). Gann **61**, 297-298.
330. Takayama, S., and Oota, K. (1963). Gann **54**, 465-471.
331. Takayama, S., and Oota, K. (1966). Cited in ref. 295, pp. 677-694.
332. Tannenbaum, A., and Silverstone, H. (1953). Advan. Cancer Res. **1**, 452-505.
333. Telford, I. R. (1955). Tex. Rep. Biol. Med. **13**, 515-521.

334. Temple, L. A., Marks, S., and Bair, W. J. (1960). *Int. J. Radiat. Biol.* **2**, 143–156.
335. Temple, L. A., Willard, D. H., Marks, S., and Bair, W. J. (1959). *Nature (London)* **183**, 408–409.
336. Terracini, B., and Testa, M. C. (1970). *Brit. J. Cancer* **24**, 588–598.
337. Toth, B. (1968). *Cancer Res.* **28**, 727–738.
338. Toth, B. (1972). *Eur. J. Cancer* **8**, 341–345.
339. Toth, B. (1972). *Int. J. Cancer* **9**, 109–118.
340. Toth, B. (1973). *J. Nat. Cancer Inst.* **50**, 181–194.
341. Toth, B., Magee, P. N., and Shubik, P. (1964). *Cancer Res.* **24**, 1712–1721.
342. Toth, B., and Rustja, M. (1967). *Int. J. Cancer* **2**, 413–420.
343. Toth, B., and Shimizu, H. (1974). *J. Nat. Cancer Inst.* **52**, 241–251.
344. Toth, B., and Shubik, P. (1966). *Cancer Res.* **26**, 1473–1475.
345. Toth, B., and Shubik, P. (1966). *Science* **152**, 1376–1377.
346. Toth, B., and Shubik, P. (1967). *Cancer Res.* **27**, 43–51.
347. Trainin, N., and Linker-Israeli, M. (1969). *Cancer Res.* **29**, 1840–1845.
348. Trainin, N., and Linker-Israeli, M. (1970). *J. Nat. Cancer Inst.* **44**, 893–900.
349. Trainin, N., and Linker-Israeli, M. (1971). *In* "Immunological Parameters of Host-Tumor Relationships" (D. W. Weiss, ed.), pp. 36–41. Academic Press, New York.
350. Trainin, N., Linker-Israeli, M., Small, M., and Boiato-Chen, L. (1967). *Int. J. Cancer* **2**, 326–336.
351. Truhaut, R., Lesca, P., Dechambre, R. P., and Gerard-Marchant R. (1966). *Pathol. Biol.* **14**, 955–959.
352. Tsubura, Y., and Kimura, I. (1966). Cited in ref. 295, pp. 737–754.
353. Turusov, V. S., Breslow, N. E., and Tomatis, L. (1974). *J. Nat. Cancer Inst.* **52**, 225–232.
354. Tye, R., and Stemmer, K. L. (1967). *J. Nat. Cancer Inst.* **39**, 175–186.
355. Unnewehr, F. (1959). *Strahlentherapie* **108**, 421–427.
356. Usunov, P. V. (1964). *Vop. Onkol.* **10**(6), 72–78.
357. Vlahakis, G., and Heston, W. E. (1959). *J. Hered.* **50**, 99–102.
358. Walters, M. A. (1966). *Brit. J. Cancer* **20**, 148–160.
359. Walters, M. A., and Roe, F. J. C. (1964). *Brit. J. Cancer* **18**, 312–316.
360. Walters, M. A., and Roe, F. J. C. (1965). *Food Cosmet. Toxicol.* **3**, 271–276.
361. Walters, M. A., and Roe, F. J. C. (1966). *Brit. J. Cancer* **20**, 161–167.
362. Wattenberg, L. W. (1973). *J. Nat. Cancer Inst.* **50**, 1541–1544.
363. Wattenberg, L. W., and Leong, J. L. (1968). *Proc. Soc. Exp. Biol. Med.* **128**, 940–943.
364. Wattenberg, L. W., and Leong, J. L. (1970). *Cancer Res.* **30**, 1922–1925.
365. Weibel, E. R., and Elias, H., eds. (1967). "Quantitative Methods in Morphology," pp. 253–268. Springer-Verlag, Berlin and New York.
366. Wells, H. G., Slye, M., and Holmes, H. F. (1941). *Cancer Res.* **1**, 259–261.
367. White, M. R., Grendon, A., and Jones, H. B. (1970). *Cancer Res.* **30**, 1030–1036.
368. White, M. R. (1971). *Proc. 6th Berkeley Symp. Math. Statist. Probabil.*, pp. 287–307.
369. White, M. R., Grendon, A., and Jones, H. B. (1967). *Proc. 5th Berkeley Symp. Math. Statist. Probabil.*, pp. 721–743.
370. Wieder, R., Wogan, G. N., and Shimkin, M. B. (1968). *J. Nat. Cancer Inst.* **40**, 1195–1197.
371. Yamamoto, R. S., and Weisburger, J. H. (1970). *Life Sci.* **9**, Part 2, 285–289.

372. Yamamoto, R. S., Weisburger, J. H., and Weisburger, E. K. (1971). *Cancer Res.* **31**, 483–486.
373. Yamane, Y., Sakai, K., and Amemiya, Y. (1972). *Gann* **63**, 153–159.
374. Yasuhira, K. (1967). *Acta Pathol. Jap.* **17**, 475–493.
375. Yuhas, J. M. (1973). *J. Nat. Cancer Inst.* **50**, 69–78.
376. Zweifel, J. R. (1966). *J. Nat. Cancer Inst.* **36**, 937–946.

CELL DEATH IN NORMAL AND MALIGNANT TISSUES

E. H. Cooper, A. J. Bedford, and T. E. Kenny

The Department of Experimental Pathology and Cancer Research,
School of Medicine, University of Leeds, England

I. Introduction	59
II. Cell Loss in Embryogenesis	61
III. Transmission Electron Microscopy	65
IV. Microcinematography	68
V. Scanning Electron Microscopy	71
VI. Chromosome Aberrations as a Cause of Cell Loss	74
VII. Identification of Dead Cells *in Vitro*	77
VIII. Assessment of Tumor Cell Death *in Vivo*	78
IX. The Blood Supply of Tumors and Tumor Cell Necrosis	80
X. Immune Elimination of Cancer Cells	82
A. Quantification of Toxic Effect upon Target Cells	83
B. Lymphoid Infiltration and Cell Destruction in Human Tumors	88
XI. Phagocytosis and Autolysis	90
XII. Tumor Cell Loss by Differentiation	93
XIII. Cell Loss in Experimental Tumors	96
XIV. Cell Loss in Human Tumors	100
XV. Cell Loss and the Treatment of Tumors	106
Addendum: Mathematical Treatment of Cell Loss in Tumors	108
References	114

> "In the midst of life we are in death."
> *Burial of the dead, First Anthem*

I. Introduction

It is only in recent years that the cell loss from tumors has been realized to be a major factor controlling their growth. An equation attempting to act as a model for growth must include suitable expressions to allow for tumor cell loss. But, despite this obvious piece of logic, we are still a long way from understanding why cells are lost, and how we can quantify this process and exploit this aspect of tumor biology by improvements in the design of therapy.

In 1962, Mendelsohn proposed the concept that tumors contained two populations, dividing and nondividing tumor cells, the fraction of proliferating cells is being termed the growth fraction (Mendelsohn, 1962). It was later that Steel (1967, 1968) drew attention to cell loss as a vital factor in cell kinetic analysis, a theme to be emphasized later by others, and Bagshawe (1968) reviewed the importance in the response of tumors to therapy. It is in human tumors that cell loss becomes most evident. Iversen (1967) considered that cell loss can account for 95–97% of tumor cell proliferation. On the other hand, although this seems a very high figure it must be remembered that in normal renewal tissue in steady state the whole of cell production is matched by an equal cell loss. The reasons for loss of cells from the proliferating pool can be classified into a number of general headings; sometimes these causes act alone, but usually they act in concert.

Intrinsic
　1. Cell aging
　2. Differentiation
　3. Chromosome abnormalities
　4. Biochemical errors

Physical Displacement
　1. Migration
　2. Exfoliation

Extrinsic
　1. Inadequate oxygenation and nutrition
　2. Host immune defenses

These factors operate continuously in varying degrees from the earliest stages that tumors can be recognized.

In this review we will attempt to consider cell death and cell loss as it affects tumor cells, but to bring it into its correct context it is necessary to look at cell death in normal multicellular animals.

The definition of the moment of cell death poses the same type of questions as the definition of death of the animal as a whole. Clearly, our knowledge of transplantation surgery has indicated that individual organs can survive in a suitable host after the death of the donor. Likewise, microsurgical nuclear transplantation at the single cell level has shown how parts of the cell can survive in the environment of cytoplasm produced originally under the control of another nucleus. Hence, parts of the body, or the nucleus of the cell can live after the body or cell as a whole has died. Perhaps the best way to define cell death is to paraphrase that given by Bessis (1964): "The moment of death coincides with the loss of a certain percentage of the cell organisation or the interrelation between vital cell organelles."

The difficulty that faces the experimentalist is the phase of irreversible injury prior to cell death. The moment and mode of death and the necrosis of the cell corpse may show widely different patterns according to the nature of the cell and the mode of its death. In some instances, the cell corpse may be preserved by mummification or calcification, but as a rule its constituent parts will disintegrate either spontaneously or as the result of ingestion by phagocytic cells. The ability of multicellular organisms to replace individual cells, yet maintaining the integrity of the population as a whole, is an enormous step forward in evolution. Excluding accidents that can produce the premature death of normal cells, the time of death in normal cells is widely different. Cells of the renewal tissues, such as erythrocytes, gut, and skin, die as the result of maturation and senescence. Compared to the life of the organism their life-span is short whereas other cells, i.e., neurons, live as long as the organism. Between these extremes there are many other variants of life-span. The regularity of the timing of death indicates that it is under genetic control, and this is particularly well demonstrated in embryogenesis, where the timing of cell death is precise and critical.

The mechanisms of cell death in normal tissues are still shrouded in mystery, so it is of little surprise that there is still much conjecture about cell loss and cell death in malignant tumors. An orderly sequence may be detectable in small solid tumors or the leukemias and ascitic tumors. Once the tumor has become well established its individual cells are then subjected to the vagaries of blood supply and the superimposition of catastrophic events, such as the random occlusion of main blood vessels that overrides all the other factors influencing cell death or survival.

In the main we shall try to consider cell death and loss at the single cell level though we shall be looking at its wider consequences. Both aspects of this problem are relevant to cancer research, as the decision on whether cells are alive or dead is central to many topics, such as tumor immunology, chemotherapy, and cell kinetics, to name but a few.

II. Cell Loss in Embryogenesis

The study of morphogenesis in the chick embryo has focused attention on the importance of cell death as a normal vital process in ontogeny (see reviews by Glücksmann, 1951; Saunders, 1966). The following examples from avian and mammalian embryology illustrate the theme of programmed necrosis.

Hinchliffe and Ede (1973) studied the wingless conditions resulting from the action of the sex-linked wingless (*ws*) gene, which causes a precocious appearance of cell death in the anterior necrotic zone (ANZ) of the forelimb bud at stage 19 and its progressive extension beyond its normal area during stages 20–23 of embryogenesis. Electron microscopic and histochemical analyses of the wing buds during their destruction revealed the presence of both isolated dead cells and macrophages, which exhibited an intense acid phosphatase activity. These findings are interpreted as showing that isolated dead cells are ingested by neighboring mesenchymal cells which thus become transformed into macrophages.

Mitotic figures in "wingless" wing mesenchyme are rare. Preliminary counts suggest that at 3 and 3.5 days, the mitotic index is 3–6 times lower than in normal embryos, which supports the argument that cells due to die are no longer in cycle.

The established concepts of embryology often imply that cell death in development is associated with remodeling and reshaping processes, but in fact in the limb the role of cell death in the ANZ is obscure. It might be that the ANZ represents a region of a particular sort of stress which results in cell death in the fowl but not in other species. These zones may represent "end-stops" to the apical ectodermal ridge and in their absence, as in the talpid mutant, the ridge is abnormally long.

Hammar and Mottet (1971) have studied degeneration and necrosis in interdigital areas of developing hind limb buds of chick embryos. Using enzyme specific tetrazolium salts and electron microscopy, they found that the enzyme succinic dehydrogenase was absent in cells in the interdigital areas one or two days before morphological evidence of degeneration and cell death was present. They postulated that the mechanism of cell death results from a decreased activity and/or loss of strategic cellular enzymes. This allows the intracellular ATP levels to fall and the resultant compromise of vital cellular processes, eventually leading to cell death, occurs. They suggested that biochemical degeneration occurred prior to morphological changes in the cells. Their electron microscopic studies showed that the final destruction of the cells appeared to be due to the action of phagocytes.

O'Connor and Wyttenbach (1974) have studied cell death of visceromotor neurons in the cervical region of the chick embryo spinal cord and have compared it to degeneration which occurs in lumbosacral cord induced by the removal of peripheral organs. The initial changes are a decrease in nuclear size, a clumping of chromatin beneath the nuclear envelope, an increase in electron opacity of the cells, the disappearance of Golgi bodies and disaggregation of polysomes. These changes are followed by loss of the nuclear envelope and most of the endoplasmic reticulum, the appearance of bundles of filaments and the formation of many ribosome crystals. These crystals are only seen in dying cells and they suggest that a drastic reduction in RNA synthesis may be one of the initial events which leads to the death of these neurons. The dying neurons are finally broken up and engulfed by cells of the normal glial population and the cell fragments are digested in large phagocytic vesicles.

Webster and Gross (1970) have considered the possible mechanism of programmed cell death in the chick embryo. They examined the cytological effects of DNA cross-linking agents, such as mitomycin C, nitrogen mustards, diepoxides, and dialkyl sulfonates, on 4-day-old chick embryos. At low doses, 12 of the 14 agents tested produced cells morphologically identical with those found in naturally occurring areas of cellular death (e.g., the PNZ and the presumptive interdigital spaces). Monofunctional analogs of the dysfunctional agents failed to produce the same type of cells at equivalent or higher doses. Other metabolic poisons, including actinomycin D, colchicine, and cyanide, were also negative; puromycin and hydroxyurea were exceptions, both of which at moderate doses had the same cytological effects as the alkylating agents. Examination of DNA isolated from presumptive interdigital spaces revealed no increase in cross-linked DNA. However, the number of cross-links per cell could be well below the level of detection of assay. Thus the cross-linking hypothesis as a mechanism for programmed cell death cannot be eliminated. Since cross-linking agents, daunomycin and hydroxyurea, are known to cause cycle arrest, perhaps the cause of programmed cell death might involve a similar block. Tritiated thymidine (Tdr-^{3}H) labeling experiments indicate that the cessation of DNA synthesis is an early event in the sequence leading to cell death in the formation of the chick wing bud (Held and Saunders, 1965).

Ballard and Holt (1968) have looked at physiological cell death and degeneration in the interdigital mesenchyme of the hind foot of the rat fetus and found that individual cells in the mesenchyme die and shrink as the result of an unknown mechanism. Acid phosphatase and esterase levels are approximately the same as in viable mesenchymal cells. The dead cells are engulfed by neighboring cells which resemble other loose mesenchymal cells. Cells showing phagocytic activity then differentiate and become macrophages. This differentiation is accompanied by a change of nuclear shape and expansion of the cytoplasm and an increase in acid phosphatase and esterase activities. Many dead cells may be engulfed by a single macrophage and are digested by its acid hydrolases. No evidence has been found suggesting that cell death might be initiated by the intracellular release of lysosomal enzymes.

Firth and Hicks (1972) investigated the membrane specialization and synchronized cell death in developing rat transitional epithelium. Differentiation of bladder epithelium in the rat is characterized by the production of a short-lived generation of differentiated superficial cells during the last week of gestation. These cells undergo necrosis during the perinatal period and desquamate into the bladder lumen. The unaffected basal cells proliferate to give rise to the definitive superficial layer which matures during the third week after birth. Necrosis of the first generation of superficial cells is likely to be a predetermined step in development. This necrosis is not caused by lysosomal autolysis but mitochondrial damage is evident in the dying cells. The effect is highly specific, and the less differentiated basal cells remain undamaged. The authors suggested that this is an example of developmentally determined cell death. The structural changes seen by these authors are suggestive of a failure of mitochondrial phosphorylase to be the immediate cause of necrosis.

Modak and Perdue (1970) have analyzed embryonic and postembryonic changes of the chick eye histologically and noted changes in the structure of the lens epithelium, the annular pad, and the lens fiber area. Pycnotic nuclei appear in the center of the fiber area by day 8 of development. An increasing number of fiber cell nuclei degenerate, undergo pycnosis, and finally disappear. The wave of pycnosis spreads peripherally, causing massive localized degeneration and disappearance of fiber cell nuclei. These events follow a strict temporal and spatial pattern. Relative amounts of DNA in nuclei of various lens cell populations were estimated by Feulgen and ultraviolet microspectrophotometry. During pycnosis, fiber cell nuclei gradually lose their DNA. In comparison with sperm (1C) the chick lens epithelium populations fall within the 2C–4C range of DNA content. They did not find any higher ploidy in any part of the lens at any stage of its development and growth. In the lens, cell death, as defined by a loss of cellular structure and function, does not occur. However, in the lens cells, the nuclei degenerate according to a strict temporal and spatial pattern. The loss of nuclear structure and function is probably accompanied by a loss of other cellular organelles. The anucleate cells, along with the previously synthesized lens-specific proteins, remain intact and are maintained throughout the life of the animal. The shortest time possible between the entrance of the prospective fiber cells into the terminal cell cycle and the first appearance of pycnotic nuclei is estimated to be 5.5–6 days.

III. Transmission Electron Microscopy

The ultrastructure of cells can show a series of abnormalities associated with the irreversible phase of dying and the subsequent necrosis. Many of these features cannot be resolved in the light microscope. Electron microscopy can be helpful in suggesting the likely sequence that is leading to the death of the cells, and it is particularly valuable for studying the death of cells when they appear discretely in well-vascularized parts of a tumor. Our experience has been gained from a study of lymphomas, particularly Hodgkin's disease (Cooper and Quaglino, 1973), as well as bladder and colon cancer (Fulker et al., 1971). Hodgkin's disease is a tumor in which tumor cells usually die discretely, although in large tumors there may be areas of confluent necrosis. Furthermore, the morphology of the tumor cells is sufficiently specific to distinguish them from macrophages, which might be a source of confusion in some other forms of tumor. A study of cell kinetics (Peckham and Cooper, 1973) indicated that the tumor cell population in Hodgkin's disease is expected to have a high turnover rate. The main abnormality in the dying Hodgkin's cells appears to be a progressive vacuolation of the cytoplasm, eventually leading to the rupture of membranes and the loss of cell contents. Small vacuoles can be seen in the cytoplasm as the early sign of this change and these eventually coalesce. Perinuclear vacuolation is a fairly typical procedure, which appears to isolate the nucleus from the rest of the cytoplasm. On the other hand, in this tumor, lysosomal activation and the formation of phagosomes appear to be late events and probably occur only after total disruption of the cytoplasmic organization. Shrinkage necrosis, as described by Kerr (1971) seemed to be an alternative mode of cell death in these lymphomas (see Figs. 1-4). Archibal and Frenster (1973) have reported an association between the closeness of the adherence of lymphocytes to the tumor cell membranes in Hodgkin's disease and damage to the cells. Their criteria for damage were mitochondrial swelling, nuclear edema, inequalities of the plasma membrane and disruption of endoplasmic reticulum. We have not been convinced of these observations, as they depend on very subjective criteria particularly when assessed in a pleomorphic tumor cell system (Dorfman et al., 1973). We are on the side of caution when interpreting electron micrographic evidence of cell damage, particularly as tumors are liable to have a wide range of mitochondrial morphology and the presence of lysozymes which necessarily indicate irreversible damage. Furthermore, it is important to assess whether the changes could be due to fixation artifacts. In the

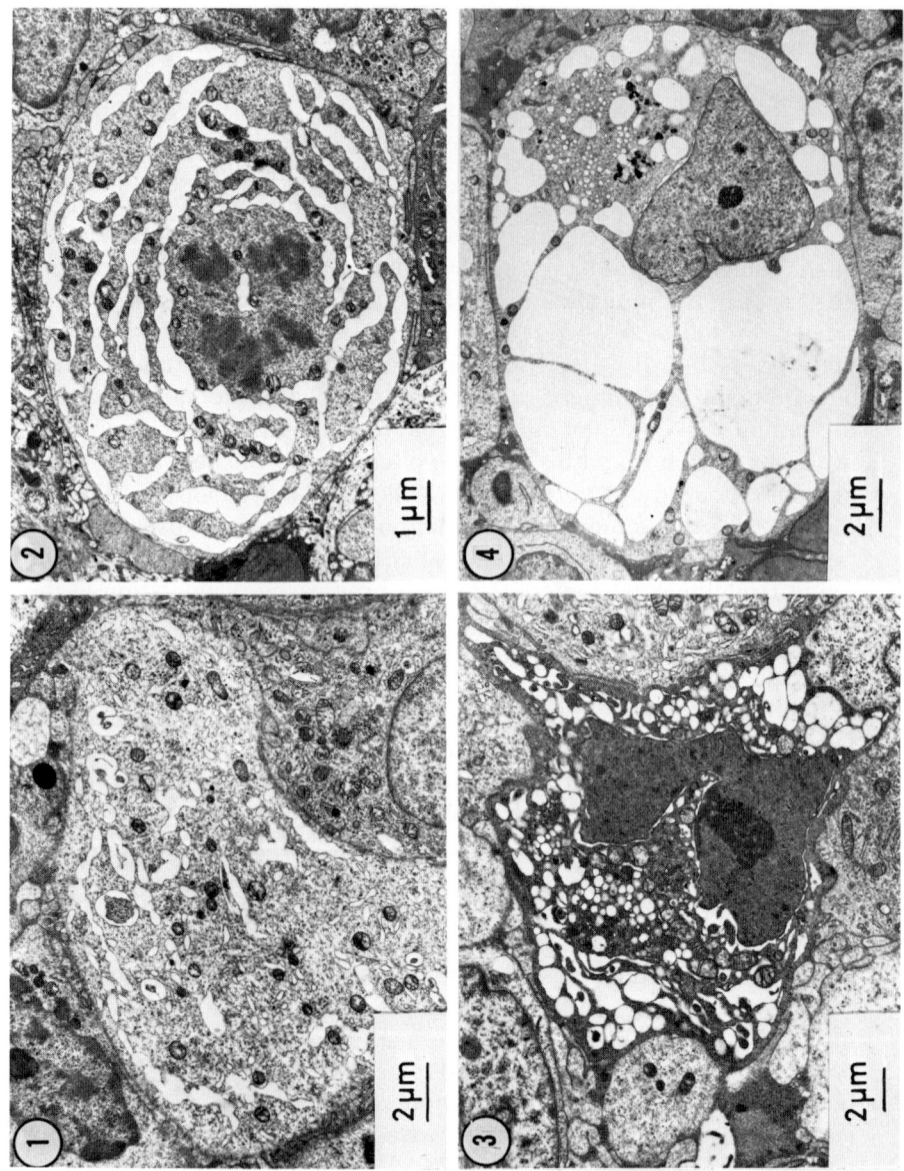

lymphomas the morphology of the surrounding tumor cells indicated that the damage that is seen is probably a genuine reflection of the abnormalities of permeability of tumor cell membrane rather than an artifact. Electron microscopy of of solid tumors has been unable to demonstrate that blebbing processes are a typical antecedent of cell death of cells in tissue culture. It is probable that for physical reasons this cannot occur except when the cell is lining a tissue space or a body cavity.

Shrinkage necrosis (Kerr, 1971; Wyllie, 1974) is characterized by the condensation of cytoplasm and compaction of the nuclear chromatin; the organelles are well preserved. This is followed by the budding of the cell to produce fragments of varying sizes that are phagocytosed by histiocytes or epithelial cells. This would seem to be a very common mode of death in both experimental and human tumors.

Cells that appear unusually dark when examined under the electron microscope are a characteristic feature in many tumors and have been reported in a number of healthy tissues (Wellings and Deome, 1963). Izard and de Harven (1968) described electron dense reticulum cells in the thymus and lymph nodes of both normal and leukemic mice. Cells of this character have been found in human lymph adenitis and in various lymphomas (Mollo et al., 1969). In our own experiences of bladder and colon cancer, it would seem that the majority of dark cells are in fact damaged cells and are probably dying (Fig. 5), possibly falling within the concept of shrinkage necrosis. On the other hand, in the lymphomas and lymphoid tissues many of the cells which had this dark staining appear to have an otherwise normal morphology. These dark cells can be recognized in semithin sections stained with toluidine blue and are independent of the method used for fixation.

In summary, recognition of cells in various forms of advanced degeneration presents no problem for the electron microscopist. However, great care must be taken in deciding whether a certain abnormality in the cytoplasm or nucleus constitutes sufficient damage for the cell to be in an irreversible phase of injury or whether these abnormalities are transient; being purely an expression of

FIGS. 1–4. Electron micrographs illustrating cell death in Hodgkin's disease.
FIG. 1. Early cytoplasmic vacuolation.
FIG. 2. Confluent cytoplasmic vacuolation in a mitotic figure.
FIG. 3. Vacuolation associated with condensation of cytoplasm in a Reed-Sternberg cell.
FIG. 4. Vacuolation in the compression of the cytoplasm, but showing no abnormality of the nucleus.

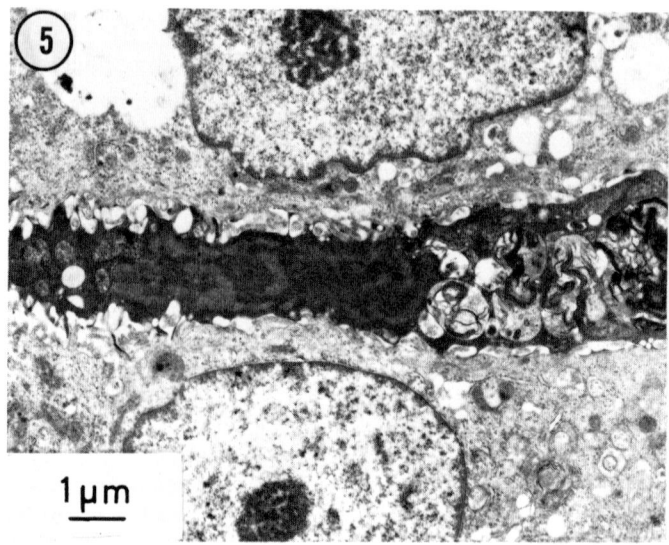

Fig. 5. A dark cell in mouse colon cancer induced by dimethylhydrazine injections. Note the typical myelin whorls in telolysosomes of the cytoplasm, indicating advanced degeneration.

simple stress or bizarre form of metabolism which is not necessarily lethal to the cells.

IV. Microcinematography

Time-lapse microcinematography provides a continuous record of the behavior and movements of cells *in vitro*. Analysis of the films enables quantitative assessment to be made of (a) the cell generation cycle, (b) the duration of mitosis, (c) multipolar mitoses, (d) cell fusion and giant cell formation, and (e) the antecedent events of such phenomena. Furthermore, pedigrees of cells derived from a common mother cell allow a clonal analysis of death, and this is of particular value when observing the latent effects of irradiation (Thompson and Suit, 1967, 1969; Hurwitz and Tolmach, 1969) and chemical insults (Katsumata *et al.*, 1973; Bedford *et al.*, 1974).

The advantage of using time-lapse cinematography to study cell death is that the whole sequence of changes is permanently recorded. The artificial speeding up of what are normally very slow processes enables the total pattern of events to be appreciated readily. Such studies are invaluable in describing the way in which cell behavior changes as it passes from normality through irreversible damage to death and subsequent necrosis. The use of analyzing projectors (permitting the frames to be viewed one by one) in conjunction with a frame counter enable the timing of the various events to be recorded accurately. Bessis (1964) and Showacre (1968) have been strong advocates for this method of the study of cell physiology. Bloom, Zirkle, and Uretz (1955), Freed and Engle (1963), and Bessis (1964) have used microcinematography to describe the pattern of death after microbeam irradiation of parts of the cell nucleus or cytoplasm.

The mode of death seems to be related to the physical or chemical event which has damaged the cell. In many cells the loss of coordinated movement of the cell membrane and the formation of large protrusions of the cytoplasm is characteristic. This process was originally called zeiosis by Costero and Pomerat (1951). Our own studies of HeLa cells (Bedford et al., 1975a) has shown that when this phenomenon occurs in cells in interphase it is accompanied by an inability of the cell to remain spread out and attached to glass. This may reflect the failure to produce sufficient energy or to convert that energy into a form suitable for maintaining the flattened state.

Single-frame analysis shows that these protrusions take only a few minutes to extend. They may be considerably longer than the diameter of the cell, and may be sustained for several hours. Occasionally the end portion of the extruded cytoplasm is lost into the medium. This process of cytoplasmic extrusion is not always a prelude to cell death, as it can be induced reversibly by a number of agents. Dornfeld and Owczarzak (1958) have reported that such reversible activity may be induced by ethylenediamine tetraacetic acid (EDTA) in chick fibroblast cells. On the other hand, in cells that will die, this is a common prelude to death. The final phase is often a short-lived, particularly violent movement of the cytoplasmic extrusions followed by stillness; followed by the sudden shrinkage of the cell, or by progressive vacuolation and rupture of the condensation of the remnants of the cell, which remain attached to glass for a variable length of time and then float off.

Electron microscopic examination of the cytoplasmic extrusions seen in zeiosis indicates that they are direct extensions of the cytoplasm containing ribosomes but no organelles (Price, 1967), and our own observations confirm this finding. This marked deformation of the cytoplasmic membranes without rupture is an interesting phenomenon; active movement in the medium is probably an energy-requiring process, but as yet there is no biophysical explanation as to the underlying mechanism involved. Belkin and Hardy (1961) found

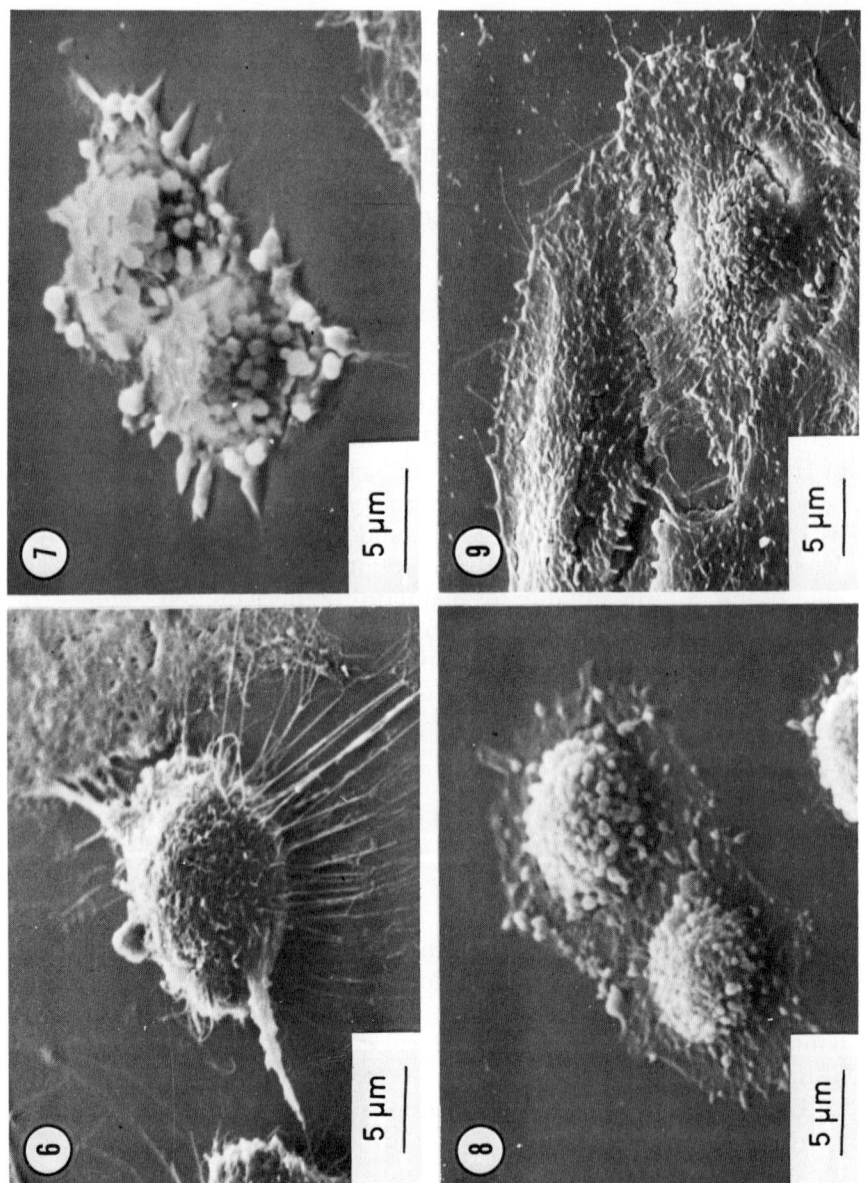

that various sulfhydryl binding agents induce blebbing of the cell membrane, but Price (1967) has suggested that such blisters have to be differentiated from true zeiosis. Cell death in the absence of this zeiosis has been described by other workers. Bessis (1964) describes the overhydration of cells with marked vacuolation and rupture; Hurwitz and Tolmach (1969) found that after irradiation interphase death could occur either with violent blebbing or by a sudden collapse and disintegration of the cell into debris without being preceded by observable signs that death was imminent.

V. Scanning Electron Microscopy

Scanning electron microscopy enables the detail of cell surfaces to be studied at high magnification. Recent technological advances, in particular the application of critical-point drying (Anderson, 1951) to specimen preparation has enabled many of the original artifacts to be overcome. It would appear from the study of synchronized Chinese hamster ovary cell populations (Porter et al., 1973) that the surface of cells undergoes a progressive change as they move through interphase. The start of G_1 is associated with a spherical shape, the cell surfaces having many microvilli. As cells progress through interphase, they flatten and the microvilli give way to small blebs on the surface. Cells in the S phase of the cell cycle tend to be flat, and their surfaces appear to be covered with fine microvilli. As cells move into mitosis, they round up, and the characteristic long, very fine extensions of the surface (filopodia) develop and remain throughout mitosis. Immediately after anaphase a short burst of blebbing of the cytoplasm is a characteristic feature (postmitotic bubbling). These appearances seem to differ from one cell line to another (Pugh-Humphries and Sinclair, 1970). Our own observations

---

FIGS. 6–9. Scanning electron micrographs showing the changes of surface structure of HeLa cells as they progress through the cell cycle. The preparations were made using critical point drying.

FIG. 6. Metaphase: the cell has taken a spherical shape and remains attached to the substratum by numerous microextensions (filopodia).

FIG. 7. Post mitotic blebbing; a typical feature commencing in telophase at the moment of cell separation.

FIG. 8. Cells showing spreading of the cytoplasm but still retaining an irregular surface over the central portions. Using synchronous cultures, it can be shown that this corresponds with the G_1 phase.

FIG. 9. Flattened and quiescent-appearing cells that are typical of the S and G_2 phases. They pass rapidly from this state to a similar state as in Fig. 6, at the commencement of prophase.

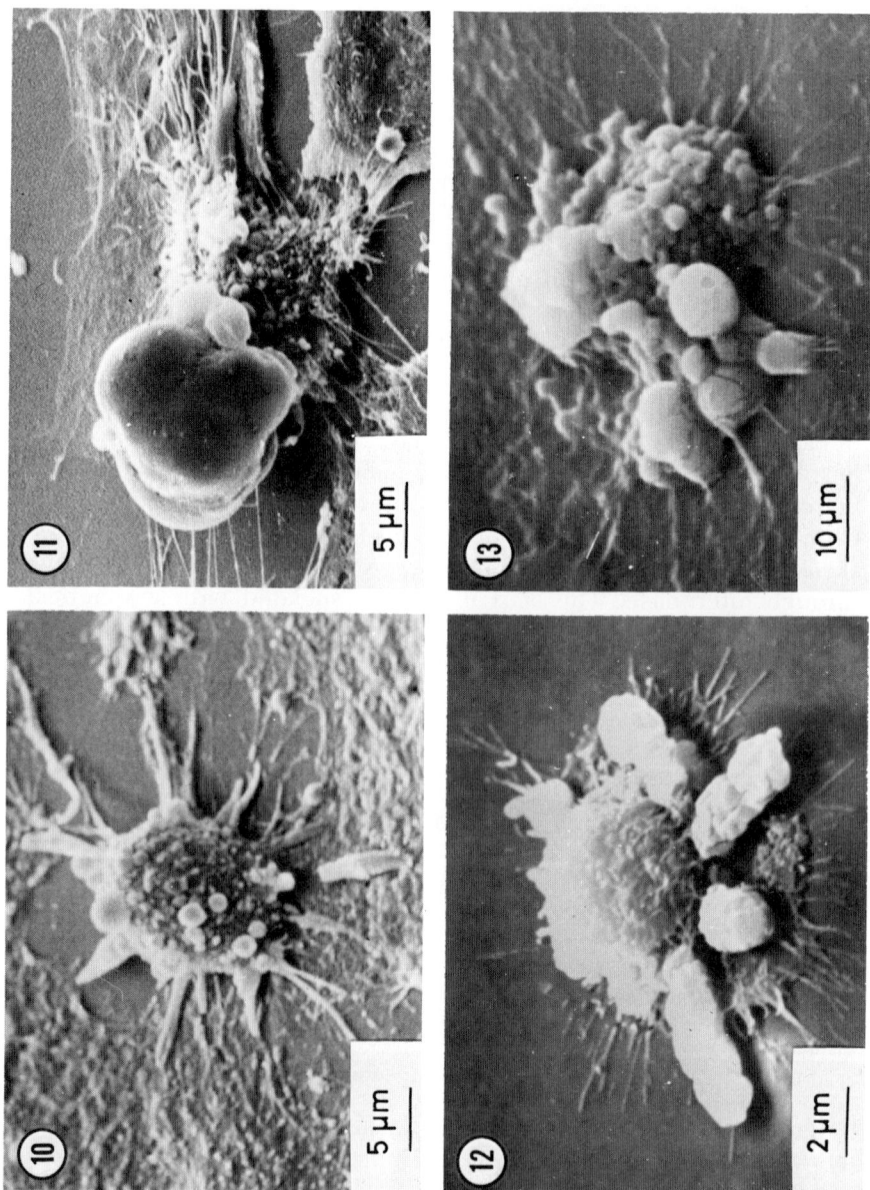

on the cell surface of HeLa cells as they progress through the cell cycle are shown in Figs. 6–9. Scanning electron microscopy can help to show some of the events associated with the terminal phases of cell death and the subsequent collapse and disintegration of the dead cell (see Figs. 10–13).

Bedford et al. (1974) studied the reaction of HeLa cells exposed to methylazoxymethanol acetate (MAM acetate) and found that the earliest sign of impending cell death was the presence of cytoplasmic blebbing either over the nucleus or the periphery of the cell. These progress to produce typical large cytoplasmic extrusions. The dead cells either disintegrate leaving patches of debris, or condense, often remaining attached to the glass by one or more thickened filopodia. However, caution must be exercised when coming to conclusions from scanning electron microscopy which takes a random static view of a dynamic process. It appears that the cell density and their ability to make contact with one another may have a profound influence on their morphology. Rubin and Everhart (1973) observed that cells plated at low density retained their G_1 morphology throughout interphase. Furthermore, certain drugs may produce considerable change in the morphology of cell surfaces and the spread of the cell on its substrate. For example, the addition of dibutyryl cyclic AMP converts the shape of Chinese hamster ovary cells from an epithelium-like appearance to a fibroblast-like appearance. Likewise the surface membrane of the fibroblastic cells could be made to produce many more blebs by the addition of either Colcemid or cytochalasin B, and this process could be abolished by the addition of dibutyryl cAMP (Puck et al., 1972). Prednisolone has been reported to alter the frequency and shape of very fine processes extruded from HeLa cells in culture (Fiskin and Melnykovych, 1972). Consequently, it is of great importance to study carefully the normal sequence of events in cells as well as the reversible changes in cell membrane behavior induced by the compound under study, before one can prescribe any particular event as being part of the sequence that inevitably will cause cell death.

FIGS. 10–13. Scanning electron micrographs of HeLa cells dying after exposure to methylazoxymethanol acetate.

FIG. 10. Abnormally thickened attachments to glass in a rounded up cell and several small cytoplasmic blebs on the surface.

FIGS. 11 and 12. Extrusion of the cytoplasm as vermiform protrusions (Fig. 12) or balloonlike extensions as in Fig. 11. At this stage, the general outlines of the cell are visible; later, (Fig. 13) the structure becomes completely disorganized and may rupture or collapse.

VI. Chromosome Aberrations as a Cause of Cell Loss

Cytogenetic analysis of malignant tumors in man has indicated the individuality of histologically apparently identical cancers. Apart from the leukemias, tumors usually show a wide spectrum of abnormalities within their cell populations. Solid tumors are composed of heterogeneous cell populations with very few members having a completely normal diploid karyotype; see the reviews by Levan (1956), Sandberg and Hossfeld (1970, 1973), and Bishun (1973).

As solid tumors become less differentiated and more anaplastic there is often a tendency for their chromosome number to rise, moving from a near diploid modal number to near tetraploid or higher. This rise in chromosome number is often accompanied by a wider dispersion about the modal number accentuating the heterogeneity of the population. The direct correlation between chromosome morphology and cell loss cannot be established, since it is only one of many factors influencing cell loss from tumors. The rearrangements of chromosomes caused by breakage and rearrangement can be classified into stable and unstable. The unstable forms are easily recognized cytologically, the stable forms may need complex analysis to detect minor changes in the karyotype. Nevertheless, it seems reasonable to assume that certain types of chromosome aberrations lead either to the loss of the cell in mitosis, or some or all of its progeny.

Chromosome damage can be produced by a great variety of chemical, viral, and physical factors (Shaw, 1970). The ephemeral nature of severe damage in rapidly dividing cell populations, such as bone marrow or experimental tumors, when exposed to agents such as cytosine arabinoside suggests the damaged cells are quickly eliminated from the population. On the other hand, lymphocytes may retain damage for months or even several years and express the abnormality only when stimulated to divide by culture with a mitogen *in vitro*. Ring chromosomes, multiple breaks with translocations, and dicentrics that cause crisscross bridges in anaphase can be expected to be associated with a loss of genetic material during mitosis (Levan, 1956; Shaw, 1970).

Carrano (1973) from a detailed study of irradiated Chinese hamster cells concluded that, although a symmetrical chromosome exchange and a chromosome deletion were equally capable of causing cell death, translocation or inversion do not necessarily cause the cell to be lost. After exposure to X-rays of 300 rad, he found that 45% of the total cell death occurred in the first two postirradiation generations, and this was mainly associated with the formation of anaphase bridges. In subsequent generations it was the loss of a fragment of the chromosome that seemed to be an important factor causing cell death. It appeared that when a cell loses a single acentric fragment it will survive for probably one generation. Some lesions are so severe, i.e., pulverization, that the cell dies in mitosis. Koller (1956) has described the cytological appearances in malignant effusions, in indicating the bizarre abnormalities of mitosis that are frequent in tumor cells of high ploidy, many of which are associated with cell degeneration. It is this type of lesion that is rapidly cleared from a population, most probably by elimination of the affected cells. Changes in chromosome number, or the relocation of chromosome material to produce marker chromosomes is not necessarily lethal and often appears to give cells a biological advantage for a particular microenvironment. The local conditions of growth may be operative in causing the spontaneous breaks and their sequelae. Koller (1960) found a higher incidence of abnormal mitoses in the necrotic parts of tumors compared with the healthy areas.

The selective deprivation of single amino acids from the growth medium of Chinese hamster cells in culture can initiate a wide variety of breaks and combinations including pulverization in the chromosome (Freed and Schatz, 1969). It is possible that the intrinsic instability of the tumor cell chromosomes may make them particularly susceptible to secondary damage.

Another, though probably less important, abnormality leading to cell loss is the formation of multinucleate cells. These arise either by failure of the cytoplasm to divide during mitosis or by cell fusion. Repeated cycles of cell replication can result in very high chromosome numbers, but in all probability this is a sterile line of cell evolution. In some human tumors, in particular acute leukemia and Burkitt's tumor, gross chromosome abnormalities of the types described above are rare. Yet in both these tumors there is strong evidence for a high cell loss rate (Cooper *et al.*, 1966). Does this mean that elimination is not connected with abnormalities in mitosis and that, if cytogenetic effects are important, they are acting through gene expression rather than instability of the chromosomes usually seen in solid tumors?

Sandberg and Hossfeld (1973) have suggested that translocations between acrocentric chromosomes could lead to a loss of the nucleolar organizer regions and alter the DNA and RNA metabolism. The detailed recognition of chromosomes has taken a major step forward with the metachromatic banding techniques (Caspersson *et al.*, 1970); no doubt this will help to resolve whether particular com-

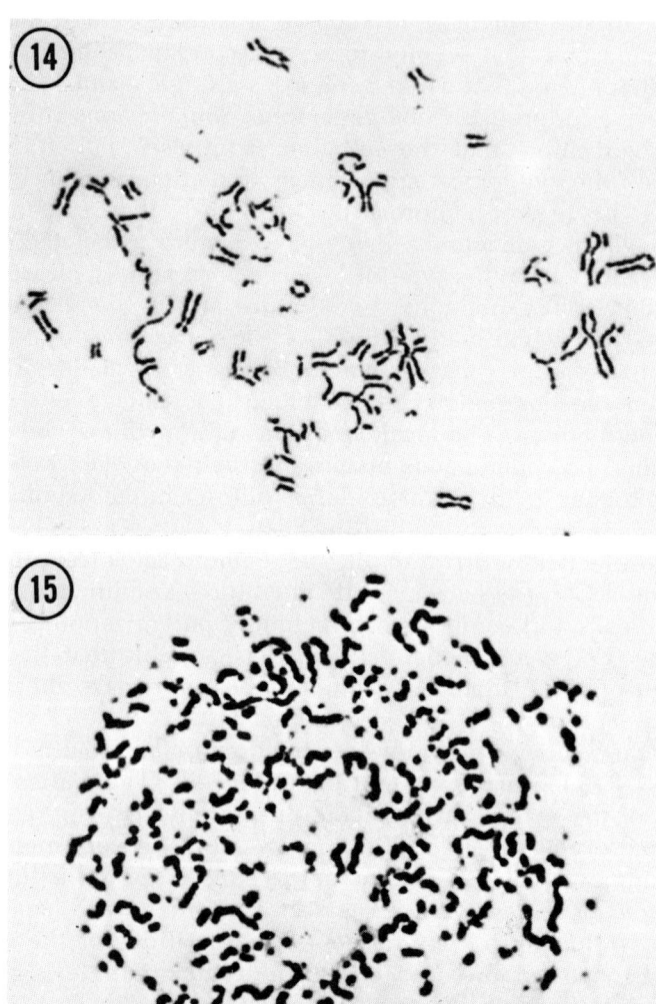

Fig. 14. Part of a mitotic spread in a HeLa cell, exposed to methylazoxymethanol acetate. Typical multiple breaks and fusions of chromosomes are present.

Fig. 15. Chromosome pulverization caused by exposure to methylazoxymethanol acetate. Both this and the lesion illustrated in Fig. 14, are expected to cause death in mitosis.

plements of chromosome can have an immediate or long-term lethal effect owing to genetic imbalance or insufficiency. In pernicious anemia there is good evidence that many of the erythrocyte precursors die in the bone marrow; arrest of cells with partially replicated DNA has been described (Cooper and Wickramasinghe, 1969). Chromosome abnormalities have been recorded in pernicious anemia, particularly giant chromosomes and breaks (Keller et al., 1970), which disappear after B_{12} therapy. In this instance cell death is entirely due to intrinsic abnormalities of DNA metabolism caused by B_{12} deficiency; whether the particular chromosome abnormality and the death in interphase are related remains unproved.

Hermens (1973) has studied the cell cycle time in rhabdomyosarcoma cells with severe mitotic abnormalities and compared them to normal tumor cells with normal mitoses. His approach was to construct percentage labeled mitosis curves for labeled and unlabeled normal mitotic figures and damaged mitotic figures. He found that there was no difference between cell cycle times of two types of cells. A similar conclusion was reached by Firket and Hopper (1970) for HeLa cells cultured *in vitro* in which there were spontaneous chromosome abnormalities. On the other hand, many drugs can produce slowing of the cell cycle as well as abnormalities of mitosis leading to cell death. Hermens (1973) calculated that the spontaneous death of cells in mitosis was a very important source of cell loss in the microscopic growth phase of the tumor; as it became bigger, other modes of cell loss predominated, i.e., interphase death and migration. He reported that in a rhabdomyosarcoma of 300 mm^3, 15.6% of the cell loss is related to death in mitosis and 84% to other causes.

Time-lapse studies of cells in tissue culture bearing chromosome aberrations have clearly demonstrated that arrest and death mitosis has a distinct morphological sequence. In our series following exposure to MAM acetate the arrest may be for 10–12 hours in mitosis before the cell eventually dies (Bedford et al., 1974). The severity of induced damage which was observed is illustrated by Figs. 14 and 15.

VII. Identification of Dead Cells *in Vitro*

After irreversible damage, cells show a permeability to several anionic dyes that are excluded from the cytoplasm of living cells. The more commonly used dyes include trypan blue (Hoskins et al.,

1956); eosin 7 (Hanks and Wallace, 1958); methylene blue (Schrek, 1936); erythrosin B (Philips and Terryberry, 1957); and nigrosin, a nontoxic dye that stains only dead cells, giving a good contrast (Kaltenbach et al., 1958). Lissamine green has been suggested to have the added advantage that it is nontoxic and can be present in the incubation medium for 48 hours without causing damage (Holmberg, 1961). The main drawback to all these dyes is their variable staining of the "damaged" cells — which is far less reliable than the staining of dead cells.

Trypsin has been proposed as a method of determination of viability of cells in culture. Damaged and dead cells are lysed, but healthy cells are resistant to the lytic action of trypsin. This method could be used for studies of the rate of loss of viability (de Luca, 1965). Scaife and Brohee (1967) have described how damaged cells show an increased binding of $^{51}Cr_3$ compared to healthy cells. This might be of value when attempting to assess methods for production of discrete cells from solid tumors. These authors make the point that the penetration and binding of chromic cations ($^{51}Cr_3$) is more sensitive than ^{51}Cr-chromate binding. Acridine orange (AO) fluorescence has been claimed to be a test for cell viability. This depends on an increased absorption of AO after injury, but unlike the dye exclusion tests it is not an all-or-none phenomenon. It has been reported that living, injured, and dead cells can be recognized on the basis of their fluorescence colors (Hathaway et al., 1964). On the other hand, Vinegar (1956) was unable to detect injury by X-ray, nitrogen mustard, and bromine ion by AO fluorescence. This method would appear to have no advantages over the simpler dye exclusion tests.

VIII. Assessment of Tumor Cell Death in Vivo

The first attempts at studying the fate of tumor cells labeled with ^{32}P (Ambrus et al., 1956) or ^{51}Cr (Selecki, 1959; Vincent and Nicholls, 1962) were unsuccessful owing to the loss of label for reasons other than cell death. The introduction of ^{125}I-labeled iododeoxyuridine (IUdR) as a radioactive DNA precursor opened up new possibilities for studying the distribution and fate of tumor cells. IUdR-^{125}I is incorporated into DNA in place of thymine during DNA synthesis and does not leave the cell until it dies. This property of IUdR-^{125}I coupled with its low reutilization, about 5% (Purschen and Feinendegen, 1969) makes it suitable for the study of cell loss. Leukemic, ascitic, or solid tumors can be labeled in vivo with IUdR-^{125}I and transferred to a suitable host. The loss of radioactivity can be measured by whole-body counting of the animal (Hofer et al., 1969) or by a suitably constructed gamma scintillation counter placed over a solid tumor growing in the leg (Purschen and Feinendegen, 1969). Hofer et al. (1969) have examined the fate of IUdR-^{125}I labeled Ehrlich ascites cells. Cells were transplanted into mice by various routes; living cells lost about 15% of their radioactivity per day, killed cells lost 60% per day for 2–3 days. Higher rates of loss of ^{125}I occurred when the cells were given intramuscularly, subcutaneously, or intravenously. After intravenous administration most of the radioactivity could be found in the lungs.

The authors consider that, if the total radioactivity used for labeling is less than 5 μCi per mouse, the radiobiological effects on the L1210 cells will be minimal. The excretion rate of ^{125}I liberated from dead cells is slower than that after a simple injection of the radioiodine. This suggests that phagocytosis and DNA liberation is the rate-limiting factor. Dethlefsen (1971) has used a IUdR-^{125}I labeling method to examine cell loss from a slow growing transplanted C_3H "spontaneous" mammary tumor. This method gave a losss function with a $T_{1/2} = 121.7 \pm 23.2$ hours. The same tumor had been analyzed previously by Mendelsohn and Dethlefsen (1968) using an autoradiographic method which indicated a loss function of 10% of the volume per day. This gave a $T_{1/2}$ of about 158 hours. However, the author felt that the close agreement was more apparent than real owing to the "noise" in both systems of measurement.

A similar technique has been used by Purschen and Feinendegen (1969) for the study of solid tumors, i.e., sarcoma 180. They recorded an hourly cell loss of 0.35% and 0.53% per hour in Ehrlich carcinoma. Hofer (1969) examined the effects of various anticancer agents on the rate of cell loss, using the IUdR-^{125}I labeled cell system to try to analyze their relative cytostatic and cytocidal activity. Methotrexate, BCNU, and cyclophosphamide increased the life-span of the mice and greatly accelerated the rate of cell death. However, when the cell kill was very high the procedure is unable to measure the cytocidal effect of the drug quantitatively. This system also suffers from the drawback that these 3 drugs slow the excretion of ^{125}I liberated from dead tumor cells. But it is uncertain whether this is due to an increase of IUdR-^{125}I reutilization, decreased phagocytosis, depressed renal function, or a combination of these factors. These experiments have shown that cell death *in vivo* is a continuous process throughout the development of a tumor. The site of growth profoundly influences these results, indicating a poor colonizing ability of cells in the blood stream or muscle compared to an intraperitoneal site.

IX. The Blood Supply of Tumors and Tumor Cell Necrosis

Some form of necrosis whether it be at the single-cell level, in microscopic zones, or larger macroscopic areas is a universal feature of all forms of malignant tumor. The relation between blood supply to tumors and necrosis has attracted the attention of a number of workers, mostly from the point of view of trying to understand the dynamic changes that take place within tumors as they grow but also to attempt to assess the oxygenation within various parts of tumors which has great significance in radiotherapy. It is now well established that hypoxic cells are more radio resistant than fully oxygenated ones. Thomlinson and Gray (1955) from their examination of the histology of bronchial carcinoma in man suggested there was a relation between oxygen concentration and tumor necrosis. They observed that the tumor cells often grew in cords fed by peripheral capillaries. Central necrosis occurred when the cords were between 100 and 180 μm thick. From this observation, they constructed various theoretical arguments about the diffusion of oxygen from the capillary through the tumor cells. Tannock (1968, 1970) investigated this problem using a transplantable mammary adenocarcinoma in mice. This tumor produced cords of tumor cells arranged about a central vessel, the cords being separated from each other by intervening necrotic areas. On average the distance from the blood vessel in the center of the cord to the peripheral necrotic edge was about 90 μm. He measured the cell proliferation in three zones—close to the blood vessel, an intermediate zone, and close to the necrotic area—and found that cell cycle time appeared to be unchanged as the cells migrated from close to the blood vessel toward the area of necrosis. On the other hand, the growth fraction fell from 100% to 50%, and the labeling index fell from 74% to 30%, as the cells became progressively more hypoxic. In later studies (Tannock, 1970), he also looked at the proliferation of stromal elements within this tumor, capillary endothelium, and fibroblasts. He came to the conclusion that if the extension of the capillary network is dependent upon proliferation of the capillary endothelial cells, then this appeared to be a limiting factor for the rate of tumor growth.

In normal tissues the labeling index (LI) of capillaries is 0.0–0.04% with a turnover time of 2 months or more; after injury it rises to about 11%. A similarly raised LI was found in the capillaries of the C3H breast tumors, suggesting that the capillaries were under continuous stimulus to divide (Tannock and Hayashi, 1972). Folkman et al. (1971) have isolated an angiotropic factor for human and animal neoplasms that induces cell division in capillary endothelium. This factor appears to arise from the tumor cells, not from the supporting stroma. Earlier, Greenblatt and Shubik (1968) had demonstrated that tumors grown in Millipore membranes placed in hamster cheek pouches produced a factor that induces capillary vascularization and capillary formation in the vicinity of a tumor. In this context it is interesting to note that Greene (1941) observed that when tumors were placed in the anterior chambers of guinea pig eyes they failed to grow, owing to the lack of vascularization of the tumor. However, when he transplanted them into muscle they grew to a large size and were well vascularized. From these observations and the earlier histological studies of Thomlinson and Gray (1955), it seemed logical that there was a fairly straightforward correlation between the distance of a cell from a blood vessel and the probability of it dying, so that as the cell migrated progressively from the blood vessel it would be increasingly deprived of oxygen and essential nutrients as well as exposed to the consequences of the buildup of waste products and fluctuation of pH in its own microenvironment. However, there seemed to be a number of alternatives to this simplistic view.

Fulker et al. (1971) observed that in a well differentiated fronded capillary tumor of human bladder of which the fronds are about 20 cells wide supplied by a central blood vessel, the mitotic index showed no difference between the inner half of the frond close to the blood vessels compared to the outer half. Rubin and Casarett (1966) reviewed those methods that had been proposed to study the microcirculation of tumors and they argued that more information can be obtained by various microangiographic techniques compared to the limited view obtained in a histological section which can give no impression of the complex vascular arborization that is normal in tumor vasculature. Their work clearly indicates that there are a number of different types of vessel arrangement in tumors that need to be taken into account when proposing a general hypothesis about the anatomical arrangements of capillaries and tumor necrosis. They divided vascular patterns into three main types: (1) peripheral vascularization with penetrating vessels; (2) peripheral vascularization without penetrating vessels, and (3) central vascularization. The first two of these types are often associated with central necrosis of the tumor mass as the tumor enlarges but the third type, which may be encountered in tumors such as lymphomas, tends to be associated with a pattern of necrosis that is essentially at the single-cell level.

Rubin and Casarett considered that from an examination of the histology it is possible to detect areas of recent and old necroses. In the recent necrosis, the vascular pattern may be preserved whereas in long-standing necrosis it will be destroyed. This led them to suggest that certain types of necrosis may be attributable to a local change in the blood flow through the vessel rather than the orderly movement of cells on the oxygenated to the hypoxic zones. There are many reasons why the microcirculation can change, such as local thrombosis, external pressure on the capillary, and the effect of pharmacologically active molecules on the capillary released from the tumor cells. All may be part of a change in hemodynamics resultant on the thrombosis of a larger feeder vessel leading to temporary or permanent reduction of blood flow through particular capillaries. Tannock and Steel (1969) studied the perfusion of tumors with radioactive chromium-labeled red cells and found evidence of capillary stasis from autoradiographic examinations of histologic sections. The hemodynamics of experimental tumors have been measured by Gullino (quoted in Mendelsohn, 1970). Using several types of transplantable tumors, he demonstrated that the vascular space is characteristic of the tumor type and does not change with the site of transplantation. The blood flow through the tumor is considerably lower than that of normal tissues and correlates poorly with tumor growth rate whereas the interstitial space of tumors is much larger than that of normal tissues. Gullino was unable to demonstrate the relationship between tumor growth and oxygen consumed, glucose utilized, and the lactate eliminated, although the glucose utilization in tumors was very high compared to normal tissues. He did not consider that the oxygen lack was compensated for by an increase in glucose utilization or by a shift in the level of lactate produced by glycolysis (Gullino et al., 1967).

X. Immune Elimination of Cancer Cells

It is now widely accepted that tumor cells possess tumor-associated antigens on their surfaces which can evoke an immune response in the autochthonous host. This response can influence tumor growth. The end point of this immune reaction is the death of the tumor cell; this is probably the result of the interplay of both humoral and cell-mediated immunity although the relative contributions of these two areas of the immune system is still a matter for debate.

Within a review of this character it is inappropriate to attempt to give a detailed account of the role of lymphocytes, macrophages, and monocytes as well as antibody and complement in the immune cytolysis of cancer cells. For these matters and for how the tumor cells are recognized, the reader must refer to the literature of tumor immunology; a special supplement published in the *British Journal of Cancer* (Moore et al., 1973) provides a useful starting point. Instead, we shall concentrate our attention on some aspects of the cytotoxic effect per se, although it will soon become evident that it is a subject still shrouded in mystery. The general problem of cell-mediated cytotoxicity has been reviewed by several authors (Henney, 1973a; Berke and Amos, 1973; Lohmann-Matthes and Fischer, 1973), who have set the topic against the wider context of allograft and tumor immunity.

Detailed knowledge of how tumor cells are killed can be obtained only from study of *in vitro* systems, and even they have their limitation at the single-cell level. The implications of various conditions of immune competence of the host upon tumor cell kinetics is one way of looking at tumor cell kill *in vivo;* the other approach is to study tumor regression with the host survival or prolongation of life as the objective criteria.

The basic design of many experiments *in vitro* has an underlying similarity though the experiments tend to differ in many subtle points of detail. Target cells, often tumor cells, are exposed to sensitized lymphocytes or macrophages with and without various added serum factors, and the cytotoxic effect upon the target cells is observed. Several methods have been proposed to quantify the toxic effect upon the target cells, and these can be divided into two broad groups.

A. Quantification of Toxic Effect upon Target Cells

1. *The Release of Radioactive Marker Substances from Target Cells at the Time of Cytolysis*

Radioactive chromium supplied as $Na_2\ ^{51}CrO_4$ binds to target cells, and on the death of the cell by immune cytolysis it is released and not neutralized by either the lymphoid or target cells (Berke et al., 1971). The ^{51}Cr is incorporated as chromate, but on subsequent release it is probably in a hexavalent or trivalent form bound to proteins (Berke and Amos, 1973). A simple formula for calculating the extent of cytolysis can be based on the counts per minute (cpm) released from the target cells (TC) in the presence of immune lymphoid cells, cpm released from the TC in the presence of normal cells or when TC are incubated alone. There is a difference of opinion whether the denominator of the equation should be the total ^{51}Cr incorporated in the TC (Henney, 1973a) or the ^{51}Cr recoverable after lysis of the TC by sonication, freeze-thawing, or detergents (Berke and Amos, 1973). Typical formulas used to calculate are given below:

$$\text{Percent specific cytolysis} = \frac{(^{51}\text{Cr release with immune lymphocytes}) - (^{51}\text{Cr release with normal lymphocytes}) \times 100}{\text{Total cell-associated }^{51}\text{Cr}}$$

(From Henney, 1973a)

$$\text{Percent specific cytolysis} = \frac{(^{51}\text{Cr released with immune lymphocytes}) - (^{51}\text{Cr released by normal lymphocytes}) \times 100}{(^{51}\text{Cr released by freeze-thaw}) - (^{51}\text{Cr released by normal lymphocytes})}$$

(From Brunner et al., 1968)

The validity of ^{51}Cr release as an indicator of cytolysis is supported by the demonstration that it is reasonably well correlated with the uptake of trypan blue by the killed TC and estimates of the numbers of surviving TC (Sullivan et al., 1972; Berke et al., 1969). Measurements of the release of ^{125}I from TC labeled with UdR-^{125}I, a compound that specifically labels DNA, is an alternative to the ^{51}Cr method; the ^{125}I released does not become reincorporated (Forman and Britton, 1973). Likewise, the release of labeled amino acids from the proteins of lysed TC has also been used in this fashion.

2. Colony Inhibition and Microcytotoxicity Tests

When suitable TC are plated in petri dishes, they will grow and form colonies that can be counted 3–5 days later. If the TC are damaged, the yield of colonies falls in proportion to the extent of the damage. This approach is well known in radiobiology and has been used in studies of immune cytolysis of tumor cells (Hellström, 1967; Hellström and Sjörgen, 1965). However, in recent years this has been largely replaced by the microcytotoxicity test introduced by Takasugi and Klein (1970) and is widely used for the study of the immune reactions against tumors in man (Hellström et al., 1971). This test uses several numbers of TC and can be set up to have several replicates and various combinations of cells and sera to indicate the cytotoxic activity of the cells and both cytotoxic and blocking factors in the sera.

As a general rule, it is true that thymus-derived (T) lymphocytes are responsible for cell-mediated immunity and bone marrow-derived (bursal equivalent) (B) lymphocytes act as the progenitors of antibody-producing cells (Miller and Mitchell, 1969; Davies, 1969). Cell-mediated cytotoxicity is effected mainly by T lymphocytes (Cerottini et al., 1970; Goldstein et al., 1972). Although macrophages carrying cytotoxic factors can kill tumor cells (Evans and Alexander, 1972; Lohmann-Matthes and Fischer, 1973) and non-T lymphocytes, possibly B cells, can attack and lyse antibody-coated tumor cells (Forman and Möller, 1973).

Berke and Amos (1973) have suggested that lymphocyte-mediated cytolysis is a cyclic process in which three main events can be resolved: (1) binding of the cytotoxic lymphocyte (CL) to the target cell; (2) cytolysis of the target; (3) recycling of the CL. The initial contact of the CL and the target cell depends on the random movement of the lymphocytes. The binding of the CL to the target cells is reversible, active CL can be recovered after they have been detached from the target cells by trypsinization (Goldstein et al., 1971) or spontaneously (Berke et al., 1969). The precise nature of the binding is unknown, although the most widely held view is that a specific cell-recognition structure is responsible. Magnesium and calcium ions play an important role (Berke and Amos, 1973). The organization of the cell membrane of the effector and target cells are probably the most important factor in the binding. Intimate contact between the cytotoxic lymphocyte and the target cell is essential for cytolysis.

Various metabolic inhibitors interfere with cell-mediated cytolysis. Cytochalasin B prevents the interaction between the effector and target cells while prostaglandin E_2 also inhibits cytolysis to the same extent, but apparently at a later stage in the lytic sequence. Cytochalasin B is known to disturb the cytoplasmic microfilaments that are important in cytoplasmic contractility essential for cell movement. Colchicine also inhibits lymphocyte cytotoxicity; this agent disrupts the microtubular framework of the cell, possibly affecting cell secretion. Inhibitors of protein synthesis, cycloheximide, pactamycin, and emetine acting at different stages in the protein biosynthetic pathway, all reduce the cytotoxic effect of the lymphocytes, but active protein synthesis in the target cells does not appear to be a prerequisite for their eventual cytolysis (Henney, 1973a). The mechanism of immune cytolysis itself is still largely a matter for speculation. Microcinematography has shown that a hypergranulation and accelerated cytoplasmic flow precede the destruction of the target cell membrane and the formation of cytoplasmic blebs surrounding an apparently intact nucleus (Ginsburg et al., 1969).

DBA/2 mastocytoma cells, a target cell frequently used in studies of cytolysis, have an intensive phosphorylase activity. The activity of this enzyme is increased 2- to 3-fold when these target cells are brought into contact with cytotoxic spleen cells (Koren et al., 1971). The phospholipid degradation could not be ascribed to the cytolysis alone. Henney (1973b) has reported that the initial reaction between

C57BL lymphocytes against DBA_2 mastocytoma cells were very fast, but loss of macromolecules of the target cells took place after several hours. There was a gradual and progressive increase of the target-cell permeability; an increase of low molecular weight indicators, ATP and ^{86}Rb could be detected 20 minutes after adding the effector cells. On the other hand, the loss of indicators associated with the cytoplasmic and nuclear components, ^{51}Cr- and ^{3}H-labeled DNA did not become apparent until after a much longer period of incubation. The rate of efflux of the different indicators varied considerably, the number of effector lymphocytes required to initiate a specific release was comparable.

Berke and Amos (1973) have put forward a hypothesis to explain immune cytolysis as the end result of alterations of charge on the target cell membrane. They drew attention to the fact that both lymphocytes and target cells are negatively charged. However, the charge on the lymphocytes is distributed asymmetrically, being greatest on the "uropod" region which is a spurlike extension of the cytoplasm. If this strongly charged tip came into close proximity with the target cell membrane it could induce a local change in the membrane potential. The final step in this hypothesis is that the local change of membrane charge would reverse the normal asymmetric distribution of permeable and impermeable ions, leading to the death of the cell. This hypothesis sounds logical, but it will no doubt be hard to prove. Although the exact steps are still unknown, at least it will be seen that attention is focused upon two main features—the intimate contact of effector and target cell and the disruption of the integrity of the target cell membrane.

Lymphocytes, as the result of contact with antigen whether on a cell surface, or independent of cell contact, are stimulated to divide and produce several soluble factors. These affect macrophage mobility and lymphocyte blast cell transformation and have direct effects upon tumor cells (see Oettgen and Hellström, 1973). The macrophage cytotoxicity factor (MCF) is of particular interest, as it confers specific cytotoxicity to macrophages (Lohmann-Matthes and Fischer, 1973). Hence, the armed macrophage can attack living tumor cells whereas the unarmed macrophage will phagocytose only dead cells. Chalmers and Weiser (1973) have made an electron microscopic examination of the behavior of armed macrophages as they attack and kill target cells. In their system using sarcoma cells as the target, adherence of the macrophage to the TC is usually followed by contact destruction of the membrane in the absence of cytophagocytosis. The macrophages spread over the surface of the TC, and this is followed by the enclosure of the TC in a phagocytic vacuole. Later there is fusion of the phagocyte granules with the phagosome membrane and the liberation of granule contents into the phagosome. It is likely that this process leads to the mutual death of both TC and macrophage (Granger and Weiser, 1966).

Lejeune and Evans (1972) have compared the behavior of syngeneic immune macrophages (IM) when challenged with L5178Y cells *in vitro*. During the 22 hours of their cocultivation distinctive changes took place in the macrophages, but not in the target cells. IM contained more lysosomes than nonimmune macrophages (NM), both types of macrophage showed an increase in lysosomes within 2 hours of being put in contact with the target cells. After 6 hours an increase of acid phosphatase activity could be detected biochemically which continued to rise for 22 hours, in both NM and IM. These studies indicate that the immune or "armed macrophage" has no specific lysosome response but the IM cells exhibit a far more active cytoplasm; this could mean they are better adapted for phagocytosis of dying cells or debris, especially at the time of tumor rejection *in vivo*.

These authors have suggested that the study of the macrophage membrane phospholipase and cyclic adenosine monophosphate(cAMP)-associated adenyl cyclase would be a logical step; this would bring it into line with the present focus on the target cell membranes, although it would probably have to be studied at the electron microscopic level, owing to the rapid response of the target cells. The macrophages may also play an important role in the loss of cancer cells in lymph nodes and could be a factor in determining whether metastases become established. Carter and Gershon (1966) have described two transplantable lymphosarcomas in Syrian hamsters, one metastasizing (ML), the other nonmetastasizing (NML). In NML homografts the draining lymph nodes developed sinus histiocytosis. Cancer cells appeared in the sinuses within 1 week but remained localized to superficial sinuses, where they were destroyed by histiocytes. The ML homografts did not cause any proliferation of the sinus littoral cells, and cancer cells were seen in the cortical regions of the node after 3 weeks and formed metastatic foci. More recently Birbeck and Carter (1972) have examined the macrophages that infiltrate these two forms of lymphoma. In the NML the macrophages were active at all times and contained products of degenerate tumor cells. The ML contained macrophages, but they appeared to be activated only during the initial stages of growth after transplantation and in the latent phases; their presence was appreciated as the result of electron microscopic identification of their primary lysosomes.

B. Lymphoid Infiltration and Cell Destruction in Human Tumors

It is well recognized that many malignant tumors in man may be associated with cellular infiltration. Sometimes this infiltration is of an inflammatory nature, typified by polymorphonuclear leukocytes, but in other tumors there are pronounced lymphocytic infiltration.

Several authors have drawn attention to this lymphoid infiltration and tried to assess its prognostic significance. Naturally, their work was usually retrospective and the histological analyses relatively crude compared to the information that can be gained from *in vitro* tests or transplantation experiments in animals. Yet this information is still valuable, as it provides a link between the speculations raised by the *in vitro* studies that cancer cells can be killed immunologically and the possible contribution of this process in the evolution of cancer in man. It is not possible to make any direct accurate quantitative assessment of cell necrosis in tumor specimens, and even if it were possible, the causes of the tumor cell death are manifold.

Lymphocytic infiltration has been found in association with carcinoma of the stomach (Black *et al.*, 1954), carcinoma of the breast (Black *et al.*, 1956; Hamlin, 1968), seminoma (Dixon and Moore, 1953), malignant melanoma (Cochran, 1969), and neuroblastoma (Lauder and Aherne, 1972). All these authors have indicated that lymphoid infiltration is a good prognostic sign, though it has not always been confirmed; for example, Weidner and Hornstein (1973) failed to detect any advantage to the patient of lymphocytic infiltration in malignant melanoma. Because of the recurrent nature of bladder cancer and treatment being frequently aimed to preserve the bladder, study of this cancer has given some additional clues. Tanaka, Cooper, and Anderson (1970) found that there was a significantly higher association between lymphoid infiltration and bladder cancer compared to all forms of diseases of the bladder mucosa, but they could not show any correlation between this infiltration and three-year survival. However, they drew attention to the variability of the infiltration in some of their series of recurrent tumors. Sarma (1972) examined biopsy and cystectomy specimens and considered lymphocytic infiltration to be a sign favoring a good prognosis. Pomerance (1972) from her study of cystectomy specimens felt that plasma cell infiltration was a more accurate indicator. Prognosis was poor when they were few or absent, but a heavy infiltration did not necessarily imply a better prognosis.

It is known that the *in vitro* cytotoxic activity of lymphocytes from bladder cancer patients against bladder cancer cells varies with the tumor load, being depressed in the presence of large amounts of tumor (O'Toole *et al.*, 1973). This may explain some of the discrepancies in the correlation of histologic lymphocytic infiltration and prognosis in bladder cancer. Elston and Bagshawe (1973) have examined gestational choriocarcinomata invasive moles and lymphocytic infiltration in teratomatous choriocarcinoma. Response to chemotherapy was significantly better in gestational choriocarcinomata with a marked lymphocytic infiltration. There was no relation between the behavior of the invasive moles and infiltration. Teratomatous choriocarcinoma were usually associated with a weak infiltration and their response to chemotherapy is usually poor, but this relation may not be a simple one of cause and effect. Perhaps the clearest correlations have come from the study of gestational trophoblastic tumors, in particular choriocarcinoma which, being derived from fetal tissues, provides a special immunological challenge. Choriocarcinoma is a malignant allograft presenting a combination of specific antigens of the trophoblast, probably the specific antigens associated with transformation to the malignant state and transplantation antigens inherited from the male parent. About 70–80% of gestational choriocarcinomata can be eradicated successfully with chemotherapy, whereas 95% of invasive moles die out spontaneously (Bagshawe, 1973). Lymphocytic infiltration has to be assessed in relation to survival or other clinical criteria.

All these studies have shown that lymphoid infiltration is a variable phenomenon. The way in which lymphocytes accumulate in a tumor is not clear. It is probable that their interaction with tumor antigen may cause the release of factors that enhance the buildup of lymphocytes in the tumor vicinity. Dumonde *et al.* (1969) have described an inflammatory factor that increases vascular permeability. The lymphocytes could then be further influenced by the mitogenic and chemotactic factor as proposed by Mackler (1971). Excess of antigen with the production of blocking factors could be one explanation for the absence of infiltration in some tumors or it could be due to individual differences in the tumor-associated antigens and the host's responsiveness to a particular antigenic stimulus.

Immune elimination of cancer cells by experimental animals *in vivo* is well established (see Old and Boyse, 1966; Oettgen and Hellström, 1973). In man, despite the strong evidence for cell-mediated cytolysis *in vitro*, we still are uncertain about the role of immune cytolysis *in vivo*. Most of the evidence is circumstantial and lacks proof. Currie (1973) has briefly summarized the evidence, which includes a number of unexplained properties of certain tumors. Rare cases of spontaneous tumor regression have been reported (Everson and Cole, 1966). The changes in the cutaneous metastases of melanoma, with some getting larger at a time when others are decreasing, suggests a local immunological defense. The possibility that small tumors may regress spontaneously is supported by the finding at postmortem of an unexpectedly high incidence of prostate and thyroid carcinomata and neuroblastomas. However, the criterion of what constitutes a latent cancer must be assessed critically before taking this type of evidence at its face value. There is a possibility that some immunological mechanism may determine the duration between excision of a primary tumor and the growth of its metastases to reach a clinically detectable size. A few years' gap is commonplace, and there are many well-recorded incidences of periods of 20 years or more. It is not known whether the cells lie dormant during this time or whether there is a slow turnover balanced by random loss to prevent an expansion of the population. Such a balance could break down either owing to selection of tumor cells with new properties or a failure of the immunological defenses.

XI. Phagocytosis and Autolysis

The removal of dead cells depends on the mode of their death, and the place where they die. In some instances, they are lost from the body by desquamation from the skin, bronchial tree, alimentary or urinary tract. However, the majority are disposed of by combinations of autolysis and phagocytosis. The end products may be able to be absorbed, but in avascular zones they tend to accumulate either as solid areas of necrotic cells that slowly collapse or as an amorphous liquid that is seen typically in the centers of certain types of tumors in man, i.e., in bronchial carcinoma or in the center of a large Walker tumor in the rat. The first-line mechanism for the removal of dead cells or parts of dead cells is phagocytosis. The phagocytes consist of polymorphonuclear neutrophilic leukocytes, monocytes, tissue macrophages (histiocytes), and alveolar macrophages in the pulmonary alveolar septa and air spaces. Many of these macrophages can be attracted toward dead tissue or cells by chemotactic factors, which appear to be of low molecular weight (Stossel, 1974). Furthermore, there is a wide range of macromolecules, both cationic and anionic and including polynucleotides, heparin, and polypeptides that can stimulate the rate and apparent efficiency of phagocytosis (Simson and Spicer, 1973). The method of recognition of a particle or cell that is to be phagocytosed and its distinction from healthy cells is not fully understood. There is good reason to suppose that the coating of the particle or cell with serum proteins assists their engulfment; this process being called opsonization. Antibodies of the IgG class, when in high concentration, are opsonically active; the Fc portion of the antibody molecule and the Fab segment that attaches the molecule to the particle are required for the opsonization (Quie, 1972). Normal serum contains opsonic activity that is a function of its complement proteins, in particular C_3. These opsonins increase the rate of phagocytosis from slow to rapid but do not increase the affinity of the macrophage for the substrate (Stossel, 1974). The specific manner in which the particles, recognized by the macrophage, elicit ingestion is unknown. Some clues come from observations that divalent cations, magnesium, and calcium alter the ingestion, and drugs that increase the levels of intracellular cAMP inhibit the rate of digestion (Stossel, 1974).

The sequence of lysosomal activation and the destruction of the dead cells and parts of cells within the macrophage is beyond the scope of this review. The recent analyses of the literature by Stossel (1974) and by Simson and Spicer (1973) are valuable guides to the events leading up to the engulfment by phagocytes and the destruction of the ingested material. Apart from macrophages and histiocytes, epithelial and tumor cells may exhibit phagocytic activity. Kerr, Wyllie, and Currie (1972) have drawn attention to a sequence involving the condensation and breakup of cells followed by their ingestion and digestion by neighboring cells (Fig. 16). They have introduced the term apoptosis (Greek = to fall off, of leaves from the trees) to describe the sequence. This cycle of events occurs in the programmed cell death in embryonic tissues, in normal tissues, spontaneously in tumors, and following cell injury. Cell debris ingested by epithelial cells undergoes the same sequence of degradation as seen in macrophages and histiocytes. They include material that can be seen in membrane-bound phagosomes which fuse with cellular lysosomes. In tumors this process would appear to be fairly common and may account for some of the various inclusion bodies, particularly those that are Feulgen positive, that have been recorded in the early literature. However, care must be taken to distinguish various phagosomes and telolysosomes that are the consequence of ingestion of cell debris from those occurring as an autolytic phenomenon. Both tumor cells and healthy normal cells may show degenerative changes in organelles, the production of autolytic vacuoles, and the

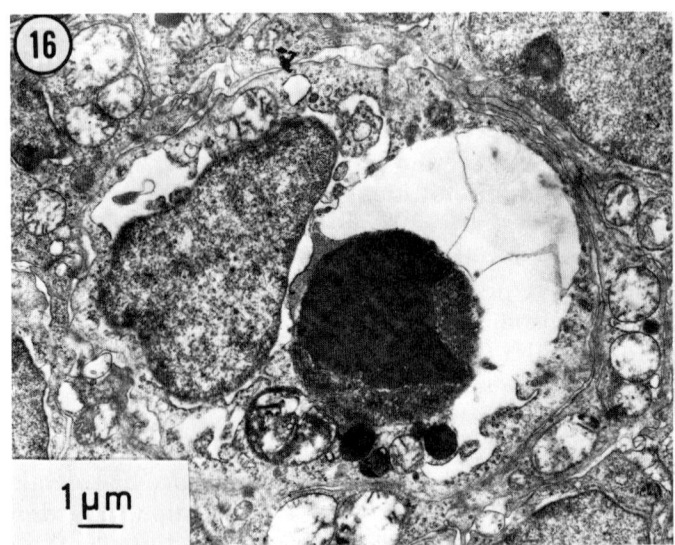

FIG. 16. Carcinoma of the colon showing apoptosis, with a dead cell containing a condensed nucleus within a phagolysosome, inside a healthy tumor cell.

formation of the end products of digestion, i.e., myelin whorls. These are all probably part of organelle turnover in long-lived cells and may not necessarily imply that the cell has phagocytosed parts of its neighbor or is itself dying. Increase in the load of dead cells by inducing a remission in a tumor, for example after oophorectomy in Huggins rat mammary tumors, causes a widespread uptake of dead cells by the surviving cancer tissue (Kerr et al., 1972). Phagocytosis of one tumor cell by another may account for some of the increase of lysosomal enzymes that have been reported after hormonal (Shamberger, 1969), spontaneous (Fodor et al., 1955; Kampschmidt and Wells, 1968), chemotherapeutic (Ambellan and Hollander, 1966; Niitani et al., 1966; Studzinski and Cohen, 1966) and radiotherapeutic (Paris et al., 1969) regression of tumors.

Hormonal-dependent mammary tumors provide a useful system to study tumor regression. Lanzerotti and Gullino (1972) investigated the changes in lysosomal activity during the rapid regression of MTWg tumors in rats deprived of mammotropic factor and castrated. Using immunoquantitation and biochemical assays they found that four acid hydrolases (acid phosphatase, arylsulfatase, β-galactosidase, and β-glucuronidase) increased during tumor regression. These workers were able to show increased amounts of enzyme as well as increased activities, which suggested de novo synthesis of β-galactosidase and β-glucuronidase in regressing tumors. Sylven and Niemi (1972) using a histochemical approach found that the enzymes that hydrolyze aminonaphthylamides at pH 5.5 were increased in dying cells of various types of tumors. These results agree with their observations in normal and ascites cells undergoing autolysis (Niemi and Sylven, 1969). They suggested that this enzyme activity is lysosomal, and although they were unable to cast much light on its biological significance, they considered it a useful marker. However, lysosomal enzymes are not always increased in the phase of irreversible damage. In some tissues, a decrease of succinic dehydrogenase activity, a marker of mitochondrial activity, is an indicator of impending cell death (Hammar & Mottet, 1971). It is apparent that the release of acid hydrolases is a fundamental process in the self-destruction of dead cells as well as their destruction within the phagosomes of scavenger cells. On the other hand, current evidence suggests that they are not concerned in the initiation or the execution of events that bring about the death of the cell, their role being to help to dispose of the corpse (Van Lancker, 1970). The autolytic processes that are valuable for removing effete organelles in the living cell and those which cause the destruction of the dead cell are in all probabilities similar except for their extent. The key to the initiation of cell death is still elusive although events in the plasma membrane changing its biophysical properties would seem to be the most likely starting point. The subsequent events will be dependent upon many factors within and outside the cell that condition the biochemical reactions to irreversible injury and the state of the enzyme systems at the moment of death.

XII. Tumor Cell Loss by Differentiation

In several forms of normal tissue the suppression of cyclic division is part of the final steps of cell differentiation. The differentiated end cell does not divide again for the remainder of its life-span. The polymorphonuclear granulocytes are a typical example; these cells do not divide, but undergo a number of morphologic changes, in particular, segmentation of the nucleus. The keratinizing cell layers in the prickle cell layer of the skin do not divide, though their keratin content increases as they approach the skin surface. The cells of the upper third of the intestinal villi are nondividing and highly specialized in the small intestine for the complex biosynthetic processed associated with absorption. These examples are all relatively short-lived; i.e., 126×10^9 granulocytes are produced per day in a 70-kg man (Cartwright *et al.*, 1964), and the intestinal mucosa has a turnover of only a few days in man (Lipkin, 1971). Erythrocytes represent an extreme form of cell differentiation in mammals, with loss of the nucleus, yet they have a life-span of about 120 days in man. The neurons are at the far end of the scale, for they do not divide during the animal's entire life-span, and are incapable of doing so. Hence, the cessation of division does not set the life-span of the cell; this is determined by its function and the different evolutionary selection pressures from one species to another. In the renewal tissues, these highly differentiated cells are end cells and represent the product of cell proliferation, which will inevitably be lost. In other tissues, e.g., liver, lymphoid tissue, and some epithelia, such as the bladder mucosa, the cells are in G_0 or a prolonged G_1 from which they can be recalled into cycle by a suitable stimulus. This simple division of cells into two function compartments — dividing or potentially able to divide, and unable to divide — shows a reasonable correlation with structure. The end cells usually have specialized organization that makes them readily distinguishable from their precursors, but this is not always the case; i.e. the ultrastructure of dividing and non-dividing chief cells in the intestine are essentially the same.

There is a growing appreciation that tumors are composed of many different subpopulations with a varying ability to differentiate and imitate the normal sequence in their tissue of origin. The most striking example is a testicular teratocarcinoma, and study of these tumors by Pierce and his group (Pierce and Wallace, 1971; Pierce, 1972) has raised a number of important questions in tumor biology. Within these highly malignant tumors, well differentiated glands, bone, brain, teeth, and other tissues may coexist with malignant blast cells. The differentiated tissues completely mirror their normal counterparts, but their arrangement, one with another, is completely random. In this tumor, some cells can express virtually any differentiation pathway of the genome and produce the controlled sequence of events and orderly intercellular relationship necessary to elaborate a tooth or the formation of hair. Yet others retain their malignant potential. Pierce (1972) has been able to cast some light on this form of tumor cell behavior. Using a spontaneous murine testicular teratoma that had been converted into an ascitic form it was possible to obtain small embryoid bodies composed of a core of embryonal sarcoma covered by endoderm. As these grew in the peritoneal cavity they formed mesenchyme, and the largest were cystic and lacked embryonal carcinoma cells. On transplantation the smallest and intermediate embryoid bodies produced typical teratocarcinomas. On the other hand, the largest embryoid bodies that lack embryonal carcinoma cells produced a tumor resembling a benign dermoid cyst.

Transplantation of single embryonal carcinoma cells confirmed that they were multipotential, as they gave rise to teratocarcinomas containing many different tissues (Kleinsmith and Pierce, 1964).

More recently, Pierce and his team have examined less exotic tumors, and their findings have a direct bearing on cell loss as the result of squamous metaplasia and in well differentiated squamous carcinomata. When rats carrying a well differentiated transplantable squamous cell carcinoma were injected with TdR-^{3}H the initial labeling was exclusively in undifferentiated cells. By 96 hours, many cells in well differentiated pearls were labeled. Pierce and Wallace (1971) confirmed the differentiation of the labeled cells by electron microscopic autoradiography. Transplantation of 78 epithelial pearls, containing 10% nonviable keratin, isolated by microdissection was not followed by any tumor takes. By contrast, 27 out of 62 transplants of undifferentiated cells gave rise to tumors. These authors drew attention to other examples in the literature suggesting that some cell clones within tumors have a phenotypic expression that causes them to differentiate — probably with the loss of their proliferative capacity.

Among these tumors are seminomas showing various forms of abortive spermatogenesis (Pierce, 1966; Rosai et al., 1969); rhabdomyosarcomas with cells ranging from embryonal myoblasts to long striated muscle fibers (Friedmann and Bird, 1969). A murine rhabdomyosarcoma has been described by Nameroff et al. (1970) which has a cellular differentiation pathway similar to normal myogenesis. In this transplantable tumor, multinucleated myotubes arose from mononucleated cells; it was only the latter that proliferated and could be labeled with TdR-^{3}H. It would appear that in this tumor the formation of myosin and the depression of DNA synthesis are linked in a similar fashion as in normal multinucleate muscle fibers (Stockdale and Holtzer, 1961). This model suggests that the malignant element of the tumor is an undifferentiated mononuclear cell, and the cells which gives the tumor its histological identity may not be involved in the tumor proliferation.

Basal cell carcinoma is a common form of skin cancer in man. It invades, destroying tissue, but rarely metastasizes. The tumors fail to differentitate *in vivo* as indicated by their lack of keratinization. Keratinization can be seen when tumors are autotransplanted (Van Scott and Reinertson, 1961) or cultured *in vitro* (Flaxman, 1972). Similar development of differentiation by cancer cells *in vitro* has been reported in other tumors. Mouse neuroblast cells take on the form and behavior of mature neurons (Augusti-Tocco and Sato, 1969). This suggests that the expression of differentiation may be suppressed as the result of reaction with the stroma. Unfortunately, with few exceptions, i.e., the keratinized cells of epithelial pearls, in most common forms of carcinomata it is not possible to state, by simple histological examination, whether the cells have differentiated. Well differentiated tumors of organs, such as the colon, stomach, or bladder, do not carry readily recognized markers to indicate differentiation to a sterile or even benign state. It can only be supposed that it is probable that the findings of nondividing cells in experimental tumors can in theory at least be extrapolated to many human solid tumors with low labeling indices.

XIII. Cell Loss in Experimental Tumors

The method used most widely to estimate the total cell loss from a tumor is based on a comparison between the observed doubling rate and that expected from the cell production rate. The approach has been used most effectively by Steel (1968), who wrote the definitive paper on the mathematics of this concept (see Addendum). He introduced the term "potential doubling time," which is the expected doubling time in the absence of any cell loss (Steel and Bensted, 1965). He argued that in a kinetic study of tumor growth the fraction of cells lost in unit time is a basic parameter, but gives little indication how the tumor growth rate is affected by this loss. As an alternative, the cell loss factor was proposed as a parameter that gives the rate of cell loss as a fraction of the rate at which cells are added to the tumor volume by mitotic division. In this way a cell loss factor of 100% describes a tumor in which there is neither growth nor regression. The general growth patterns of tumors are complicated by minor fluctuations in rate as well as a progressive overall change with time. The Gompertz equation $V = V_0 \exp[A/\alpha(1 - e^{\alpha t})]$ can often be used to describe the growth rate of tumors. This states that the exponential growth progresses with a doubling time that increases exponentially (Laird, 1964). This alone suggests that various estimates of the cell loss factor can be expected to differ as the tumor increases in size (see Fig. 17).

Examples of calculations of cell loss factors are given in Tables I and II, taken from the papers of Steel (1968) and Hermens (1973), respectively. Skipper (1972) has also made similar calculations for several experimental tumors and related their growth patterns to their sensitivity of chemotherapeutic agents.

There are a number of factors that can influence these calculations, which can only, at best, be guides to the degree of cell loss and must be treated with some reservation. The use of tumor doubling time will tend to give an underestimate of cell loss due to the

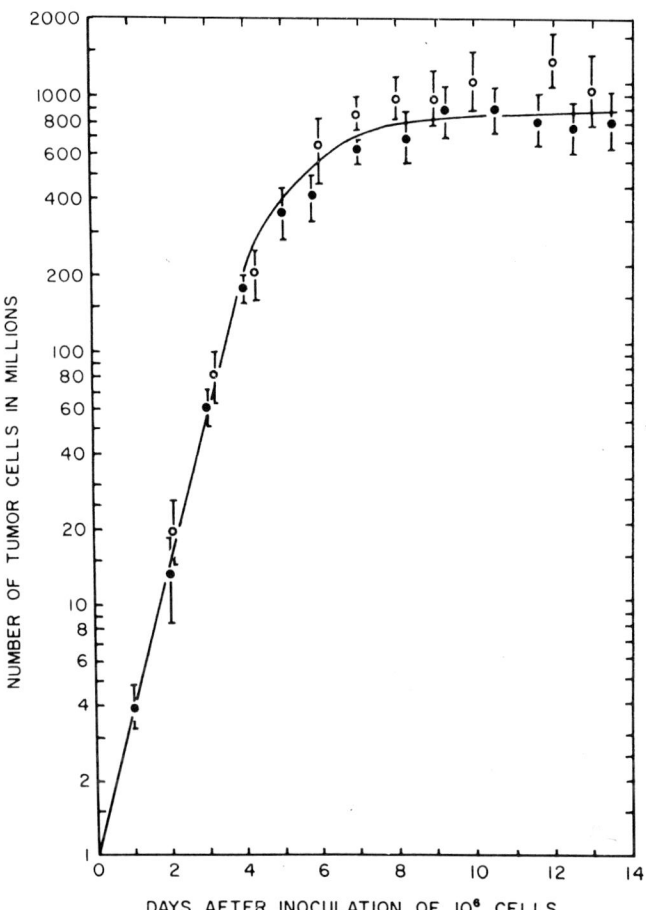

FIG. 17. Growth curve of Ehrlich ascites tumor produced with 10^6 cells. Vertical bars represent standard errors. Taken from Lala (1972), with permission.

inclusion of blood, tissue fluid, and necrotic material in the measurements of tumor volume. Histologic studies have indicated the ratio of necrotic to viable cells increases as the tumor increases in size. Large tumors are most liable to be affected by the random vagaries of alterations of their microcirculation.

Variations in the labeling index at different points within the same tumor has been reported by several workers (Frindel *et al.*, 1969). These may be related to the blood supply (Tannock, 1968) and apparently without effect on the cell cycle time. Rabes (1965) observed differences in the shape of the fraction of labeled mitoses

TABLE I
CELL LOSS FROM EXPERIMENTAL TUMORS[a]

Tumor	Labeling index, LI (%)	DNA synthetic period, ts (hours)	G_2 period, tG2 (hours)	Measured volume doubling time (hours)	Potential doubling time (hours)	Rate of cell loss, kL (per hour)	Cell loss factor (%)	Reference
Ehrlich ascites	47	8.5	6.6	18.0	18.6	0[b]	0[b]	Edwards et al. (1960)
Ehrlich ascites	40	8.8	4.8	19	21.4	0[b]	0[b]	Kim and Evans (1964)
Ehrlich ascites								
4-Day tumor	54	11	6	20.6	20.6	0[b]	0[b]	Baserga
7-Day tumor	49	11	6	38.4	22.2	0.0131		(1963)
13-Day tumor	27	11	6	336	35.7	0.0173	89	
Ehrlich ascites								
1-Day tumor	67	6	2	11	9	0.0139	18	Lala and
4-Day tumor	55	13	4	40	23	0.0126	42	Patt
7-Day tumor	46	18	4	120	35	0.0127	71	(1966)
NCTC								
3-Day tumor	26	10	2	30[c]	30.2	0[b]	0[b]	Frindel
7-Day tumor	24	10	2	38	34	0.0020	10	et al.
20-Day tumor	20	12.5	2	110	49	0.0078	55	(1967)
BICR/MI	34.2	8.0	3.0	22.7	20.7	0.0031	9[b]	Steel et al.
BICR/A2	3.5	10	3.0	190	205	0[e]	0[e]	(1966)
WAG/Rij	19.2	9.5	(2)	60	39	0.0062	35	Hermens and Barendsen (1967)
C3H mammary tumor	18.5 12.0[d]	10	3	204	43 64	0.0127 0.0075	79 69	Mendelsohn (1960a,b, 1965)
C3H mammary tumor	14.1	11.6	(3)	(204)	64	0.0075	69	Bresciani (1965)

[a] From Steel (1968).
[b] Not significantly different from zero.
[c] Value from growth curve; author's table gives 24 hours.
[d] Labeling index of autotransplants.
[e] Large possible error in LI; not significantly different from zero.

(FLM) curves when cells in the periphery of tumors were compared to cells from all regions. More recently, Steel (1970), has analyzed the form of FLM curves from experimental tumors, in particular drawing attention to their well pronounced second wave, and concluded that there is not a great deal of spread of cell cycle times within the population. No doubt this is the effect of genetic selection associated with recurrent transplantation. It will be seen from Tables

TABLE II

DATA ON GROWTH PARAMETERS FOR VARIOUS TYPES OF SOLID TUMORS STUDIED AT SUCCESSIVE STAGES OF GROWTH[a]

Host animals	Tumor cell-type	Stage of growth			Growth parameters[b]					Reference
		Age (days)	Weight (mg)	Volume (mm³)	α	T_c (hr)	$T_{d(Pot)}$ (hr)	T_d (hr)	Percent	
C3H-mice	NCTC-2472 fibrosarcoma	3	—	10.7	1.45	16.5	30.7	24.0	"0"	Frindel et al. (1968)
		7	—	80.0	1.40	17.5	36.1	38.0	5	
		20	—	2100.0	1.24	17.5	56.4	56.4	49	
BDF-1- mice	755-adeno- carcinoma	4	46.0	—	1.51	12.0	20.4	17.7	"0"	Simpson-Herren and Lloyd (1970)
		8	378.0	—	1.45	14.0	26.0	31.2	17	
		14	2660.0	—	1.28	16.0	44.8	132.0	66	
Hamsters	Fortner plasmacytoma	6	493.0	—	1.23	13.8	46.2	38.4	"0"	Simpson-Herren and Lloyd (1970)
		7	310.0	—	1.16	15.1	70.7	33.6	"0"	
		10	1990.0	—	1.21	15.0	54.5	57.6	5	
		10	2270.0	—	1.28	16.8	47.2	60.0	21	
		19	10700.0	—	1.32	16.5	41.1	153.6	73	
CF1-mice (female)	Ehrlich ascites cells	6	300.0	—	1.44	16.4	31.2	67.0	53	Lala (1972)
		14	900.0	—	1.37	17.8	39.2	156.0	75	
		26	2200.0	—	1.32	18.3	45.7	312.0	85	
WAG/Rij rats (female)	R-1 rhabdomyo- sarcoma	—	—	1 to 5	1.485	19.6	41.4	60±10[c]	31±10	Hermens (1973)
		—	—	300.0	1.410	20.5	50.7	50.4	0	
		—	—	1500.0 to 3000.0	1.322	20.5	59.7	87.6	32	

[a] From Hermens (1973). Summary of data on growth parameters for different types of tumors published in the literature. Each of these tumors was studied at different time intervals after transplantation of cells into host animals in order to obtain information on the natural variations in cell kinetics, in rates of cell production, and in rates of cell loss. The values on cell loss, between quotation marks, refer to a negative difference between T_o and $T_{d(Pot)}$.

[b] α, average number of newly produced P cells per cell division; T_c, median cell cycle time; $T_{d(Pot)}$, potential volume doubling time, T_d, measured volume doubling time.

[c] The standard deviation is specified here, because the real curve at this stage of growth is uncertain.

I and II that several transplantable tumors have apparently no cell loss in their earlier phases of growth. It probably starts to become important when the tumor has reached 10^9 cells or 0.1 gm in the mouse (Steel, 1968). This may be a further reflection of genetic selection so that intrinsic cell death and immunologic cell elimination is unimportant, or that the methodology is incapable of appreciating these losses when the tumor is expanding at its maximum growth rate.

The slowing of the growth rate is probably due to a combination of two major factors: (1) a decrease of the proportion of proliferating cells produced at each division, in other words decline of the growth fraction, and (2) cell loss. In the most important transplantable tumors, loss by exfoliation or migration into lymphatics or the blood stream is slight, but exfoliation can be an important factor in primary tumors arising in the gastrointestinal tract, the urinary tract, and the skin. Lala (1972), from his studies of the mode of death of cells in

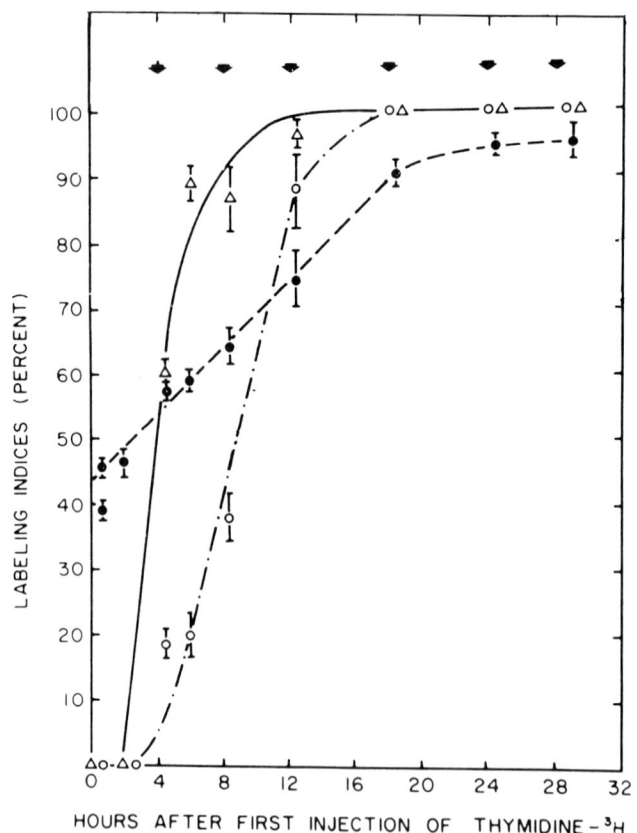

Fig. 18. Temporal changes with labeling indices of tumor cells scored in various morphological categories, following repeated injections of ^{3}H-labeled thymidine (arrowheads at top of figure). Arrows indicate intervals when TdR-^{3}H was repeated. —, Mitotic tumor cells; –·–, fragmented pycnotic tumor cell nuclei; ---, total tumor cell population, excluding pycnotic nuclei. Taken from Lala (1972), with permission.

Ehrlich ascites cell tumor, came to the conclusion that the main loss was from the nonproliferating part of the population. Analysis of various kinetic parameters and the labeling pattern after repeated injections of TdR-^{3}H (Fig. 18), indicated that the loss was age dependent. However, no light was shed on the mechanism of this aging.

XIV. Cell Loss in Human Tumors

The general principles outlined for the calculation of cell loss from experimental tumors hold true for similar calculations in man. There are a number of important factors that must be borne in mind before any attempt is made to interpret the published data. Estimates of the growth rate of the human tumors are difficult to obtain. First, the occasions in medicine during which it is justified to observe undisturbed tumor growth in man are few. The majority of observations have been made on suitable metastatic tumors in which it was judged to be ethical to leave untreated. The nature and site of many types of cancers in man make them unsuitable for recurrent measurement so that our knowledge is based on selected groups of tumors. With very few exceptions the tumor size during the period of observation is considerably larger than that in experimental animals, which may be one explanation of the marked differences in behavior.

It has been assessed that human tumors must have passed through about 30 cell-doubling times for them to be visible clinically (Iversen, 1967). Direct observations of skin tumors has been used by some workers to study their growth (Frindel et al., 1968). However, in practice it has been found that repeated radiologic examinations of tumors, especially when growing as pulmonary metastases, have provided the most useful information about their doubling time. Charbit, Malaise, and Tubiana (1971) have made an analysis of 546 human tumors that have been well described in the literature in terms of their pathology and doubling times. The doubling times within each group of tumors had a log normal distribution. There was a marked difference between primary and secondary adenocarcinomata and the correlation between the histologic type and the mean doubling time. Charbit et al. considered that the difference between the doubling times of primary and metastatic adenocarcinoma could be due to (1) a different composition of tumors in the two groups; (2) reduction of the loss by exfoliation when a tumor grows in the lung and the advantages of the environment of the lung to support tumor growth.

The slow progress of certain human tumors has been well illustrated by observation of colorectal cancer by repeated barium enemas (Welin et al., 1963). They give a mean doubling time for primary tumors of 620 days with a calculated spread of 138–1155 days. On the other hand, metastatic colon cancer growing in the lung had a mean doubling time of 109 days. It must be remembered that certain primary tumors in man may grow relatively slowly and, if they are not located in a site producing immediate damage to vital tissue by invasion, they are obviously compatible with prolonged life-span. The outcome of these patients, however, will depend mainly upon the behavior of the metastatic growth. It is well recognized that sometimes in human tumors the primary growth may be very small at a time when the metastases may weigh several kilograms.

Measurement of cell proliferation in human tumors offers more difficulty than the measurement of doubling time. A formal cell kinetic analysis using TdR-^{3}H-labeling *in vivo* followed by multiple biopsies of the tumor to construct a FLM curve is rarely feasible or ethically justified. Such an analysis has been made in a small number of solid tumors in man, particularly squamous cell carcinomas (Frindel et al., 1968; Bennington, 1969), melanomas (Young and de Vita, 1970; Shirakawa et al., 1970), and adenocarcinomas (Young and de Vita, 1970) as well as a larger number of leukemias (see Gavosto and Pileri, 1971), where the technical problems of tissue sampling are not so formidable, being those of recurrent bone marrow aspiration. These studies have given good evidence about the duration of G_2, mitosis, and the S phase in human tumors, but, unlike the FLM curves of tumors in experimental animals, the second peak is often indistinct or absent indicating a wide dispersion of cell cycle times (Steel, 1973).

Estimates of the percentage of cells synthesizing DNA have been made in many human tumors by incubation of suitable pieces with TdR-^{3}H *in vitro*. In loosely packed tissues, such as bone marrow or some of the lymphomas, the labeling index probably corresponds closely to that found *in vivo*. Diffusion of TdR-^{3}H through more solidly packed tumor specimens is often restricted and the labeling may be uneven for technical reasons. By using a combination of an injection of TdR-^{3}H into the tumor *in vivo* and the subsequent labeling of a biopsy specimen with TdR-^{14}C *in vitro*, estimates of the duration of DNA synthesis have been made in Hodgkin's tumor tissue (Schiffer, 1971) and in human melanoma (Hagemann and Schiffer, 1971).

Refsum and Berdal (1967) obtained an indication of proliferation in laryngeal cancer from an analysis of the rate of accumulation of mitotic figures in tumors following the injection of the patient with a colchicine derivative, demecolcine (Colcemid®, CIBA). In this stathmokinetic method, cells entering mitosis are blocked in metaphase by the drug; by counting the number of mitoses in a biopsy before and 3–4 hours after giving the drug, the rate of entry of cells into mitosis can be calculated. Vincristine has a similar stathmokinetic effect, but it is not without hazard. Refsum and Berdal (1967) found that, on average, laryngeal carcinomata have 12.4 cells arrested in mitosis per hour per 1000 cell. Comparing this with an average doubling time for human tumors of 60 days (Steel and Lamer-

TABLE III
LABELING INDICES AND POTENTIAL DOUBLING TIMES OF HUMAN TUMORS[a,b]

Lymphomas	Number of tumors measured	Median labeling index (LI)	Potential doubling time (days)	Reference
Hodgkin's disease[c]	10	25.0	1.8	Peckham and Cooper
Reticulum cell sarcoma[c]	13	28	1.6	(1969)
Lymphatic lymphoma[c]	12	28	1.6	Peckham and Cooper
Histiocytic-lymphocytic[c]	5	11.6	4.0	(1970)
Burkitt tumor	26	32	1.4	Iversen (personal
	23	24	1.9	communication)
Carcinoma of bladder	32	3.2	15.0	Levi et al. (1969)
Carcinoma of the colon	31	4.5	10.4	Wolberg (1964; Lieb and Lisco (1966)
Carcinoma of the breast	38	1.1	43	Wolberg and Brown (1962)

[a] Adapted from Steel (1967).
[b] Calculated $T = \lambda(ts/LI)$; $\lambda = 0.75$; $Ts = 15$ hours.
[c] Tumor cells only.

ton, 1966), they estimated a cell loss of 96%. This technique has been applied to the study of human bladder cancer (Spooner and Cooper, 1972) and to colon cancer (Bottomley and Cooper, 1973; Camplejohn et al., 1973).

Unfortunately, in all these situations there is no reliable method of estimating the tumor doubling time. In bladder and colon cancer, stathmokinetic tests have drawn attention to the wide variation of cell proliferation that may be found within tumors of apparently similar histologic type. This suggests that the loss, particularly by exfoliation, must vary considerably, and it is not known whether a tumor alters its stability in response to various external causes, such as infection. Steel (1968) calculated the potential doubling time for a number of human tumors based on their labeling indices in a collection of 170 tumors from all sites: the mean labeling index was 3.0%, and the potential doubling time was 15.6 days. In Table III we show a calculation of this type illustrating tumors that have been investigated by one of the authors and additional material for comparison. It will be seen that there is a considerable discrepancy between the potential doubling time for any tumor and the observed doubling time for tumors of similar histologic class. In Steel's series, taking the mean labeling index in bladder and a doubling time of 66 days and an S period of 15 hours, he calculated a medium cell loss of 77%. An

TABLE IV
CELL KINETICS AND CELL LOSS FROM HUMAN TUMORS[a]

Tumor	Actual DT (days)	Labeling index (LI) (%)	Potential DT[c]	Estimated GF	Cell loss factor (%)	Rate of cell loss (per 10^9 cells per day)
Embryonal tumors	27 (22–33)	30 (22–41)	1.66	90	94	487×10^6
Hematosarcoma	29 (23–37)	29 (22–38)	1.70	90	94	437×10^6
Mesenchymal sarcomas	41 (35–50)	3.8 (2.5–5.9)	13.2	11	68	37×10^6
Squamous cell carcinoma	58 (48–70)	8.3 (6.4–10.9)	6.0	25	90	111×10^6
Adenocarcinoma	83 (72–96)	2.1 (1.7–2.7)	23.8	6	71	21×10^6

[a] From Malaise et al. (1973).

[b] For each pathological type, the mean value and, in parentheses, the 95% confidence intervals, are given.

[c] $DT_{pot} = L(Ts/LI)$; $L = 0.75$; $GF = \overline{LI}(Tc/Ts)$. DT = doubling time; GF = growth factor.

increase in the mean S period to a value of 20 hours gave a figure of 70% , and for 30 hours 54%.

Recently, Malaise, Chavaudra, and Tubiana (1973) have given further attention to the relation between the mean labeling index and the mean doubling time (DT) of the 5 histologic classes of tumors. They took 156 labeling indices from the literature and added 86 of their own; their most recent calculations, based on these data, are shown in Table IV.

It can be seen that there is no correlation between the labeling indices and the actual DTs. The growth fraction would appear to be the main parameter of the tumor kinetics that explains the differences in growth rate. The growth fraction is nearly 100% for embryonal tumors and lymphomas (hematosarcomas) and much lower for sarcomas, squamous cell tumors, and adenocarcinomata. The cell loss factor, on the other hand, is not as high in one of the slower growing tumors, squamous cell carcinoma, as in adenocarcinoma. These estimates of loss are more accurate than those forecast by the earlier work of Iversen (1967) and Refsum and Berdal (1967) and suggests that Steel's figure of about 60% is about right for adenocarcinoma. Although it must be accepted that calculations of this character are bound to be inaccurate, they repeatedly confirmed the suspicion that cell loss is a major factor by the time a tumor becomes clinically detectable. Studies of the rate of growth of very small metastatic Burkitt tumors in the skin followed by their excision and the termination of the proportion of labeled cells and the duration of S indicated a loss of about 75% (Iversen, personal communication).

In some tumors high rates of loss can be suspected from their histologic appearance. Burkitt tumor has many characteristic large macrophages interspaced between tumor cells, and these macrophages are loaded with the debris from a dying tumor cell. Basal cell carcinomas frequently have a high mitotic rate but grow slowly. Histologically, many of the tumor cells contain so-called Councilman bodies. Kerr and Searle (1972) have demonstrated that one method of cell loss in this tumor is shrinkage necrosis followed by the ingestion of the remnants by healthy tumor cells and the digestion in their phagolysosomes. The Councilman bodies have been demonstrated to be either dead cells lying outside or within basal carcinoma cells. The loss of cells by exfoliation can readily be appreciated in transitional cell carcinoma of the urinary bladder in which single cells or groups of cells break free from the tumor and can be recovered from the urine. In colon cancer, desquamated cells can be seen within the lumen of the tumor acini (Fig. 19). As we have said earlier, necrotic areas within a tumor are obvious histologic indicators that cell loss must have taken place.

In human tumors the loss of cells into the lymphatics and the

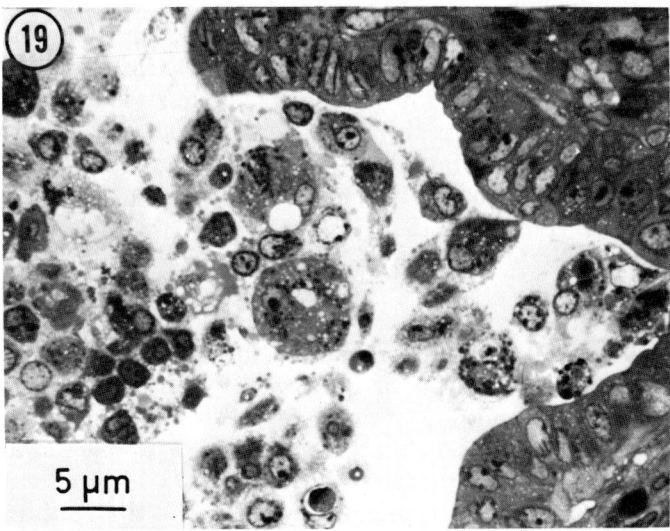

FIG. 19. Section of carcinoma of the colon growing as a transplantable tumor in a mouse and illustrating cell loss by desquamation into a tumor acinus which contains necrotic cancer cells and viable macrophages.

blood stream is probably a more important mode of loss of cells than in many experimental tumors. Carcinoma of the kidney and Wilms tumors are well known to have direct extensions into the blood vessels. Direct invasion of tumor through the walls of a blood vessel can be followed by massive hematogenesis, spread, for example, in carcinoma of the bronchus. Cancer cells can be found circulating in the blood in many forms of neoplastic disease. It would seem that only very few of them can form metastatic growth, and the majority are probably destroyed.

XV. Cell Loss and the Treatment of Tumors

Bagshawe (1968) has made a theoretical analysis of the action of chemotherapeutic drugs in tumors and related his theories to the responses in sensitive human tumors, such as lymphoma and choriocarcinoma. He concluded that it is the additive effect of the chemotherapeutic agent, and the spontaneous loss, that results in tumor elimination. It was proposed that the spontaneous loss rate needs to exceed a critical value for any particular chemotherapy regimen to be able to reduce the tumor population size. This critical rate will vary according to the therapy used. Denekamp (1970) made a comparison between the volume change in experimental sarcomas and carcinomas 24 hours after irradiation and in their cell loss factor (ϕ). As a rule she found that the carcinomas had a higher ϕ than sarcomas. Only the carcinomas showed tumor shrinkage within 24 hours of irradiation. The sarcomas were unchanged for at least 48 hours, but in her series of tumors, while it was true that the shrinkage pattern and the histology were related, they did not seem to be well correlated to the cell loss factor. Tumor shrinkage depends not only on the radiosensitivity of the tissue, but also the rate of removal of the dead cells by autolysis and phagocytosis, and the latter in part depend on the blood supply. Hermens (1973) made a comparative study of the growth parameters of irradiated and nonirradiated tumors in several species of laboratory animals. He demonstrated that there was a marked difference in their reactions to irradiation. The type-specific differences were likely to be related to (a) intrinsic radiosensitivity and oxygen status of the tumor cells, which will be the main factor determining the proportion of dead cells in the tumor after irradiation; and (b) differences in the kinetics of cell production and cell loss by cells that will survive and those that will eventually die.

Breur (1966) observed a relationship between the doubling time (DT) of human tumors prior to irradiation and the response to fractionation irradiation. Tumors characterized by short DT were more radiosensitive. Although this applies to lymphoma and embryonal tumors with short DTs and bowel and kidney with long DTs, there are some obvious exceptions: osteogenic sarcomas and fibrosarcomas have short DTs and are radioresistant, and breast cancers are slow growing but are radiosensitive.

Tumors are composed of several elements apart from tumor cells. Macrophages, blood vessels, fibroblasts, and blood both within and outside vessels as well as dead cells, are the usual components, to which must be added a variable amount of inflammatory and lymphoid cells. The RIB 5 fibrosarcoma in rats has been the subject of considerable investigation, particularly in relation to its radiosensitivity and oxygenation (Thomlinson, 1960). Peel and Cowen (1972, 1973) examined the response of this tumor to cyclophosphamide using morphometric analysis whereby the constitution of tumor was analyzed at various times before and after treatment using the multiple random point method as first described by Chalkley (1943) and later developed by Weibel, Kistler, and Scherle (1966). From this analysis and previous studies of the cell kinetics using autoradiographic, cytophotometric, and cytological methods, these authors were able to describe some of the main sequences that follow the treatment of this tumor. Morphologically, the tumor cells swell, followed by a wave of karyorrhexis and pycnosis associated with an increased hemorrhage beginning at about 12 hours and lasting for 48 hours. At 72 hours after a single dose of cyclophosphamide the tumor has returned to its pretreatment state. Those studies indicated that the initial response to injury is associated with an abortive wave of DNA synthesis which produces cells at 24 and 48 hours with gross chromosome abnormalities, but these are quickly removed from the population, suggesting that they do not contribute to cell proliferation. The other feature that was marked was a change in the distribution of the proliferative areas within the tumor. In the controls, the maximum number of labeled cells were at the periphery and the maximum necrosis in the center of the tumor. By the third day after treatment, cell proliferation appeared to be fairly evenly distributed through the tumor mass. These experiments and those of other workers clearly demonstrate that major, although quite often short-term, disturbances of tumor populations are produced by chemotherapy or radiotherapy, and that the precise moment at which they are sampled after the damage may considerably influence the overall morphological picture and indeed can give rise to quite false interpretation. For example, the induction wave of mitosis may be taken as a sign of increased cell proliferation whereas a more detailed study will often indicate that these mitoses are in no way contributory to the expansion of tumor mass.

Addendum: Mathematical Treatment of Cell Loss in Tumors

In the mathematical analysis of a real problem it is usually necessary to make simplifying assumptions and develop an idealized model. Sometimes the assumptions may be suggested by experimental evidence, but often there is no prior justification. The latter is very much the case with mathematical models for tumor growth, particularly in man.

This note presents some of the theoretical treatments of cell loss in tumors and emphasizes the assumptions involved.

1. *Mathematical Models of the Cell Cycle*

Over recent years an enormous literature concerning theoretical models for cell population growth has developed. Many treatments have been based on the theory of branching processes (see Harris, 1963; Jagers, 1969) or renewal theory (see Cox, 1962). In particular, considerable attention has been given to models for the synthesis of fraction-labeled mitosis (FLM) curves (e.g., see Barrett, 1966; Trucco and Brockwell, 1968; Brockwell et al., 1970; Takahashi, 1968; MacDonald, 1970). The present discussion will deal with those features of the models relevant to the treatment of cell death.

It is usually assumed that the sojourn time of a cell in each of the four phases, G_1, S, G_2, and M, may be represented by the independent probability density functions, $F_i(t)$, $i = 1, \ldots 4$. The probability density function for the whole cycle is then given by the convolution

$$F(t) = F_1(t) * F_2(t) * F_3(t) * F_4(t)$$

The special case where correlations are allowed to exist between the $F_i(t)$, $i = 1, \ldots 4$, has been studied by MacDonald (1970) and Barrett (1974).

Data concerning the form of $F_i(t)$, $i = 1, \ldots 4$, cannot be obtained from experimental techniques presently available, and assumed forms must be used. Some information concerning $F(t)$ for cells *in vitro* may be obtained using time-lapse cinematography (e.g., see Hsu, 1960; Sisken and Kinosita, 1961; Norrby, 1970). However, Norrby et al. (1967) have pointed out that the small sample sizes analyzed in such studies do not represent accurately the true population distribution. Jagers and Norrby (1974) have described a statistical method which enables $F(t)$ to be calculated from observations on a small sample of cells, provided the culture is in steady-state exponential growth. Data concerning $F(t)$ for cells *in vivo* are not available.

For a cell population in steady-state exponential growth where each cell upon division produces, on average, A new cells which enter the proliferative cycle (P cells) and 2-A nonproliferative cells (Q cells), the number of cycling cells present at time t is

$$N(t) = N_0 \exp(Kt) \qquad (1)$$

where K is the Malthusian parameter and is given by the nonnegative root of

$$A \int_0^\infty \exp(-Kx) F(x)\, dx = 1 \qquad (2)$$

(see Trucco and Brockwell, 1968).

Such a cell population has a stable age distribution, with the density of cells with age between u and $u + du$ given by

$$g(u) = \left(\frac{A}{A-1}\right) K \exp(-Ku) \left[1 - \int_0^u F(x)\, dx\right] \qquad (3)$$

(see MacDonald, 1970).

From (1) the population doubling time is obtained as

$$T = \ln 2/K \qquad (4)$$

For the simple case when the cell cycle time is assumed to be a constant, t_c, for all cells, Eq. (2) gives

$$K = \ln A/t_c \qquad (5)$$

The age distribution density function may then be written

$$g(u) = A/(A-1)\, (\ln A/t_c) \exp[-(\ln A/t_c)]u \qquad (3a)$$

If cell loss occurs at random throughout the cycle, i.e., if the probability of loss is the same for every cell in the population at a given time, Eq. (1) may be rewritten.

$$N(t) = N_0 \exp(K - \lambda)t \qquad (1a)$$

where λ represents the rate of cell loss.

It should be noted that Eqs. (3) and (3a) are still valid if this type of loss occurs. However, for age-dependent loss, this equation is no longer valid. The latter situation has been examined by Bartlett (1969).

Mendelsohn (1960a) introduced the concept of growth fraction (GF) and defined this as the ratio of proliferating to total cells in a population. For a cell population in steady-state exponential growth and assuming a constant value for A, then

$$GF = A - 1 \qquad (6)$$

Furthermore, the doubling time for such a population is equal to that of the proliferating compartment alone and is given by Eqs. (4) and (5).

2. Cell Loss and FLM Curves

Brockwell, Trucco, and Fry (1972) drew attention to the fact that, provided cell loss is random, i.e., is represented by the term λ in Eq. (1a), then λ has no effect on the FLM curves. The FLM curve therefore, is of no value in the direct estimation of cell loss (but see later).

3. Growth Fraction and FLM Curve

Barrett (1966) in a Monte-Carlo simulation of the cell cycle assumed a steady-state population with $A = 1$ and produced synthetic FLM curves. Brockwell, MacLaren, and Trucco (1970) used a similar method, except that A was variable $(1 \leq A \leq 2)$. The simulated FLM curve that they obtained, using the same cell cycle parameters as Barrett but with $A = 2$, did differ slightly. For practical purposes, however, this difference would probably lie well within the experimental error of measured FLM curves, so this technique cannot give any information about growth fraction.

4. Application to Tumor Growth

Steel (1967, 1968) has used the ideal model of cell proliferation described above to obtain an estimate of cell loss in tumors. For such a population the rate of growth depends on: (a) cell cycle time distribution; (b) growth fraction; (c) rate of cell loss, and these components are difficult to separate.

From Eqs. (4) and (1a) we obtain

$$N(t) = N_0 \exp[(\ln 2/T) - \lambda]t \tag{7}$$

where T is the "potential doubling time" as defined by Steel and Bensted (1965).

Furthermore, if the population is in exponential growth, then the growth equation may also be written

$$N(t) = N_0 \exp[(\ln 2/T_D)]t \tag{8}$$

where T_D is the measured doubling time of the tumor. Therefore

$$\lambda = \ln 2/T[1 - (T/T_D)] \tag{9}$$

From Eq. (4) $K = \ln 2/T$.

Steel (1967, 1968) then defines the cell loss factor, ϕ, by

$$\phi = \lambda K = 1 - (T/T_D) \tag{10}$$

Note that in deriving this equation, no assumptions have yet been made about the distribution of cell cycle times, but it has been assumed that cell loss occurs with equal probability for all cells in the cycle. As Steel pointed out, an age-dependent loss occurring immediately after mitosis might be regarded as altering A, so that the value for the potential doubling time given by Eq. (4) is underestimated. In order to apply Eq. (10) the value of T must be estimated. If it is further assumed that (a) the cell cycle time and individual phase duration are constants, and (b) the duration of G_2 is known, then the iterative procedure given by Steel (1968) can be applied and T can be estimated from the measurement of labeling index and t_s (S phase duration) alone. Note that this method is fairly insensitive to the value of A and does not require data concerning the growth fraction. This value of T may then be used in Eq. (10) to calculate ϕ. However, since this estimate of T is based upon labeling index, it has to be assumed that no cell loss occurs after labeling. Thus, an age-dependent loss is implied, so the distribution given in Eq. (3a) and used by Steel (1968) does not apply strictly.

5. *Some Limitations of the Model*

A number of assumptions, apart from those discussed above, are implied in this model. For example, the model assumes that change in tumor volume is due entirely to change in the number of cells. No account is taken of possible changes in cell size with either position in the tumor or time, or indeed both. No allowance can be made for the possibility of cystic or hemorrhagic areas in the tumor. Furthermore, it is not possible to allow for random events like thrombosis and subsequent necrosis with reabsorption of areas in the tumor. Also, it is assumed that the cell cycle time is a constant in all regions of the tumor, regardless of nutrient supply. Nevertheless, this model has become very popular and has been used by a number of workers (e.g., see Tannock, 1968; Denekamp, 1970).

6. *Variation of Cell Cycle Parameters within a Tumor*

Some information about how the cell cycle parameters vary with position in a tumor is given by Tannock (1968). In this study, a mouse mammary tumor in which the viable tumor tissue was arranged in cylindrical cords around central blood vessels was used as a model. The labeling index and mitotic index decreased with increasing distance from the central vessel, while the mean cell cycle time showed little variation with position, except in the immediate vicinity of a blood vessel. It is suggested that the growth fraction probably decreases with increasing distance from the central vessel.

7. Cell Loss and Continuous Labeling Data

Steel et al. (1966) have used data from continuous labeling experiments to calculate A and estimate, to a limited extent, the degree of cell loss in transplanted rat tumors. Three models of the cell cycle are proposed:

a. All cells are proliferative, and no cell loss occurs. This model is used to estimate the cell cycle parameter from the measured FLM curve. The Monte Carlo procedure developed by Barrett (1966), assuming log-normal distributions for $F_i(t)$, $i = 1, \ldots 3$, is used to produce synthetic FLM curves. The parameters are then altered until a satisfactory fit is obtained between the synthetic FLM curve and the experimental data.

b. Proliferative cells (P cells) and nonproliferative cells (Q cells) are produced with a constant probability at each division. The P cells have $F_i(t)$, $i = 1, \ldots 3$, defined by the parameters obtained in (a) above. There is no cell loss.

c. As in (b) but with cell loss occurring in the following modes: (i) Q cells being assigned a particular life-time; (ii) cell death at mitosis; (iii) random cell loss throughout the P and Q cell compartments.

Using the cell cycle parameters calculated from model a, the age density distributions, and hence the continuous labeling curves, may be calculated for each of the models above. The continuous labeling curve obtained using model a does not fit the data satisfactorily in either of the two tumor types investigated. Model b, with suitable choice of A, gives an adequate fit to the experimental data for one case. However, in order to obtain a satisfactory fit for the second tumor, it is necessary to use model c, with cell loss. Steel et al. (1966) pointed out that, although this model fits the data well, as good a fit might have been obtained using an alternative model; e.g., if it were assumed that some cells have a particularly long cycle time, a similar result might have been obtained. Cell loss is, therefore, a possible but not the unique explanation in this case. Steel and Hanes (1971) have described an automated procedure for estimating the cell cycle parameter described in model a above and producing synthetic continuous-labeling curves. In particular, the effects of the modes of cell loss described in c above on the continuous labeling curve have been investigated.

8. Alternative Mathematical Method for Estimating Cell Loss

One of the most rigorous mathematical treatments of cell population kinetics is that of Jagers (1970), based on the theory of branching processes. In particular, a remarkable formula for calculating cell loss is obtained. Unfortunately, this formula is applicable to *in vitro* systems only, since direct observations of the durations of mitosis for a sample of cells is required. Nevertheless, this result is extremely valuable and is outlined below.

It is assumed that the cell population is in steady-state exponential growth with a growth fraction of unity and that cell loss occurs with equal probability for all cells. For this system, Jagers obtains limits for λ as,

$$\frac{m}{m + (1 + m)\overline{M}(K) - 1} \leq \lambda \leq \frac{1 - (1 - m)\overline{M}(K)}{2m\overline{M}(K)}$$

where m is the mitotic index and $\overline{M}(K)$ is the Laplace transform of the measured mitotic time distribution function. This result is independent of $F_i(t)$, $i = 1, \ldots 3$ and depends only on the observable quantities m and M, where M represents the measured distribution of mitotic durations.

Norrby (1970) has applied this result to the estimation of cell loss in monolayer cultures, where M has been measured directly by time-lapse cinematography.

9. *Modes of Cell Loss in Tumors*

So far in this discussion, no distinction has been made between the various types of cell loss that may occur in tumors. Several authors, however, have discussed the mathematical treatment of specific modes of cell loss. Blumenson (1970) has studied the local spread of endometrial cancer, using a model based on a modified diffusion process (see below). The results obtained are potentially extremely valuable because they allow an estimate to be made regarding the extent of invisible invasion on the basis of visible tumor size.

The spread of tumor cells is assumed to occur by two mechanisms: (a) migration through the interstitial spaces; (b) local vascular dissemination.

In addition, the tumor cell number is allowed to increase at a rate defined by the doubling time, T. Blumenson shows that the process defined in mechanism a above may be described by an equation analogous to the well-known diffusion equation in three dimensions and that mechanism b can be regarded as diffusion under a constant external force in one dimension. The spatial/time density distribution function for the cells is then given by the solution of a partial differential equation similar to the diffusion equation but with terms to allow for diffusion under the influence of an external force and increase in cell number with time. Blumenson gives examples of the deciding whether spread has extended beyond the uterine wall are also given. Blumenson, Bross, and Slack (1971) have used clinical data concerning endometrial tumor growth to estimate the parameters of the model.

Williams and Bjerknes (1972) have simulated the spread of tumor cells through the basal zone of an epithelial layer and produced computer pictures of the growth pattern. The cells are assumed to occupy a honeycomb distribution, and initially a single cell is assigned a "carcinogenic advantage" κ; i.e., this cell divides κ times faster than the normal cells ($\kappa > 1$). The simulated invasion patterns resulting from this model are extremely interesting because those patterns that look the most invasive are in fact obtained with low κ values. The pattern obtained with a high κ value ($k = \infty$) appears more like a carcinoma *in situ*. It is suggested that the highly infiltrating pattern of some tumor growths may be due to a counterinvasion of the abnormal by the normal cells.

Acknowledgments

The authors gratefully acknowledge the assistance of Mrs. M. C. Birdsall in preparing this manuscript, and Mrs. J. C. Knowles for the transmission electron microscopy.

References

Ambellan, E., and Hollander, V. P. (1966). *Cancer Res.* 26, 903–969.
Ambrus, J. L., Ambrus, C. M., Byron, J. W., Goldberg, M. E., and Harrison, J. W. E. (1956). *Ann. N. Y. Acad. Sci.* 63, 938–961.
Anderson, T. F. (1951). *Trans. N. Y. Acad. Sci.* 13, Sect. 11, 130–134.
Archibal, R. B., and Frenster, J. H. (1973). *Nat. Cancer Inst., Monogr.* 36, 230–243.
Augusti-Tocco, G., and Sato, G. (1969). *Proc. Nat. Acad. Sci. U. S.* 64, 311–315.
Bagshawe, K. D. (1968). *Brit. J. Cancer* 22, 698–713.
Bagshawe, K. D. (1973). *Brit. J. Cancer Suppl.* 1, 28, 250–253.
Ballard, K. J., and Holt, S. J. (1968). *J. Cell Sci.* 3, 245–262.
Barrett, J. C. (1966). *J. Nat. Cancer Inst.* 37, 443–450.
Barrett, J. C. (1974). *J. Theor. Biol.* 44, 319–336.
Bartlett, M. S. (1969). *Biometrika* 56, 391–400.
Baserga, R. (1963). *Arch. Pathol.* 75, 156–161.
Bedford, A. J., Cooper, E. H., and Kenny, T. E. (1974). *Eur. J. Cancer* 10, 713–720.
Bedford, A. D., Adamthwaite, S. J., and Fulker, M. J. (1975b). In preparation.
Belkin, M., and Hardy, W. G. (1961). *J. Biophys. Biochem. Cytol.* 9, 733–745.
Bennington, J. L. (1969). *Cancer Res.* 29, 1082–1088.
Berke, G., and Amos, D. B. (1973). *Transplant. Rev.* 17, 71–107.
Berke, G., Ax, W., Ginsberg, H., and Feldman, M. (1969). *Immunology* 16, 643–657.
Berke, G., Ginsberg, H., and Feldman, M. (1971). In "Cell Mediated Immunity" (P. Revillard, ed.), pp. 103–129. Karger, Basel.
Bessis, M. (1964). *Cell. Injury Ciba Found. Symp., 1963*, pp. 287–316.

Birbeck, M. S. C., and Carter, R. L. (1972). *Int. J. Cancer* **9**, 249–257.
Bishun, N. P. (1973). *In* "Modern Trends in Oncology–I" (R. W. Raven, ed.), Part I, pp. 145–162. Butterworth, London.
Black, M. M., Opler, S. R., and Speer, F. D. (1954). *Surg., Gynecol. Obstet.* **98**, 725–734.
Black, M. M., Speer, F. D., and Opler, S. R. (1956). *Amer. J. Clin. Pathol.* **26**, 250–265.
Bloom, W., Zirkle, R. E., and Uretz, R. B. (1955). *Ann. N. Y. Acad. Sci.* **59**, 503–513.
Blumenson, L. E. (1970). *J. Theor. Biol.* **27**, 273–290.
Blumenson, L. E., Bross, D. J., and Slack, N. H. (1971). *Cancer (Philadelphia)* **28**, 735–744.
Bottomley, P., and Cooper, E. H. (1973). *Proc. Roy. Soc. Med.* **66**, 1183–1184.
Bresciani, F. (1965). *In* "Cellular Radiation Biology," M. D. Anderson Hospital Symposium, pp. 547–557. Williams & Wilkins, Baltimore, Maryland.
Breur, K. (1966). *Eur. J. Cancer* **2**, 173–188.
Brockwell, P. J., MacLaren, M. D., and Trucco, E. (1970). *Bull. Math. Biophys.* **32**, 429–443.
Brockwell, P. J., Trucco, E., and Fry, R. J. M. (1972). *Bull. Math. Biophys.* **34**, 1–12.
Brunner, K. T., Mauel, J., Cerottini, J. C., and Chapuis, B. (1968). *Immunology* **14**, 181–196.
Camplejohn, R. S., Bone, G., and Aherne, W. (1973). *Eur. J. Cancer* **9**, 577–582.
Carrano, A. V. (1973). *Mutat. Res.* **17**, 355–366.
Carter, R. L., and Gershon, R. K. (1966). *Amer. J. Pathol.* **49**, 637–655.
Cartwright, G. E., Athens, J. W., and Wintrobe, M. M. (1964). *Blood* **24**, 780–803.
Caspersson, T., Zech, L., Johansson, C., and Modest, E. J. (1970). *Chromosoma* **30**, 215–227.
Cerottini, J. C., Nordin, A. A., and Brunner, K. T. (1970). *Nature (London)* **228**, 1308–1309.
Chalkley, H. W. (1943). *J. Nat. Cancer Inst.* **4**, 47–53.
Chalmers, V. C., and Weiser, R. S. (1973). *J. Nat. Cancer Inst.* **51**, 1367–1371.
Charbit, A., Malaise, E. P., and Tubiana, M. (1971). *Eur. J. Cancer* **7**, 307–315.
Cochran, A. J. (1969). *J. Pathol.* **97**, 459–468.
Cooper, E. H., and Quaglino, D. (1973). *Ricerca* **3**, 1–41.
Cooper, E. H., and Wickramasinghe, S. (1969). *Ser. Haematol.* **11**, 65–89.
Cooper, E. H., Frank, G. L., and Wright, D. H. (1966). *Eur. J. Cancer* **2**, 377–384.
Costero, I., and Pomerat, C. M. (1951). *Amer. J. Anat.* **89**, 405–468.
Cox, D. R. (1962). "Renewal Theory," Methuen, London.
Currie, G. A. (1973). *In* "Modern Trends in Oncology–I" (R. W. Raven, ed.), Part I, pp. 127–143. Butterworth, London.
Davies, A. J. S. (1969). *Transplant. Rev.* **1**, 43.
de Luca, C. (1965). *Exp. Cell Res.* **40**, 186–188.
Denekamp, J. (1970). *Cancer Res.* **30**, 393–400.
Dethlefsen, C. A. (1971). *Cell Tissue Kinet.* **4**, 123–138.
Dixon, F. J., and Moore, R. A. (1953). *Cancer (New York)* **6**, 427–454.
Dorfman, R. F., Rice, D. F., Mitchell, A. D., Kempson, R. L., and Levine, G. (1973). *Nat. Cancer Inst. Monogr.* **36**, 221–238.
Dornfeld, E. J., and Owczarzak, A. (1958). *J. Biophys. Biochem. Cytol.* **4**, 243–249.
Dumonde, D. C., Wolstencroft, R. A., Panay, G. S., Mathew, M., Morley, J., and Howson, W. T. (1969). *Nature (London)* **224**, 38–42.
Edwards, J. L., Koch, A. L., Youcis, P., Freese, H. E., Laite, M. B., and Donaldson, J. T. (1960). *J. Biophys. Biochem. Cytol.* **7**, 273–282.

Elston, C. W., and Bagshawe, K. D. (1973). *Brit. J. Cancer* **28**, 245–256.
Evans, R., and Alexander, P. (1972). *Immunology* **23**, 615–626.
Everson, T. C., and Cole, W. H. (1966). "Spontaneous Regressions of Cancer." Saunders, Philadelphia, Pennsylvania.
Firket, H., and Hopper, A. F. (1970). *J. Cell Biol.* **44**, 675–681.
Firth, J. A., and Hicks, R. M. (1972). *J. Anat.* **113**, 95–107.
Fiskin, A. M., and Melnykovych, G. (1972). *Exp. Cell Res.* **66**, 483–486.
Flaxman, A. B. (1972). *Cancer Res.* **32**, 462–469.
Fodor, P., Funk, C. L., and Tomaschefsky, P. (1955). *Arch. Biochem. Biophys.* **56**, 281–289.
Folkman, J., Merler, E., Abernathy, C., and Williams, G. (1971). *J. Exp. Med.* **133**, 275–288.
Forman, J., and Britton, S. (1973). *J. Exp. Med.* **137**, 369–386.
Forman, J., and Möller, G. (1973). *Transplant. Rev.* **17**, 108–149.
Freed, J. J., and Engle, J. L. (1963). In "Cinemicrography in Cell Biology" (G. G. Rose, ed.), pp. 93–121. Academic Press, New York.
Freed, J. J., and Schatz, S. A. (1969). *Exp. Cell Res.* **55**, 393–409.
Friedmann, I., and Bird, E. S. (1969). *J. Pathol.* **97**, 373–382.
Frindel, E., Malaise, E. P., Alpen, E., and Tubiana, M. (1967). *Cancer Res.* **27**, 1122–1131.
Frindel, E., Malaise, E., and Tubiana, M. (1968). *Cancer (Philadelphia)* **22**, 611–620.
Frindel, E., Valleron, A. J., Vassort, F., and Tubiana, M. (1969). *Cell Tissue Kinet.* **2**, 51–65.
Fulker, M. J., Cooper, E. H., and Tanaka, T. (1971). *Cancer (Philadelphia)* **27**, 71–82.
Gavosto, F., and Pileri, A. (1971). In "The Cell Cycle and Cancer" (R. Baserga, ed.), pp. 97–128. Dekker, New York.
Ginsberg, H., Ax, W., and Berke, G. (1969). In "Pharmacological Treatment in Organ and Tissue Transplantation" (A. Bertelli and A. P. Monaco, eds.), pp. 85–107. Williams & Wilkins, Baltimore, Maryland.
Glücksmann, A. (1951). *Biol. Rev. Cambridge Phil. Soc.* **26**, 59–86.
Goldstein, P., Svedmyr, E. A. J., and Wigzell, H. (1971). *J. Exp. Med.* **134**, 1385–1402.
Goldstein, P., Wigzell, H., Blomgren, H., and Svedmyr, E. A. J. (1972). *J. Exp. Med.* **135**, 890–906.
Granger, G. A., and Weiser, R. S. (1966). *Science* **151**, 97–99.
Greenblatt, M., and Shubik, P. (1968). *J. Nat. Cancer Inst.* **41**, 111–124.
Greene, H. S. N. (1941). *J. Exp. Med.* **73**, 461–483.
Gullino, P. M., Grantham, F. H., and Courtney, A. H. (1967). *Cancer Res.* **27**, 1031–1040.
Hagemann, R., and Schiffer, L. M. (1971). *J. Nat. Cancer Inst.* **47**, 519–525.
Hamlin, I. M. (1968). *Brit. J. Cancer* **22**, 383–401.
Hammar, S. P., and Mottet, N. K. (1971). *J. Cell Sci.* **8**, 229–251.
Hanks, J. H., and Wallace, J. H. (1958). *Proc. Soc. Exp. Biol. Med.* **98**, 188–192.
Harris, T. E. (1963). "The Theory of Branching Processes." Springer-Verlag, Berlin and New York.
Hathaway, W. E., Newby, L. A., and Githens, J. H. (1964). *Blood* **23**, 517–525.
Held, W., and Saunders, J. W., Jr. (1965). *Amer. Zool.* **5**, 214.
Hellström, I. (1967). *Int. J. Cancer* **2**, 65–68.
Hellström, I., and Sjörgren, H. O. (1965). *Exp. Cell Res.* **40**, 212–215.
Hellström, I., Sjörgren, H. O., Warner, G., and Hellström, K. E. (1971). *Int. J. Cancer* **7**, 226–237.

Henney, C. S. (1973a). *Transplant. Rev.* **17**, 35-70.
Henney, C. S. (1973b). *J. Immunol.* **110**, 73-84.
Hermens, A. F. (1973). Ph. D. Thesis, Univ. of Amsterdam. Publication of Radiobiological Inst. of the Organization of Health Research, TNO, Rijswijk (R. H.).
Hermens, A. F., and Barendsen, G. W. (167). *Eur. J. Cancer* **3**, 361-369.
Hinchliffe, J. R., and Ede, D. A. (1973). *J. Embryol. Exp. Morphol.* **30**, 753-772.
Hofer, K. G. (1969). *Cancer Chemother. Rep.* **53**, 273-281.
Hofer, K. G., Prensky, W., and Hughes, W. L. (1969). *J. Nat. Cancer Inst.* **43**, 763-773.
Holmberg, B. (1961). *Exp. Cell Res.* **22**, 406-414.
Hoskins, J. M., Meynell, G. G., and Sanders, F. K. (1956). *Exp. Cell Res.* **11**, 297-305.
Hsu, T. C. (1960). *Tex. Rep. Biol. Med.* **18**, 31-33.
Hurwitz, C., and Tolmach, L. J. (1969). *Biophys. J.* **9**, 1131-1143.
Iversen, O. H. (1967). *Eur. J. Cancer* **3**, 389-394.
Izard, J., and de Harven, E. (1968). *Cancer Res.* **28**, 421-433.
Jagers, P. (1969). *Skand. Aktuarie Tidskr.* 3/4, 84-103.
Jagers, P. (1970). *Math. Biosci.* **8**, 227-238.
Jagers, P., and Norrby, K. (1974). *Cell Tissue Kinet.* **7**, 201-212.
Kaltenbach, J. P., Kaltenbach, M. H., and Lyons, W. B. (1958). *Exp. Cell Res.* **15**, 112-117.
Kampschmidt, R. F., and Wells, D. (1968). *Cancer Res.* **28**, 1938-1943.
Katsumata, T., Watanabe, M., Takabe, Y., Terasima, T., and Umezawa, H. (1973). *Gann* **64**, 71-78.
Keller, R., Lindstrand, K., and Norden, A. (1970). *Scand. J. Haematol.* **7**, 478-485.
Kerr, J. F. R. (1971). *J. Pathol.* **105**, 13-20.
Kerr, J. F. R., and Searle, J. (1972). *J. Pathol.* **107**, 41-48.
Kerr, J. F. R., Wyllie, A. H., and Currie, A. R. (1972). *Brit. J. Cancer* **26**, 239-261.
Kim, J. H., and Evans, T. C. (1964). *Radiat. Res.* **21**, 129-143.
Kleinsmith, L. J., and Pierce, G. B. (1964). *Cancer Res.* **24**, 1544-1551.
Koller, P. C. (1956). *Ann. N. Y. Acad. Sci.* **63**, 793-817.
Koller, P. C. (1960). *In* "Cell Physiology of Neoplasia," pp. 9-48. Univ. of Texas Press, Austin.
Koren, H. S., Ferber, E., and Fischer, H. (1971). *Biochim. Biophys. Acta* **231**, 520-526.
Laird, A. K. (1964). *Brit. J. Cancer* **18**, 490-502.
Lala, P. K. (1972). *Cancer (Philadelphia)* **29**, 261-266.
Lala, P. K., and Patt, H. M. (1966). *Proc. Nat. Acad. Sci. U. S.* **56**, 1735-1742.
Lanzerotti, R. H., and Gullino, P. M. (1972). *Cancer Res.* **32**, 2679-2685.
Lauder, I., and Aherne, W. (1972). *Brit. J. Cancer* **26**, 321-330.
Lejeune, F., and Evans, R. (1972). *Eur. J. Cancer* **8**, 549-555.
Levan, A. (1956). *Ann. N. Y. Acad. Sci.* **63**, 774-792.
Levi, P. E., Cooper, E. H., Anderson, C. K., and Williams, R. E. (1969). *Cancer (Philadelphia)* **23**, 1074-1969.
Lieb, L. M., and Lisco, H. (1966). *Cancer Res.* **26**, 733-740.
Lipkin, M. (1971). *Cancer (Philadelphia)* **28**, 38-40.
Lohmann-Matthes, M. L., and Fischer, H. (1973). *Transplant. Rev.* **17**, 150-171.
MacDonald, P. D. M. (1970). *Biometrika* **57**, 489-503.
Mackler, B. F. (1971). *Lancet* **ii**, 297-301.
Malaise, E. P., Chavaudra, N., and Tubiana, M. (1973). *Eur. J. Cancer* **9**, 305-312.
Mendelsohn, M. L. (1960a). *Science* **132**, 1496.
Mendelsohn, M. L. (1960b). *J. Nat. Cancer Inst.* **25**, 477-484.
Mendelsohn, M. L. (1962). *J. Nat. Cancer Inst.* **28**, 1015-1029.

Mendelsohn, M. L. (1965). In "Cellular Radiation Biology," M. D. Anderson Hospital Symposium, pp. 498–513. Williams & Wilkins, Baltimore, Maryland.
Mendelsohn, M. L. (1970). *Cell Tissue Kinet.* 3, 405–414.
Mendelsohn, M. L., and Dethlefsen, L. A. (1968). *Proc. Amer. Ass. Cancer Res.* 9, 47.
Miller, J. F. A. P., and Mitchell, G. F. (1969). *Transplant. Rev.* 1, 535–538.
Modak, S. P., and Perdue, S. W. (1970). *Exp. Cell Res.* 59, 43–56.
Mollo, F., Monga, G., and Stramignoni, A. (1969). *Virchows Arch., B* 3, 117–126.
Moore, M., Nisbet, N. W., and Haigh, M. V., eds. (1973). Immunology of Malignancy. *Brit. J. Cancer* 28, Suppl. 1.
Nameroff, M. A., Reznik, M., Anderson, P., and Hanse, J. L. (1970). *Cancer Res.* 30, 596–600.
Niemi, M., and Sylven, B. (1969). *Histochemie* 18, 40–47.
Niitani, H., Suzuki, A., Shimoyama, M., and Kimura, K. (1966). *Gann* 57, 193–200.
Norrby, K. (1970). *Acta Pathol. Microbiol. Scand., Suppl.* 78, 114.
Norrby, K., Johannison, E., and Mellgren, J. (1967). *Exp. Cell Res.* 48, 582–594.
O'Connor, T. M., and Wyttenbach, C. (1974). *J. Cell Biol.* 60, 448–459.
Oettgen, H. F., and Hellström, K. E. (1973). In "Cancer Medicine" (J. F. Holland and E. Frei, III, eds.), pp. 951–990. Lea & Febiger, Philadelphia, Pennsylvania.
Old, J. L., and Boyse, E. A. (1966). *Med. Clin. N. Amer.* 50, 901–912.
O'Toole, C., Unsgaard, B., Almgard, L. E., and Johansson, B. (1973). *Brit. J. Cancer* 28, Suppl. 1, 266–275.
Paris, J. E., Brandes, D., and Anton, E. (1969). *J. Nat. Cancer Inst.* 42, 383–398.
Peckham, M. J., and Cooper, E. H. (1969). *Cancer (Philadelphia)* 24, 135–146.
Peckham, M. J., and Cooper, E. H. (1970). *Eur. J. Cancer* 6, 453–463.
Peckham, M. J., and Cooper, E. H. (1973). *Nat. Cancer Inst., Monogr.* 36, 179–189.
Peel, S., and Cowen, D. M. (1972). *Brit. J. Cancer* 26, 304–314.
Peel, S., and Cowen, D. M. (1973). *Brit. J. Cancer* 27, 72–79.
Philips, H. J., and Terryberry, J. E. (1957). *Exp. Cell Res.* 13, 341–347.
Pierce, G. B. (1966). *Cancer (Philadelphia)* 19, 1963–1983.
Pierce, G. B. (1972). In "Cell Differentiation" (R. Harris, P. Allin, and D. Viza, eds.), pp. 109–114. Munksgaard, Copenhagen.
Pierce, G. B., and Wallace, C. (1971). *Cancer Res.* 31, 127–134.
Pomerance, A. (1972). *Brit. J. Urol.* 44, 451–458.
Porter, K., Prescott, D., and Frye, J. (1973). *J. Cell Biol.* 57, 815–836.
Price, Z. H. (1967). *Exp. Cell Res.* 48, 82–92.
Puck, T. T., Waldren, C. A., and Hsie, A. W. (1972). *Proc. Nat. Acad. Sci. U. S.* 69, 1043–1047.
Pugh-Humphries, R. G. P., and Sinclair, W. (1970). *J. Cell Sci.* 6, 477–484.
Purschen, W., and Feinendegen, L. (1969). *Strahlentherapie* 137, 718–723.
Quie, P. G. (1972). *Pediatrics* 50, 264–270.
Rabes, H. (1965). *Biophysik* 3, 65–93.
Refsum, S., and Berdal, P. (1967). *Eur. J. Cancer* 3, 235–236.
Rosai, J., Khadadoust, K., and Silber, I. (1969). *Cancer (Philadelphia)* 24, 103–116.
Rubin, P., and Casarett, G. W. (1966). *Clin. Radiol.* 17, 220–229.
Rubin, R. W., and Everhart, L. P. (1973). *J. Cell Biol.* 57, 837–844.
Sandberg, A. A., and Hossfeld, D. K. (1970). *Annu. Rev. Med.* 21, 379–408.
Sandberg, A. A., and Hossfeld, D. K. (1973). In "Cancer Medicine" (J. F. Holland and E. Frei, III, eds.), pp. 151–177. Lea & Febiger, Philadelphia, Pennsylvania.
Sarma, K. P. (1972). *Invest. Urol.* 10, 199–207.
Saunders, J. W., Jr. (1966). *Science* 154, 604–612.

Scaife, J. F., and Brohee, H. (1967). *Exp. Cell Res.* **46,** 612–615.
Schiffer, L. M. (1971). *Cell Tissue Kinet.* **4,** 589–595.
Schrek, R. (1936). *Amer. J. Cancer* **28,** 389–392.
Selecki, E. E. (1959). *Aust. J. Exp. Biol. Med. Sci.* **37,** 489–498.
Shamberger, R. J. (1969). *Biochem. J.* **111,** 375–383.
Shaw, W. M. (1970). *Annu. Rev. Med.* **21,** 409–432.
Shirakawa, S., Luce, J. K., Tannock, I., and Frei, E. (1970). *J. Clin. Invest.* **49,** 1188–1199.
Showacre, J. L. (1968). *Methods Cell Physiol.* **3,** 147–159.
Simpson-Herren, L., and Lloyd, H. H. (1970). *Cancer Chemother. Rep.* **54,** 143–174.
Simson, J. V., and Spicer, S. S. (1973). *Int. Rev. Pathol.* **12,** 79–118.
Sisken, J. E., and Kinosita, R. (1961). *Exp. Cell Res.* **22,** 521–525.
Skipper, H. E. (1972). *In* "The Cell Cycle and Cancer" (R. Baserga, ed.), pp. 358–387. Dekker, New York.
Spooner, M., and Cooper, E. H. (1972). *Cancer (Philadelphia)* **29,** 1401–1412.
Steel, G. G. (1967). *Eur. J. Cancer* **3,** 381–387.
Steel, G. G. (1968). *Cell Tissue Kinet.* **1,** 193–207.
Steel, G. G. (1970). *Time Dose Relationship Radiat. Biol. Appl. Radiother., Carmel Symp., Brookhaven Nat. Lab.* **BNL 50203 (1-57),** pp. 131–135.
Steel, G. G. (1973). *In* "Cancer Medicine" (J. F. Holland and E. Frei, III, eds.), pp. 125–139. Lea & Febiger, Philadelphia, Pennsylvania.
Steel, G. G., and Bensted, J. P. M. (1965). *Eur. J. Cancer* **1,** 275–279.
Steel, G. G., and Hanes, S. (1971). *Cell Tissue Kinet.* **4,** 83–105.
Steel, G. G., and Lamerton, L. F. (1966). *Brit. J. Cancer* **20,** 74–86.
Steel, G. G., Adams, K., and Barrett, J. C. (1966). *Brit. J. Cancer* **20,** 784–800.
Stockdale, F. E., and Holtzer, H. (1961). *Exp. Cell Res.* **24,** 508–520.
Stossel, T. P. (1974). *New Engl. J. Med.* **290,** 717–724.
Studzinski, G. P., and Cohen, L. S. (1966). *Biochem. Biophys. Res. Commun.* **23,** 506–512.
Sullivan, K. A., Berke, G., and Amos, D. B. (1972). *Transplantation* **13,** 627–628.
Sylven, B., and Niemi, M. (1972). *Virchows Arch., B* **10,** 127–133.
Takahashi, M. (1968). *J. Theor. Biol.* **18,** 195–209.
Takasugi, M., and Klein, E. (1970). *Transplantation* **9,** 219–227.
Tanaka, T., Cooper, E. H., and Anderson, C. K. (1970). *Rev. Eur. Etud. Clin. Biol.* **15,** 1084–1089.
Tannock, I. F. (1968). *Brit. J. Cancer* **22,** 258–273.
Tannock, I. F. (1970). *Cancer Res.* **30,** 2470–2476.
Tannock, I. F., and Hayashi, S. (1972). *Cancer Res.* **32,** 77–82.
Tannock, I. F., and Steel, G. G. (1969). *J. Nat. Cancer Inst.* **42,** 771–782.
Thomlinson, R. H. (1960). *Brit. J. Cancer* **14,** 555–576.
Thomlinson, R. H., and Gray, L. H. (1955). *Brit. J. Cancer* **9,** 539–549.
Thompson, L. H., and Suit, H. D. (1967). *Int. J. Radiat. Biol.* **13,** 391–397.
Thompson, L. H., and Suit, H. D. (1969). *Int. J. Radiat. Biol.* **15,** 347–362.
Trucco, E., and Brockwell, P. J. (1968). *J. Theor. Biol.* **20,** 321–337.
Van Lancker, J. L. (1970). *In* "Metabolic Conjugation and Metabolic Hydrolysis" (W. H. Fishman, ed.), Vol. 1, pp. 355–418. Academic Press, New York.
Van Scott, E. J., and Reinertson, R. P. (1961). *J. Invest. Dermatol.* **36,** 109–131.
Vincent, P. L., and Nicholls, A. (1962). *Aust. J. Exp. Biol. Med. Sci.* **42,** 569–578.
Vinegar, R. (1956). *Cancer Res.* **16,** 900–916.
Webster, D. A., and Gross, J. (1970). *Develop. Biol.* **22,** 157–184.

Weibel, E. R., Kistler, G. S., and Scherle, W. F. (1966). *J. Cell Biol.* **30**, 23–38.
Weidner, F., and Hornstein, O. P. (1973). *Virchows Arch., A* **395**, 77–85.
Welin, S., Youker, J., and Spratt, J. S. (1963). *Amer. J. Roentgenol., Radium Ther. Nucl. Med.* **90**, 673–687.
Wellings, S. R., and Deome, K. B. (1963). *J. Nat. Cancer Inst.* **30**, 241–267.
Williams, T., and Bjerknes, R. (1972). *Nature (London)* **236**, 19–21.
Wolberg, W. H. (1964). *Cancer Res.* **24**, 1437–1447.
Wolberg, W. H., and Brown, R. R. (1962). *Cancer Res.* **22**, 1113–1119.
Wyllie, A. H. (1974). *J. Clin. Pathol.* **27**, Suppl. (Royal Coll. Pathol.) No. 7, 35–42.
Young, R. C., and de Vita, T. (1970). *Cell Tissue Kinet.* **3**, 285–290.

THE HISTOCOMPATIBILITY-LINKED IMMUNE RESPONSE GENES

Baruj Benacerraf and David H. Katz

Department of Pathology, Harvard Medical School, Boston, Massachusetts

I. Immune Responses Controlled by Histocompatibility-Linked *Ir* Genes.
   Species Distribution 121
   A. Guinea Pig H-Linked *Ir* Genes 122
   B. Mouse H-Linked *Ir* Genes 124
   C. Rat H-Linked *Ir* Genes 129
II. The Mapping of Mouse H-Linked *Ir* Genes 130
III. Relationship of H-Linked *Ir* Genes to Immunoglobulin Structural Genes . 133
IV. The Cell Type Where Histocompatibility-Linked *Ir* Genes Are
    Expressed 135
V. The Demonstration of Suppressor T Cells Specific for GAT^{10} in Genetic
   Nonresponder Mice 140
VI. The Role of Histocompatibility Gene Products in T–B Cell Interactions. 143
    A. Failure of Physiologic Cooperative Interactions to Occur between T
       and B Lymphocytes from Histoincompatible Donor Strains . . 145
    B. Demonstration That the H-2 Histocompatibility Gene Complex
       Determines Successful Physiologic Lymphocyte Interactions . . 149
    C. Identification of Histocompatibility Genes Involved in Control of
       T–B Cell Interactions 153
    D. Relevance of Genetic Requirements for T–B Cell Interactions . . 157
VII. Identification of *I* Region Gene Products 159
VIII. Relationship of Histocompatibility Gene Products to Each Other in
     Nature and Function 162
IX. Function of Products of H-Linked *Ir* Genes and of Other *I* Region Gene
    Products: Relationship of These Products to Activation of
    Immunocompetent Cells 165
X. The Histocompatibility-Linked *Ir* Genes and Disease 168
   References 171

I. Immune Responses Controlled by Histocompatibility-Linked *Ir* Genes. Species Distribution

In the past decade, the genetic study of the capacity to form specific immune responses has revealed that the recognition of antigens as immunogens by individual animals and inbred strains is governed by the product of individual dominant genes located in the genome in close relationship with the genes coding for the molecules bearing the major histocompatibility specificities (1–3). This has now been verified in mice (4), guinea pigs (5), rats (6–8), and rhesus monkeys

(9, 10). Those genes have been termed histocompatibility, or H-linked *Ir* genes. The presence of the relevant genes permit immune responses to be formed, characterized by cellular immunity and antibody synthesis against the determinants on the antigens concerned. Three types of antigens have been most useful in the identification of H-linked *Ir* genes: (1) synthetic polypeptides with limited structural heterogeneity; (2) alloantigens which differ but slightly from their autologous counterparts, and (3) complex multideterminant antigens administered in limiting immunizing doses in conditions where only the most immunogenic determinants are recognized. Thus the discovery of specific H-linked *Ir* genes has depended upon experiments wherein the immunological system is presented with a challenge of highly restricted heterogeneity and specificity. These conditons tend to limit the possibility of specific interactions between the antigens and clones of immunocompetent cells. This approach has permitted in a relatively short time the demonstration that the responses to a wide variety of antigens in the guinea pig, the mouse and the rat are under the control of dominant H-linked *Ir* genes. The single dominant gene control of specific immune responses has been totally unexpected for immunologists considering the complexity of immune phenomena and the numerous specificities against which antibodies can be formed. These data provide, therefore, both a challenge to the classical theory of the recognition of immunological specificity solely by preexisting immunoglobulin receptors on immunocompetent cells as well as a powerful tool to analyze the complex interactions between antigens and the various cell types—macrophages, B and T cells—concerned collectively with the development of specific immunity.

In this section we shall address ourselves to a description of the specific immune responses which have been shown to be under the control of H-linked *Ir* genes in guinea pigs, mice, and rats.

A. GUINEA PIG H-LINKED *Ir* GENES

Two inbred guinea pig strains, 2 and 13 (developed by Sewall Wright from a small closed colony) as well as random-bred lines, have been used to study the genetic control of specific immune responsiveness. The synthetic polypeptide antigens used in those studies are described in Table I.

The gene which controls the response to poly-L-lysine (PLL) was the first specific immune response gene identified (*11*). It controls responsiveness to PLL, poly-L-arginine (PLA), to copolymers of L-glutamic acid and L-lysine (GL) and to hapten conjugates of these

TABLE I
POLYPEPTIDE ANTIGENS THE RESPONSES TO WHICH ARE CONTROLLED
BY SPECIFIC GUINEA PIG *Ir* GENES

A. Homopolymers	
1. Poly-L-lysine	PLL
2. Poly-L-arginine	PLA
B. Copolymers of	
1. 60% L-Glutamic acid / 40% L-Lysine	GL
2. 60% L-Glutamic acid / 40% L-Alanine	GA
3. 50% L-Glutamic acid / 50% L-Tyrosine	GT
4. 60% L-Glutamic acid / 30% L-Alanine / 10% L-Tyrosine	GAT
C. Hapten polypeptide conjugates	
1. 2,4-Dinitrophenyl-poly-L-lysine	DNP-PLL
2. 2,4-Dinitrophenyl-GL	DNP-GL

polypeptides. The PLL gene is found in all strain 2 and some Hartley guinea pigs and is lacking in strain 13 animals.

The immune response of guinea pigs to the antigens, the recognition of which is under the control of H-linked *Ir* genes, is characterized by cellular immunity, and the synthesis of significant levels of specific antibody. Animals lacking the gene never develop delayed sensitivity and do not produce significant levels of antibodies under usual conditions of immunization. The activity of these immune response genes in guinea pigs is therefore responsible for clear-cut qualitative differences between responder and nonresponder animals.

As shown in Table II, the abilities of inbred guinea pigs to form immune responses to the synthetic polypeptide antigens, DNP-PLL, GA, and GT and to limiting doses of native antigens and their hapten conjugates, bovine serum albumin (BSA), human serum albumin (HSA), DNP-BSA, DNP-guinea pig albumin (DNP-GPA) are inherited according to strict Mendelian genetics, indicating that the immune responses to these antigens are controlled by distinct dominant *Ir* genes. Thus, strain 2, but not strain 13, guinea pigs respond to DNP-PLL, GL, GA and to low doses of BSA, HSA, and DNP-BSA, whereas strain 13, but not strain 2, animals respond to GT and to limiting doses of DNP-GPA. All $(2 \times 13)F_1$ animals are responders to

TABLE II

INHERITANCE OF SPECIFIC *Ir* GENES AND OF THE MAJOR HISTOCOMPATIBILITY LOCUS OF STRAIN 2 AND STRAIN 13 GUINEA PIGS BY (2 × 13)F$_1$ AND BACKCROSS ANIMALS

	Strain			(2 × 13)F$_1$ × 13		(2 × 13)F$_1$ × 2	
Antigens[a]	2	13	(2 × 13)F$_1$	50%[b]	50%	50%	50%
DNP-PLL	+[c]	−[c]	+	+	−		
GL	+	−	+	+	−		
GA	+	−	+	+	−		
GT	−	+	+			+	−
BSA 0.1 μg	+	−	+	+	−		
HSA 1 μg	+	−	+				
DNP-BSA 1 μg	+	−	+	+	−		
DNP-GPA 1 μg	−	+	+			+	−
Major H locus							
Strain 2	+		+	+	−		
Strain 13		+	+			+	−

[a] DNP, dinitrophenyl; PLL, poly-L-lysine; GL, GA, GT, copolymers of glutamic acid and, respectively, L-lysine, L-alanine, and L-tyrosine; BSA, bovine serum albumin; HSA, human serum albumin; GPA, guinea pig albumin.

[b] Column identifies the same group of backcross animals.

[c] Plus indicates responsiveness and presence of major histocompatibility specificities: minus indicates nonresponsiveness and absence of major histocompatibility specificities of the inbred strains.

all these antigens, illustrating the dominant character of these responses.

Responsiveness to DNP-PLL, GA, and low doses of BSA and DNP-BSA segregate together in 50% of (2 × 13)F$_1$ × 13 backcross guinea pigs. On the other hand, the abilities to respond to GT and to low doses of DNP-GPA are inherited together by 50% of (2 × 13)F$_1$ × 2 backcross offspring.

B. MOUSE H-LINKED *Ir* GENES

Similar to what was found in guinea pigs, specific *Ir* genes controlling responsiveness to synthetic polypeptides and to limiting doses of protein antigens have been identified in mice (1–3). In addition, in the mouse many H-linked *Ir* genes have been discovered which control responsiveness to alloantigens. The mouse has truly been the most rewarding species for the study of H-linked *Ir* genes because of the availability of: (1) numberous inbred strains developed by students of tissue transplantation; (2) congenic resistant strains which differ only at the H-2 complex; and (3) strains with documented recombinant events within the H-2 complex, precisely in the region where the *Ir* genes are located. Whereas the response to polypeptide antigens under H-linked *Ir* gene control in the guinea pig are all-or-none responses characterized both by delayed hypersensitivity and antibody synthesis, in the mouse a species which exhibits poor delayed hypersensitivity, the data have relied almost exclusively on the genetic control of specific antibody synthesis. In addition, although the responder strains possessing the relevant *Ir* genes always produced high levels of serum antibodies, the nonresponder strains, depending upon the antigen and the strain, were often characterized as "low-responders." This is particularly true for the branched multichain synthetic copolymers most extensively studied by McDevitt and Sela (*12*), (T,G)-A—L, (H,G)-A—L, and (Phe,G)-A—L. The response to these polypeptides was the first to be shown in mice to be under dominant H-linked *Ir* gene control at a locus designated *Ir-1* (*13*). Thus the ability of inbred mice to make antibodies in response to each of these antigens is a *quantitative* genetic trait. The antibody responses to other polypeptide antigens, i.e., the random copolymers of 2 or 3 of the following L-amino acids—glutamic acid, alanine, lysine, tyrosine, phenylalanine, and proline—behave as all or none responses in most inbred strains of mice (*14*) as in guinea pigs.

In Fig. 1 we have compiled all the available information on the responses of strains with 13 distinct *H-2* haplotypes to 24 antigens: (1) 8 linear copolymers and 3 branched copolymers of L-amino acids; (2) 6 mouse alloantigens; and (3) 7 conventional native antigens. The response to each of these 24 antigens was shown to be under dominant H-linked *Ir* gene control (for references, see Fig. 1). As will be shown in Section II, many of these genes have been mapped in the *I* region within the *H-2* complex.

The relatively large number of antigens and of inbred strains which have been used to obtain the data summarized in Fig. 1 in a checkerboard fashion makes some comparison meaningful. Analysis of the results demonstrates two important points: (1) Except for the H-2^K and H-2^a strains and the H-2^n and H-2^p strains, which display identical patterns, respectively, no two strains with different *H-2* haplotypes behave alike in their response patterns when a sufficiently large panel of antigens is used, which is not surprising. The strain bearing the K-2^k and H-2^a haplotypes were expected to display identical response patterns as they share the left part of the *H-2*

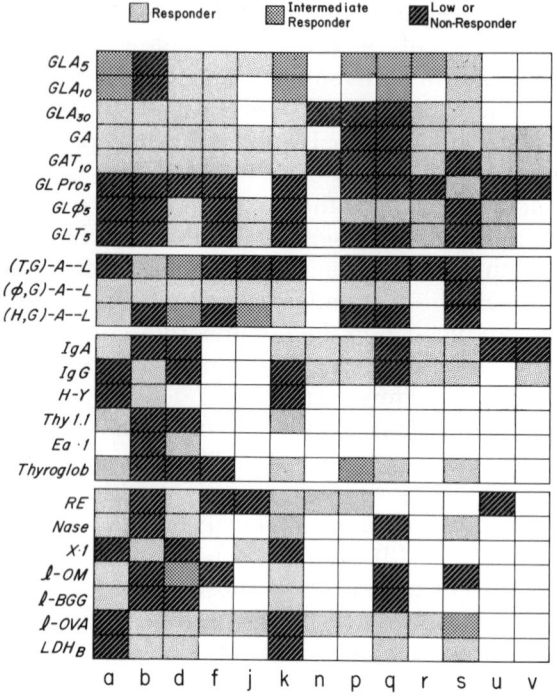

H-2 HAPLOTYPE

FIG. 1. Immune responses under H-linked *Ir* gene control of mice bearing 13 different *H-2* haplotypes to four classes of antigens. Top to bottom: (I) random linear copolymers of L-amino acids; (II) branched copolymers of L-amino acids; (III) murine alloantigens; (IV) foreign antigens. References are cited by italic numbers in parentheses.

I. Random linear copolymers of L-amino acids (superscript numbers are percentages; these are shown in figure by subscripts) $GLA^5 = (Glu^{57}Lys^{38}Ala^5)^\eta$ (1); $GLA^{10} = (Glu^{54}Lys^{36}Ala^{10})^\eta$ (1); $GLA^{30} = (Glu^{35}Lys^{35}Ala^{30})^\eta$ (2); $GA = Glu^{60}Ala^{40})^\eta$ (2, 3); $GAT^{10} = (Glu^{60}Ala^{30}Tyr^{10})^\eta$ (2, 4, 5); $GLPro^5 = (Glu^{57}Lys^{38}Pro^5)^\eta$ (2); $GL\phi^5 = (Glu^{57}Lys^{38}Phe^5)^\eta$ (2, 6); $GLT^5 = (Glu^{57}Lys^{38}Tyr^5)^\eta$ (2, 3).

II. Branched copolymers of L-amino acids (7, 8): (T,G)-A—L = (Tyr,Glu)-Ala—Lys; (ϕ,G)-A—L = (Phe,Glu)-Ala—Lys; (H,G)-A—L = (His,Glu)-Ala—Lys.

III. Murine alloantigens: IgA = allotype determinants on BALB/c IgA myeloma (9, 10); IgG = allotype determinants on BALB/c IgG myeloma (9, 10); H-Y = histocompatibility antigen coded for by the Y chromosome (11); Thy 1.1 = mouse thymocyte antigen, theta (12); Ea.1 = mouse red blood cell antigen (13); Thyroglob = Mouse thyroglobulin (14).

IV. Foreign antigens: RE = Ragweed extract antigens (15); NASE = staphylococcal nuclease (16); X.1 = leukemia-associated transplantation antigen (17); l-OM = low dose of hen ovomucoid (18, 19); l-BGG = low dose of bovine γ-globulin (18); l-OVA = low dose of ovalbumin (18–20); LDH_B = porcine lactic dehydrophenase B (21).

Key to references for Fig 1:
1. Maurer, P. H., and Merryman, C. F. (1974). *Immunogenetics* 1, 174.

complex which comprises the *I* region where all known *Ir* genes have been mapped. With respect to the strains bearing the $H\text{-}2^p$ and $H\text{-}2^n$ haplotypes, the most recent serological analysis has raised doubts whether they could be distinguished (15). (2) More important is that most antigens for which sufficient data are available elicit different response patterns in the inbred strains with a few notable exceptions. These exceptions are of two types. Identical response patterns are observed for polypeptides with closely related structures such as GLA^5 and GLA^{10} (which differ by only 5% L-alanine residues) and GLA^{30} and $G^{60}A^{40}$. It is, therefore, very probable that the same genes control the responses to GLA^5 and GLA^{10} and to GLA^{30} and $G^{60}A^{40}$, respectively. Identical response patterns are observed also for 2 couples of unrelated antigens, i.e., for the copolymer (H,G)-A—L and ovomucoid and for ragweed extract (RE) and staphylococcal nuclease (NASE). The similarity in response patterns for these unrelated antigens is most probably fortuitous since, as shown in Fig. 3, the *Ir* genes controlling the response to RE and NASE have been mapped in different segments of the *H-2* complex. We have intentionally not considered significant patterns of similarity involving

---

2. Dorf, M. E., and Benacerraf, B. Unpublished data.
3. Merryman, D. F., and Maurer, P. H. (1973). *Fed. Proc., Fed. Amer. Soc. Exp. Biol.* **32**, 995.
4. Martin, W. J., Maurer, P. H., and Benacerraf, B. (1971). *J. Immunol.* **107**, 715.
5. Merryman, C. F., and Maurer, P. H. (1972). *J. Immunol.* **108**, 135.
6. Merryman, C. F., Maurer, P. H., and Bailey, D. W. (1972). *J. Immunol.* **108**, 937.
7. McDevitt, H. O., and Chinitz, A. (1969). *Science* **163**, 1207.
8. McDevitt, H. O., and Landy, M., eds. (1972). "Genetic Control of Immune Responsiveness: Relationship to Disease Susceptibility." Academic Press, New York.
9. Lieberman, R., and Humphrey, W., Jr. (1972). *J. Exp. Med.* **136**, 1222.
10. Lieberman, R., Paul, W. E., Humphrey, W., Jr., and Stimpfling, J. H. (1972). *J. Exp. Med.* **136**, 1231.
11. Stimpfling, J. H., and Reichert, A. E. (1971). *Transplantation* **12**, 527.
12. Fuji, H., Zaleski, M., and Milgrom, F. (1971). *Transplant. Proc.* **3**, 852.
13. Gasser, D. L. (1969). *J. Immunol.* **103**, 66.
14. Vladiutiu, A. O., and Rose, N. R. (1971). *Science* **174**, 1137.
15. Dorf, M. E., Newburger, P. E., Hamaoka, T., Katz, D. H., and Benacerraf, B. (1974). *Eur. J. Immunol.* **4**, 346.
16. Lozner, E. C., Sachs, D. H., and Shearer, G. M. (1974). *J. Exp. Med.* **139**, 1204.
17. Sato, H., Boyse, E. A., Aoki, T., Iritani, C., and Old, L. J. (1973). *J. Exp. Med.* **138**, 593.
18. Vaz, N. M., and Levine, B. B. (1970). *Science* **168**, 852.
19. Dunham, E. K., Dorf, M. E., and Benacerraf, B. Unpublished data.
20. Vaz, N. M., and Levine, B. B. (1970). *J. Immunol.* **104**, 1572.
21. Melchers, I., Rajewsky, K., and Shreffler, D. C. (1973). *Eur. J. Immunol.* **3**, 754.

the responses to hen ovalbumin, to thyroglobulin, to the transplantation antigen coded for by the Y chromosome and other antigens since data concerning these three antigens are available for only 2 to 4 H-2 haplotypes.

The distinctive strain distribution of responses observed for most antigens which have been studied in a sufficient number of strains with different H-2 haplotypes may be considered a strong argument that the Ir genes concerned with the control of most of these responses are distinct. Additional evidence will be presented in Section II in favor of this interpretation.

The most important information which can be derived from Fig. 1 concerns the specificity of the genetic control of the responses to synthetic polypeptides. Thus, the antigens GLT^5, $GL\phi^5$, $GLPro^5$, differ from each other only in the third amino acid, which constitutes only 5% of the residues of these copolymers. The antibody responses to these antigens are so cross-reactive that responsiveness to each of these three polymers could be accurately ascertained by measuring the serum antibodies to GLT^5. However, the patterns of genetic responses for GLT^5, $GL\phi^5$, and $GLPro^5$ are absolutely distinct for the different H-2 haplotypes. Similar statements can be made with respect to the antibody responses to (T,G)-A—L, (ϕ,G)-A—L, and (H,G)-A—L (2), and for the antibody response to GA and GAT^{10} (14), respectively. The genetic patterns are clearly different although the specific antibodies are very cross-reactive in both cases. Taken collectively, these findings indicate that the H-linked Ir gene control of specific immune responsiveness is not concerned with the structural genes for immunoglobulin V regions (as will be discussed in Section III) and that the specificity for individual antigens displayed by the traits controlled by the individual H-linked Ir genes is not contributed by conventional immunoglobulin antibodies. Another very interesting finding shown in Fig. 1 concerns the differences observed in the responsiveness to the copolymer $G^{60}A^{40}$ and GAT^{10} which differ only by the presence of 10% L-tyrosine residues in GAT^{10}. The pattern of responsiveness is identical for these antigens for all strains except H-2^s strains, which are responders to GA and nonresponders to GAT^{10}. The significant point is that the presence of 10% L-tyrosine has destroyed responsiveness of this antigen for strains bearing the H-2^s haplotype. It may be of some importance, therefore, with respect to the nature of the recognition process controlled by the H-linked Ir genes that H-2^s strains are nonresponders to all polypeptides containing L-tyrosine or L-phenylalanine, GAT^{10}, GLT^5, (T,G)-A—L, $GL\phi^5$, (ϕ,G)-A—L, whereas it is the only responder haplotype of the eleven tested for GLPro[5] (14). However, it is clear that mere amino acid "composition" does not determine response patterns since (T,G)-A—L and GAT[10], and GLPro[5] and GLA[5], which, respectively, have great similarities in amino acid composition, show very different response patterns in strains with different H-2 haplotypes.

C. RAT H-LINKED Ir GENES

The same phenomenon of histocompatibility-linked single gene control of specific immune responses to polypeptide and native antigens which has been demonstrated in guinea pigs and mice has also been observed in the rat (for references, see Fig. 2). The number of antigens and the histocompatibility types studied have been fewer

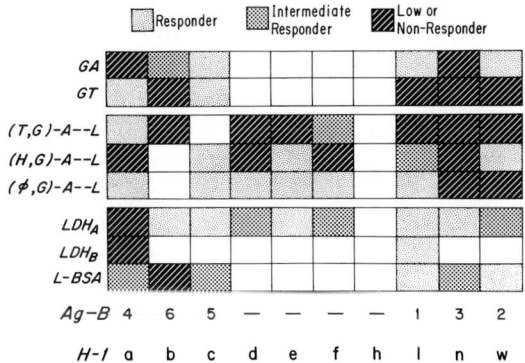

FIG. 2. Immune responses under H-linked Ir gene control of rats bearing different H-1 (Ag-B) haplotypes. References are cited by italic numbers in parentheses.
Antigens—Random linear copolymers of L-amino acids: GA = $(Glu^{60}A^{40})^\eta$ (1); GT = $(Glu^{50}Tyr^{50})^\eta$ (1).
Branched copolymers: (T,G)-A—L = (Tyr, Glu)-Ala—Lys (2); (H,G)-A—L = (His,Glu)-Ala—Lys (3); (Phe,G)-A—L = (Phe,Glu)-Ala—Lys (3).
Foreign antigens: LDH_A = porcine lactic dehydrogenase A (4, 5); LDH_B = porcine lactic dehydrogenase B (6); L-BSA = low-dose bovine serum albumin (1).
H-1, Ag-B = Major histocompatibility complex in rats (7, 8).
Key to references for Fig. 2:
1. Armerding, D., Katz, D. H., and Benacerraf, B. (1974). Immunogenetics 1, 329.
2. Gunther, R., Rude, E., and Stark, O. (1972). Eur. J. Immunol. 2, 151.
3. Rude, E., Gunther, E., Liehl, E., and Wrede, J. (1975). Eur. J. Immunol. 5.
4. Armerding, D., and Rejewsky, K. (1970). Protides Biol. Fluid, Proc. Colloq. 17, 185.
5. Wurzburg, V. (1971). Eur. J. Immunol. 1, 496.
6. Wurzburg, V., Schutt-Gerowitt, H., and Rajewsky, K. (1973). Eur. J. Immunol. 3, 762.
7. Palm, J., and Black, G. (1971). Transplantation 11, 184.
8. Stark, O., and Kren, K. (1971). Transplant. Proc. 3, 165.

than in the mouse. However, the data are of considerable interest because the results are identical and because in many cases the same antigens have been used to demonstrate H-linked *Ir* gene control of specific immune responses in the three experimental species. The results available to date for the rat have been summarized in Fig. 2. It is of interest that, with the limited number of antigens studied, distinctive patterns of responsiveness have been obtained in the rat as in the mouse for (T,G)-A—L, (H,G)-A—L, (ϕ,G)-A—L, GA, and LDHA. On the other hand, a similar strain distribution has been observed for the related antigens (T,G)-A—L and GT. The responses in the rat to antigens under H-linked *Ir* gene control are characterized as in the guinea pig by both the development of delayed hypersensitivity and the synthesis of high amounts of antibodies. On the other hand, as observed in the mouse for many antigens, rats bearing nonresponder haplotypes are able to produce low amounts of antibodies. The study of H-linked *Ir* genes in different species leads to the conclusion that these genes behave in an identical manner in all mammalian species where they have been studied and identified and that they control precisely the same process in the various species investigated. This process is essential for the development of immune responses and is determined by different genes for structurally different antigens, and presumably by the same gene for structurally related antigens.

II. The Mapping of Mouse H-Linked *Ir* Genes

From the genetic point of view, a remarkable feature of the immune response genes is their intimate linkage in several species with genes controlling histocompatibility specificities. The first evidence of such a linkage was provided in mice by the observations of McDevitt and Chinitz (4) that responsiveness of inbred mice to (T,G)-A—L, (H,G)-A—L, and (Phe,G)-A—L is determined by their *H-2* genotype. The locus controlling these responses was termed *Ir-1*. Extensive studies were then made by McDevitt *et al.* (13) to localize *Ir-1* in the *H-2* complex by studying the response of mice with known *H-2* recombinant alleles. These experiments demonstrated that *Ir-1* maps in a region distinct from the *K*, *D*, and *Ss-Slp* regions of the *H-2* complex. This region is located between *K* and *Ss-Slp*, and has been recently termed the *I* region [reviewed in Shreffler and David (16)]. As a result of the identification of *Ir-1* and of the mapping of other *Ir* genes (Fig. 3), the *H-2* complex of the mouse has indeed been subdivided into four regions; *K*, *I*, *S*, and *D* (16). All known mouse *Ir* genes which could be precisely mapped have been localized in the *I* region and have been shown to be distinct from the genes coding for the histocompatibility serological specificities which are controlled at the K and D regions. In Fig. 3 we present the available information and pertinent literature concerning the localization of mouse *Ir* genes within the *H-2* complex. Many genes are clearly located in the *Ir-1A* or *Ir-1B* subregions whereas other *Ir* genes have not as yet been formally distinguished from K because of the lack of appropriate crossover strains. However, enough *Ir* genes have been shown to map in the *I* region distinct from the K region to

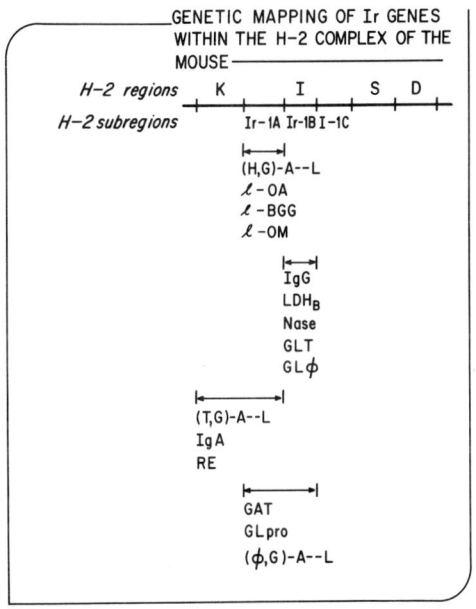

FIG. 3. Mapping of several *Ir* genes in the *I* region of the *H-2* complex (antigen abbreviations are explained in the legend of Fig. 1).

References for mapping data:
(H,G)-A—L, (Phe,G)-A—L, and (T,G)-A—L: McDevitt, H. O., Deak, B. D., Shreffler, D. C., Klein, J., Stimpfling, J. H., and Snell, G. D. (1972). *J. Exp. Med.* **135**, 1259.
I-OA, GAT[10]: Dunham, E. K., Dorf, M. E., Shreffler, D. E., and Benacerraf, B. (1973). *J. Immunol.* **111**, 1621.
I-BGG, I-OM: Freed, J. H., Deak, B. D., and Bechtol, K. B. (1973). *Fed. Proc., Fed. Amer. Soc. Exp. Biol.* **32**, 995.
IgG, IgA: Lieberman, R., Paul, W. E., Humphrey, W., Jr., and Stimpfling, J. H. (1972). *J. Exp. Med.* **136**, 1231.
LDH$_B$: Melchers, I., Rajewsky, K., and Shreffler, D. C. (1973). *Eur. J. Immunol.* **3**, 754.
Nase: Lozner, E. C., Sachs, D. H., and Shearer, G. M. (1974). *J. Exp. Med.* **139**, 1204.
GLT, GLϕ, RE: Dorf, M. E., Lilly, F., and Benacerraf, B. (1974). *J. Exp. Med.* **140**, 859.
GLPro: Dorf, M. E., Plate, J. M. D., Stimpfling, J., and Benacerraf, B. (1975). *J. Immunol.* (in press).

permit the statement to be made that *Ir* genes are distinct from the genes coding for the histocompatibility serological specificities. The important issues concerning the H-linked *Ir* genes is whether genes controlling responses to different antigens can be distinguished from each other genetically and, if this is the case, how many *Ir* genes there are in the *I* region of the *H-2* complex. The answer to these questions has depended upon the existence of strains with documented crossing-over within the *I* region between distinct immune response genes. Two such recombinants, B10.A (4R) between $H-2^k$ and $H-2^b$ and D2.GD between $H-2^d$ and $H-2^b$ have been recognized to date, and their responses to relevant antigens have been studied. These two recombinant strains have defined the two *I* subregions termed *Ir-1A* and *Ir-1B*. The B10.A (4R) strain was the first to be recognized by Lieberman *et al.* (17) as a recombinant in the *I* region between the *Ir* genes controlling the response to allotype determinants on IgG and IgGA BALB/c myelomas, respectively. More recently, the D2.GD strain was shown by Dorf, Lilly, and Benacerraf (18) to also be a recombinant between specific *Ir* genes, i.e., the gene controlling the response to ragweed extract and the genes controlling the responses to the copolymers GLT^5 and $GL\phi^5$. It is not clear, however, whether these recombinants in the *I* region between *Ir-1A* and *Ir-1B* were generated by crossover at precisely the same place in the chromosome.

The development of more recombinant strains between known specific *Ir* genes are required to better resolve the *I* region and to establish whether the *Ir* genes located in the *Ir-1A* and *Ir-1B* subregions are indeed distinct genes and to arrive at an estimate of how many *Ir* loci exist. However, on the basis of the available evidence, it is reasonable to consider that most of the specific mouse *Ir* genes controlling responsiveness to different antigens are indeed the products of distinct loci. As stated in Section I, this interpretation would better account for the unique patterns of immune responsiveness to a variety of antigens characteristic of each haplotype.

As in the mouse, guinea pig *Ir* genes have also been shown to be distinct from genes controlling histocompatibility specificities in this species also. This conclusion could be made because random-bred guinea pigs display specificities of strain 2 and 13 guinea pigs. As in inbred strain 2 guinea pigs, the PLL gene remains linked with strain 2 specificities in nearly all random-bred animals tested (19), but rare Hartley animals have been found which possess the PLL gene and lack strain 2 specificities or which display strain 2 specificities and lack the PLL gene (3). Dissociation between the GA gene and strain 2 specificities in random-bred Hartley animals is more frequent, whereas the BSA-1 gene is not significantly linked in these animals to strain 2 specificities or to the PLL gene. These data suggest that, if in guinea pigs and mice the major histocompatibility regions are analogous, the PLL gene is closest and the BSA-1 gene the farthest distant from loci controlling major serological specificities in the guinea pig.

The important conclusion which has been reached for both mice and guinea pigs is the clear distinction between *Ir* genes and the genes controlling serological specificities. This observation is of considerable importance when the significance of the inhibition of *Ir* gene controlled responses of cells from immune animals by antihistocompatibility alloantisera is discussed and evaluated in a later section (Section VIII).

It has been recently shown both in man and mice that the loci which control the mixed leukocyte reaction (MLC) are distinct from the loci coding for serological histocompatibility specificities. The data obtained in mice by Bach and associates (20) indicate that genetic differences at the *I* region are essential for positive MLC; this suggests some relationship, if not identity, between the receptors responsible for MLC and the *Ir* gene products. This relationship may have considerable significance when, as will be shown, the H-linked *Ir* genes are found to be necessarily expressed in the thymus-derived cells which are also the cells responsible for MLC reactions.

At this early stage, no simple explanation may be proposed to account for the relationship between *Ir* genes and the major histocompatibility loci of several species. Although this relationship is possibly fortuitous, in our opinion it is more reasonable, as well as more challenging, to consider it a fundamental feature of the immune mechanism and of its discriminating capacity, implying a fundamental relationship between histocompatibility molecules and the ability of a class of immunocompetent cells to recognize foreignness. We shall consider further the significance of this relationship when we discuss the process controlled by the *Ir* genes in the immune response.

III. Relationship of H-Linked *Ir* Genes to Immunoglobulin Structural Genes

In addition to the H-linked *Ir* genes, another class of specific *Ir* genes has been identified in several laboratories in the past few years. This second class of genes, which have been detected in the mouse, is not linked to histocompatibility genotype but has been shown instead to be linked to the genes controlling immunoglobulin allotype determinants on the mouse heavy chain linkage group. These "allotype-linked *Ir* genes" have been identified in responses of mice to antigens which stimulate the formation of antibodies with restricted specificity and heterogeneity such as α-3 dextran (*21*) and streptococcal polysaccharide (*22*). Furthermore, an idiotypic specificity was demonstrated by Pawlak and Nisonoff (*23*) to be very closely linked to heavy-chain allotype markers in anti-*p*-azophenylarsonate antibodies produced by all mice of the BC9 strain possessing the heavy-chain allotype of the AL/N strain on a BALB/c background. The structural gene coding for this idiotype must therefore be closely linked to genes coding for the constant regions of mouse heavy-chain immunoglobulins.

It is important to note that contrary to the methods used to study H-linked *Ir* genes, which rely on the identification of responder and nonresponder strains and animals, the discovery of allotype-linked *Ir* genes has depended upon the characterization of the antibody produced. Thus allotype-linked *Ir* genes control idiotypic determinants or the fine specificity of the antibody produced. For these reasons and since the V region and the C region of immunoglobulin chains are known to be linked, it is generally accepted that allotype-linked *Ir* genes code for immunoglobulin V regions.

In contrast, there is a compelling body of evidence which established that H-linked *Ir* genes do not code for immunoglobulin V regions. Considering that distinct H-linked *Ir* genes control responses to different antigens and therefore that the product of H-linked *Ir* genes must in some way be capable of specific recognition, this is a very crucial issue because it implies the existence of a second type of molecule and a second level concerned with immunological specificity besides immunoglobulins. The data must therefore be evaluated very critically in this respect. The strongest evidence is provided by the genetics of the two systems. The immunoglobulin V regions of H chains are closely linked to the genes encoding the C regions. The rabbit allotype data concerning recombinants between the a and the 14–15 loci is extremely convincing (*24*). In addition, as stated above, the observed linkage of idiotypic specificities to heavy-chain allotype (*21–23*), but not to *H-2* in inbred mice, identify a new class of *Ir* genes controlling immunoglobulin V regions, as well as provide the techniques to recognize and study these genes. The objection might be raised that the evidence discussed above concerns only the H chain. However, it is clear that in man the light-chain structural genes are not linked to the major histocompatibility complex, and, if more precise genetic evidence is required, McDevitt observed several years ago that the response of rabbits to (T,G)-A—L, which is under genetic control in this species as in mice, is not linked to the allotype b locus of the K chain (25). Since all current theories of immunoglobulin structure postulate that the V and C regions are linked in both H and L chains, the genetic data discussed above establish that the H-linked *Ir* genes do not code for immunoglobulin V genes, a function that should be attributed to the increasing number of allotype-linked *Ir* genes, which are being identified in several laboratories.

The different methodologies which have permitted the detection of H-linked *Ir* genes and allotype-linked *Ir* genes support these conclusions. The ease with which H-linked *Ir* genes have been detected as determining responsiveness to antigens with limited structural heterogeneity or limited number of determinants contrast with the sophisticated requirements to identify allotype-linked *Ir* genes which necessitate a detailed study of the fine specificity or structure of the antibody population synthesized. These differences have important implications for the two types of recognition systems coded by the two classes of *Ir* genes and indicate that the H-linked *Ir* genes are considerably less numerous than the immunoglobulin specificities that can be generated by the combination of H and L V regions.

IV. The Cell Type Where Histocompatibility-Linked *Ir* Genes Are Expressed

Let us consider now the cells where the H-linked *Ir* genes are expressed. In the two systems most extensively studied, the PLL gene in guinea pigs and genes at the *Ir-1* locus in mice, responsiveness can be passively transferred to irradiated nonresponder recipient strains with immunocompetent cells from animals possessing the *Ir* genes, demonstrating that the genes are indeed expressed in cells which participate in the immune response (1). It should be noted that in these chimeras, the responding cells have been found to be of donor origin (26). Thus, the *Ir* genes are expressed in immunocompetent cells. This conclusion is further supported by studies on the immune response of mouse spleen cells in culture to the terpolymer GAT^{10}. As described in Section I, mice bearing the a, b, d, f, j, k, r, u, or v *H-2* haplotypes respond to GAT with high levels of IgG antibodies whereas mice of the $H\text{-}2^{n,p,q,s}$ types do not respond to this antigen.

In vitro cultures of spleen cells from inbred and congenic-resistant strains in the presence of 1 or 10 µg of soluble GAT^{10} have shown identical results to those observed *in vivo* (27). Soluble GAT in these concentrations stimulates the development of IgG GAT-specific plaque-forming cell (PFC) responses in cultures of spleen cells from responder C57B1/6(H-2^b), F_1 (C57 × SJL) (H-$2^{b/s}$), and A/J (H-2^a) mice. Soluble GAT did not stimulate the development of GAT-specific PFC responses in cultures of spleen cells from nonresponder H-2^s mice (SJL, B10.S, A.SW) or H-2^q (DBA/1). It is of interest to note that GAT did not stimulate antibody production of the IgM class by responder or nonresponder strains either *in vivo* or *in vitro*. The GAT^{10} terpolymer differs, therefore, markedly in this respect from the branched polymers, such as (T,G)-A—L, which stimulate the synthesis of IgM antibodies in both responder and nonresponder strains.

The next question to be considered is the type of cell of the immune system, macrophages, T cells or B cells, where the product of histocompatibility-linked *Ir* genes are necessarily expressed for immune responses to develop.

Evidence will be presented that the *Ir* gene products are not expressed in macrophages and appear to be necessarily expressed in one or several classes of T cells. Many of the data on which these conclusions are based have been provided by the studies on the guinea pig H-linked *Ir* genes and on the mouse *Ir* genes at the *Ir-1* locus, which display identical properties in every respect in both species, and also from the study of the *in vitro* anti-GAT responses by mouse spleen cells. It is reasonable to conclude that H-linked *Ir* genes control the same processes in all the species where they have been identified; mouse, rat, guinea pig, and monkeys, and that all conclusions with respect to gene function or expression reached with distinct systems in different species can be generalized to the behavior of all H-linked *Ir* genes.

The following evidence has been obtained for the expression of the H-linked *Ir* gene product in T cells:

1. The presence of the relevant *Ir* gene is absolutely required for the development of cellular immunity, a characteristic T cell function. Thus, in guinea pigs, those functions which are attributed to the activity of "thymus-derived" cells, such as cellular immunity, depend exclusively upon the presence of the relevant *Ir*-gene. The reactions of cellular immunity to PLL, DNP-PLL, GA, and GT are totally under the control of the corresponding specific immune response genes. They are never observed in animals lacking the genes [reviewed in Benacerraf and McDevitt (2)].

2. H-linked *Ir* genes are concerned with the recognition and responses to the carrier molecules of hapten-carrier conjugates, not

to the haptens they bear [reviewed in Benacerraf and McDevitt (2)]. Thus, guinea pigs possessing the PLL gene and therefore capable of responding to DNP-PLL with the synthesis of anti-DNP antibodies, respond similarly to immunization with PLL conjugates of other non-cross-reacting haptens, with vigorous antihapten synthesis. Guinea pigs lacking the PLL gene and therefore incapable of responding to DNP-PLL are also incapable of responding to benzylpenicilloyl-PLL or to other unrelated hapten PLL conjugates. This experiment indicates that the PLL gene is concerned with the specific recognition of the carrier molecules, which is known to be the function of thymus-derived cells. A similar situation has been demonstrated in the genetic controls of the anti-DNP antibody responses to limiting doses of DNP_7-BSA or DNP_6-GPA. As mentioned earlier (Table II), strain 2 but not strain 13 guinea pigs synthesize anti-DNP antibodies when immunized with 1 μg DNP_7-BSA, whereas strain 13 but not strain 2 guinea pigs produce anti-DNP antibodies in response to 1 μg of DNP_6-GPA (28). The capacity to form anti-DNP antibody exists equally in both inbred strains, but it is determined by the genetically controlled recognition of the carrier, again a function of thymus-derived cells.

3. The genetic differences between responder and nonresponder mouse strains in the response to (T,G)-A—L, i.e., the production of IgG antibodies and the development of specific memory by the responder strains, are abolished by neonatal thymectomy of responder animals (29). This illustrates directly the required role of T cells in the capacity of responder mice to develop IgG responses to (T,G)-A—L.

4. An animal unable to respond to an antigen because it lacks the relevant *Ir* gene may nevertheless be stimulated to form antibodies against determinants on that antigen, when immunized with the antigen bound to an immunogenic carrier to which its helper T cells are able to respond. Thus, when a genetically nonimmunogenic molecule such as DNP-PLL (30) or GAT (27) is administered to a nonresponder animal complexed with an immunogenic carrier which is able to stimulate thymus-derived cells specific for the carrier, an antibody response is induced against DNP-PLL or GAT, and the antibody produced cannot be distinguished from those produced by responder animals with respect to amount, class, or specificity. Therefore, DNP-PLL or GAT, which are complete antigens in genetic responder animals, may behave as haptens in nonresponder strains. These observations support the conclusion that the genetic defect in nonresponder animals is not a result of the inability to synthesize antibodies to some determinants on the molecule.

5. As would be expected, nonresponder animals possess B cells capable of binding antigens to which they are genetically unable to respond in numbers comparable to those found in responder animals (31).

6. The demonstration that nonspecific T cell stimulation of B cells, by the "allogeneic effect," can stimulate strong antibody responses by genetic nonresponder strains (32) and the finding that tetraparental mice generated from responder and nonresponder strains behave as responders to (T,G)-A—L and synthesize antibody of nonresponder allotype (33) may be considered further evidence for the lack of expression of H-linked Ir gene function in B cells.

7. These conclusions were also supported by our recent studies of the genetic control of the response to GAT^{10} by spleen cell cultures. As stated earlier, soluble GAT^{10} stimulated primary IgG GAT-specific PFC responses in spleen cell cultures from C57B1/6 ($H-2^b$) mice, but not in cultures from DBA/1 ($H-2^q$), SJL, or B10.S ($H-2^s$) mice. However, GAT^{10} bound to the antigenic carrier, methylated BSA (MBSA), stimulates IgG GAT-specific PFC responses by spleen cell cultures from both responder and nonresponder strains alike (27).

The role of macrophages in responses controlled by H-linked Ir genes was then investigated (34). Macrophages were shown to be required for development of responses to GAT^{10} and GAT-MBSA in cultures of spleen cells from responder mice and for responses to GAT-MBSA in cultures of spleen cells from nonresponder mice. Macrophages from nonresponder mice supported the development of responses to GAT^{10} by nonadherent responder spleen cells, indicating that the failure of nonresponder mice to respond to GAT^{10} is not due to a macrophage defect. Furthermore, responder macrophages supported the responses of nonadherent, nonresponder spleen cells to SRBC and GAT-MBSA, but not to GAT^{10}. This indicates that the capacity to respond to GAT^{10} is a function of the nonadherent population which is composed of thymus-derived (T) helper cells and precursors of antibody-producing cells. Treatment of spleen cells with anti-θ serum and complement before culture initiation abolished PFC responses to GAT^{10} and GAT-MBSA, thus establishing the requirement for T cells in the development of PFC responses to these antigens. Since precursors of antibody-producing cells in nonresponder mice are capable of synthesizing antibody specific for GAT^{10} after stimulation with GAT-MBSA, and since the response to GAT^{10} is thymus-dependent, it appears that nonresponder mice lack GAT-specific helper T cell function.

Taken collectively, all these results demonstrate that H-linked Ir gene function is expressed in some class of T cells responsible for the development of cellular immunity and helper function, but is not necessarily expressed in macrophages for immune responses under Ir gene control to occur. The evidence for the expression of Ir gene function in T cells, but not in macrophages, is therefore compelling and clear. However, the possible expression of H-linked Ir gene function in B cells is still controversial.

Most of the data which we have discussed, i.e., the possibility to trigger B cell antibody responses in genetic nonresponder mice provided the antigen is presented coupled to an immunogenic carrier or that allogeneic T cells are injected, and the existence of antigen-binding B cells in comparable numbers in nonimmune responder and nonresponder animals indicate that in most cases the expression of H-linked Ir gene products in B cells is not essential for antibody responses to occur.

However, other data have been interpreted as suggesting the expression of H-linked Ir genes in B cells. Shearer, Mozes, and Sela (35) have presented evidence from limiting dilution cell transfer studies which suggest that in some cases H-2 linked Ir genes are expressed in B cells. However, as Shearer has indicated, these results could be due either to an actual expression of the Ir gene defect in B cell or to an effect of Ir genes or closely linked genes on T–B cell cooperation [discussed in McDevitt and Landy (36)].

Another experiment that could be interpreted as indicating the necessary expression of Ir gene products in B cells is the demonstration by Katz et al. (37) (discussed in Section VI) that GLT^5-primed T cells from (responder × nonresponder)F_1 animals are unable to cooperate *in vivo* with DNP-primed nonresponder (to GLT) B cells in an irradiated F_1 recipient, in contrast to DNP-primed responder B cells. There is, however, another possible interpretation for this finding besides the conclusion that the GLT gene is expressed in B cells, as will be discussed in Section VI. More recently, we have also observed that nonresponder B cells to GAT could be inhibited from developing IgG PFC responses in culture to macrophage-bound GAT or to GAT-MBSA in the presence of GAT-primed (responder × nonresponder)F_1 T cells by lower concentrations of soluble GAT than are inhibitory under the same experimental conditions for responder B cells, suggesting again some differences in responder and nonresponder B cells (38). These various observations, however, could be equally interpreted as indicating an absence of efficient helper function of (responder × nonresponder)F_1 T cells for nonresponder B cells, particularly since, as will be discussed in Section VI, the *I* region where *Ir* genes are located has been shown to be concerned with the genetic control of T and B cell interactions in immune responses.

The significance of the expression of H-linked *Ir* genes in T cells for an understanding of the recognition process by the products of H-linked *Ir* genes will be discussed at length in Section IX. The available data have, however, conclusively established, in our opinion, that there exists in addition to immunoglobulin antibodies a distinct class of molecules coded for by the H-linked *Ir* genes which are responsible for specificity at the level of interaction of a class of T cells with antigen. In keeping with the application of the clonal selection theory to these postulated antigen receptors, the product of H-linked *Ir* genes would be expected to be clonally expressed in T cells.

V. The Demonstration of Suppressor T Cells Specific for GAT^{10} in Genetic Nonresponder Mice

It has become increasingly apparent in the last few years that T cells are concerned with the regulation of immune responses and that, in addition to activated carrier-specific T cells capable of providing helper function for antibody responses of various classes, the administration of antigen at the appropriate time and in the appropriate form stimulates the generation of lymphocytes bearing the θ antigen and lacking surface immunoglobulin (T cells), which are capable of suppressing specific immune responses (39). In some documented cases these "suppressor T cells" appear to function by suppressing helper T cells (40), or T cells concerned with cellular immunity (41).

In view of the absence of T cell helper function in genetic nonresponder animals, it appeared relevant to explore whether an antigen, the response to which is under *Ir* gene control and which is unable to stimulate cellular immunity and T cell helper function in nonresponder animals, could nevertheless stimulate specific suppressor T cells. This possibility was first suggested by studies reported by Gershon *et al.* (42). More recently, this has indeed been shown to be the case in our laboratory for the GAT system in mice (43). We have observed that injection of GAT^{10} to mice of nonresponder strains renders them unable to mount a GAT-specific PFC response to a subsequent challenge with GAT-MBSA to which control mice normally respond. This suppressive effect may be obtained with very small doses of GAT^{10} (0.1 mg in alum), is observed as early as 3 days after GAT^{10} injection and is still detectable 5 weeks after GAT^{10} administration. Treatment of nonresponder DBA/1 or SJL mice with GAT^{10} also renders the spleen cells in culture unable to develop a GAT-specific response when incubated with GAT-MBSA although their response to sheep red blood cells (SRBC) is equivalent to that of spleen cells from normal DBA/1 mice.

To analyze the mechanism of the suppression induced by GAT^{10} in nonresponder mice, we have investigated (44): (1) the immunocompetence of T and B cells from spleens of nonresponder mice previously rendered unresponsive by injection of GAT^{10}; and (2) the effects of such populations of T and B cells on the development of GAT-specific PFC responses by normal nonresponder spleen cells incubated with GAT-MBSA. We have been able to show that B cells from nonresponder DBA/1 mice rendered unresponsive by GAT^{10} in vivo can respond in vitro to GAT-MBSA if exogenous, carrier-primed T cells are added to the cultures. The unresponsiveness was therefore demonstrated to be the result of impaired carrier-specific helper T cell function in the spleen cells of GAT-primed mice.

More important, spleen cells from GAT-primed mice specifically suppressed the GAT-specific PFC response of spleen cells from normal DBA/1 mice incubated with GAT-MBSA. This suppression was prevented by pretreatment of GAT-primed spleen cells with anti-θ serum and complement or by X-irradiation. Identification of the suppressor cells as T cells was confirmed by the demonstration that suppressor cells were confined to the fraction of lymphocytes purified on antimouse immunoglobulin columns which contained theta-positive cells and only a few nonimmunoglobulin-bearing cells (44).

The demonstration that nonresponder mice injected with GAT^{10}, the response to which is under Ir gene control, do not develop an antibody response to GAT and become specifically unresponsive to a subsequent challenge with GAT-MBSA and that this unresponsiveness is the result of an active suppressive process mediated by T cells, raises important questions concerning the mechanism of Ir gene regulation of the immune response. The first question is whether the generation of suppressor T cells in nonresponder mice is unique to this system or may be generalized to other systems and species where the response to the antigen is under the control of histocompatibility-linked Ir genes. Experiments are in progress to resolve this important issue.

What are the implications of the demonstration of GAT-specific suppressor T cells in nonresponder animals for the function of *Ir* genes and their products? We can offer three possible hypotheses for the function of H-linked *Ir* genes which could account for these observations.

1. One could postulate that nonresponder animals develop both GAT-specific suppressor and helper T cells, but that the suppressor T cells predominate. However, we feel that this is an unlikely possibility since we were never able to demonstrate GAT-specific T cell helper activity in nonresponder animals even when we took advantage of the considerably greater sensitivity to X-irradiation of GAT-specific suppressor T cells compared to helper T cells. Thus, irradiated GAT-primed nonresponder DBA/1 cells could never show GAT-specific helper activity for nonresponder B cells in anti-GAT responses *in vitro*.

2. The second hypothesis states that suppressor T cells are a normal component of all immune responses, in responder and nonresponder animals, but that *Ir* genes determine the presence or absence of helper T cells specific for the antigen and are not involved in the generation of suppressor cells. However, since GAT specifically induces suppressor T cells in nonresponders, it would be necessary to postulate two separate, antigen-specific recognition systems for helper and suppressor T cells, respectively, the former one only under *Ir* gene control.

3. The last hypothesis, and the one which we feel is the most attractive, postulates that T cells have the potential of developing into helper or suppressor cells. The manner of interaction of antigen with GAT-specific T cell receptors should determine whether the cell develops as a helper or suppressor cell. In a nonresponder animal the absence of the critical *Ir* gene would limit the differentiation of the T cells after interaction with antigen to suppressor cells, but not to helper cells or cells concerned with cell-mediated immunity.

Since suppressor T cells have been shown to be responsible for many states of specific tolerance at the T cell level, H-linked *Ir* genes could thus be intimately concerned with the development of tolerance or immunity. The manner in which a gene product with antigen recognition capacity in T cells could perform this function in responder and nonresponder mice is a matter for speculation. Several possible mechanisms may be considered. If the *Ir* gene product indeed functions as an antigen receptor on T cells, the strength of the binding and the amount of antigen bound could account for the differences between responder and nonresponder which then result in the generation of helper versus suppressor T cells according to this interpretation. Alternatively, the *Ir* gene products in responders could affect in a critical way the mode of interaction with antigen of a spatially related receptor molecule on the T cell membrane required for the stimulation of helper but not of suppressor T cells. The observations that thymocytes from responder and nonresponder strains bind in equal numbers, irrespective of responder status, antigens such as (T,G)-A—L (45) or GAT[10] (46) but that only T cells from primed responder animals are able to be stimulated by (T,G)-A—L to show increased thymidine-^{3}H incorporation (47) is in agreement with the last hypothesis (see Section VIII).

It is of interest to note when we consider the nature of the elusive antigen receptor on T cells and its relationship or identity with the products of H-linked *Ir* genes that the specific binding of antigens such as (T,G)-A—L or GAT[10] by thymocytes of both responder and nonresponder strains is only efficient at 37°C and that this binding is *totally* inhibited by alloantisera raised against lymphocytes bearing the *H-2* haplotype of the thymocytes examined, but not by anti-immunoglobulin antisera. These observations are discussed in detail in Section VIII.

VI. The Role of Histocompatibility Gene Products in T–B Cell Interactions

Delineation of the complex events involved in requisite cooperative interactions between thymus-derived (T) and bone marrow-derived (B) lymphocytes in the development of antibody responses to all but a selected class of antigens has been the subject of intensive analysis in many laboratories [reviewed in Katz and Benacerraf (48)]. Several hypotheses have been developed over the past years to explain the mechanism of T–B cell cooperation. These have included direct or indirect antigen presentation by T cells, and the active regulation of B cell responses by either direct membrane interaction with T cells or by the interaction with soluble mediators produced and released by T cells (48). The latter hypothesis stems largely from the demonstration that T cells activated by means other than the constituent determinants of the antigen employed, such as by allogeneic cell interactions, were highly effective in providing helper function for antigen-specific B cells (48). More recently, it has been demonstrated that the most optimal cell interactions occur between T and B lymphocytes bearing identical histocompatibility antigens, thus adding an additional condition to consider in the mechanism of such cell interactions. In this section, we shall review the data and observations that have pointed to the genetic restrictions of T–B cell interactions and discuss the implications of these findings with respect to control of such interactions.

Even before the question of genetic requirements for T–B cell cooperation was directly investigated, there were small pieces of evidence that bore on the issue. Indeed the observations of several investigators (49–52) can be interpreted to indicate a requirement for histocompatibility at the major locus between the two cell types. These studies were done, however, under circumstances that make definitive conclusions difficult, since potential contributions to the results of rejection reactions and/or an allogeneic effect [for reviews, see Katz and Benacerraf (48) and Katz (53)] cannot be excluded. Recently, kindred and Shreffler (54) reported results of their studies, which were designed specifically to investigate this question in backcrosses of nude and BALB/c mice. Since the nude mouse cannot reject foreign tissue grafts, this complicating feature was theoretically eliminated. In such mice T cell helper effects could be obtained with thymus cells from *H-2* compatible, but not from incompatible, donors (54).

At about the same time, studies were being conducted in our own laboratory utilizing specific T cells and hapten-specific B cells in antihapten humoral responses as an appropriate model system to investigate the possible importance of histocompatibility requirements in T–B cell cooperation. The initial experiments were planned by taking advantage of the *in vivo* radioresistance of primed carrier-specific T cells (55, 56). According to the simplest approach, allogeneic hapten-specific B cells could presumably be safely transferred to carrier-primed irradiated recipients to investigate T cell–B cell interactions. Achieving this end, however, was not without considerable technical difficulty for the following reasons: The difficulty stemmed primarily from the contribution of the "allogeneic effect" in nonspecifically enhancing adoptive immune responses in irradiated recipients under quite unexpected circumstances. The allogeneic effect is a phenomenon in which specific B lymphocytes become readily activated by antigen in the absence of antigen-specific T helper cells by virtue of a direct interaction with histoincompatible T lymphocytes recognizing surface antigen differences on such B cells (48, 53). In order to minimize possible confusion of terminology, we are distinguishing the phenomenon of the allogeneic effect from interactions between normally isologous antigen-specific T and B lymphocytes by referring to the latter, for purposes of brevity, as "physiologic" T–B cell cooperation. In our first experiments, we made the unexpected observation that a heavily irradiated mouse (600 R) possesses sufficient numbers of active residual T cells to exert this effect on a small population of adoptively transferred histoincompatible primed B lymphocytes (57).

A. Failure of Physiologic Cooperative Interactions to Occur between T and B Lymphocytes from Histoincompatible Donor Strains

The central problem was, therefore, to design an experimental scheme that specifically circumvented the possible contribution to the results of a complicating allogeneic effect. This was accomplished for *in vivo* cell transfer studies by using an F_1 hybrid as the recipient of T and B cells from the respective parental strains against which the semiallogeneic host would be genetically incapable of reacting.

The protocol is schematically illustrated in Fig. 4 (58). Spleen cells, 50×10^6, from either BGG-primed or normal parental donor

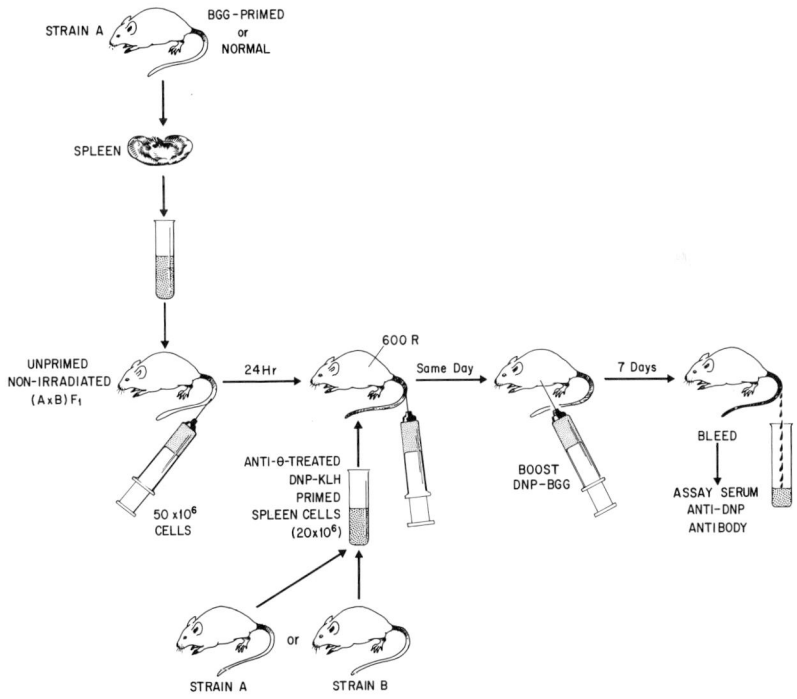

FIG. 4. Protocol for determining physiologic cooperation between histoincompatible T and B lymphocytes. See text for detailed explanation. Taken from Katz et al. (58).

mice are injected intravenously into nonirradiated, unprimed CAF_1 hybrid recipients. Twenty-four hours later, when the transferred cells have migrated to the lymphoid organs, these mice are irradiated (600 R) and then injected intravenously with a second cell inoculum consisting of 20×10^6 DNP-KLH-primed B lymphocytes derived from the same or the other parental strain. The latter cells are depleted of T lymphocytes by treatment with anti-θ serum and complement prior to transfer to eliminate development of a fatal graft versus host reaction in the irradiated F_1 recipient. Immediately thereafter, secondary challenge is performed with 50 μg of DNP-BGG intraperitoneally in saline, and the mice are bled 7 days later. This type of experiment is always performed in a simultaneously symmetrical fashion to alleviate potential variability between different pools and strain origins of carrier-primed and DNP-primed donor cells.

This protocol takes advantage of the fact that: (1) primed mature mouse T lymphocytes are relatively radioresistant when they are subjected to X-irradiation *in situ* after adoptive transfer and a suitable period for migration to the recipient lymphoid organs has elapsed (56); and (2) semiallogeneic recipients are genetically incapable of reacting against histocompatibility specificities of either parental strain lymphocytes. Since the F_1 host is genetically incapable of reacting against either parental donor cell population, and since the irradiated carrier-primed parental cells are present in restricted numbers, the allogeneic effect has been avoided. This is true for both *enhancing* and *suppressive* influences of the allogeneic effect. Furthermore, the fact that the transferred parental DNP-specific B cells in the F_1 recipient, which would be the potential target for the allogeneic effect, constitutes but a small proportion of the cells against which the T cells from the second parent can react in the F_1 environment is an additional argument for the absence of allogeneic effects in this experimental design.

The results of one such *in vivo* experiment are shown in Fig. 5 (58). Groups I–IV are controls which verify the cooperative functional capacities of the irradiated (*in situ*) BGG-primed and the anti-θ-treated DNP-primed cells of BALB/c and A/J origin in their respective totally syngeneic combinations (including recipients). Additional controls (not shown) confirmed the efficacy of anti-θ-treatment in that such T cell-depleted populations failed to respond to DNP-KLH in unprimed irradiated recipients. Groups V and VI demonstrate that BALB/c syngeneic BGG-primed (T) and DNP-primed (B) cell populations cooperate quite effectively within the environs

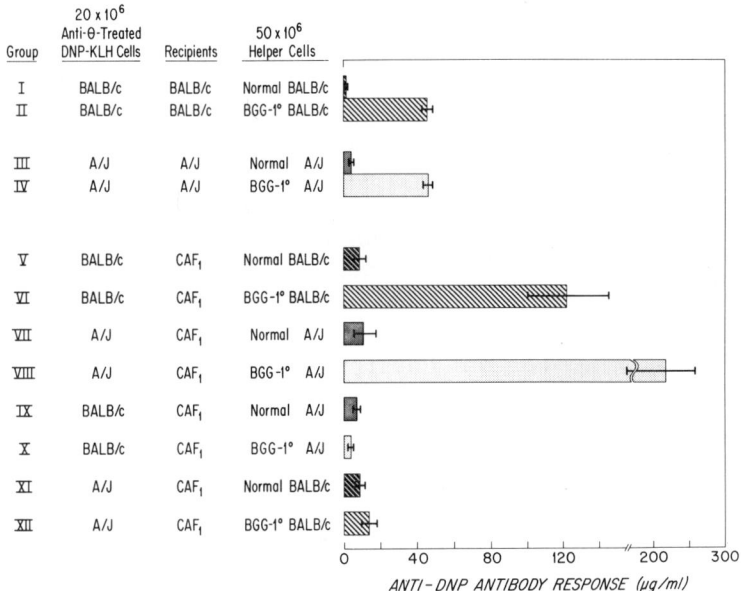

FIG. 5. Failure of physiologic cooperative interactions to occur between histoincompatible T and B lymphocytes: *in vivo*. The scheme followed is outlined in Fig. 4. The donor cell–recipient strain combinations are indicated. Mean serum anti-DNP antibody levels of groups of 5 mice on day 7 after secondary challenge with 50 μg of DNP-BGG (dinitrophenyl-bovine γ-globulin) are illustrated. Horizontal bars represent the range of the standard errors. Statistical comparisons between the various groups gave the following results: groups I and II, groups III and IV, groups V and VI, and groups VII and VIII, $0.005 > P > 0.001$ in all cases; groups IX and X, $0.30 > P > 0.20$; groups XI and XII, $0.40 > P > 0.30$; groups V and IX, $0.70 > P > 0.60$; groups VII and XI, $0.70 > P > 0.60$; groups II and VI, $0.025 > P > 0.02$; groups IV and VIII, $0.005 > P > 0.001$; groups I and V and groups III and VII, $0.40 > P > 0.30$ in both cases. Taken from Katz *et al.* (58).

of a CAF_1 irradiated recipient. Similarly, A/J syngeneic T and B lymphocytes interact very well with one another in the F_1 host (groups VII and VIII). In striking contrast, however, is the very obvious failure of the BGG-primed B cells derived from BALB/c mice (group X), and vice versa (group XII). The complete absence of a complicating allogeneic effect in this particular system is demonstrated by the lack of responses in control groups IX and XI (receiving normal allogeneic cells prior to irradiation) which are not significantly different from those in control groups V and VII (receiving normal syngeneic cells prior to irradiation).

The failure of physiologic cooperation to occur between T and B lymphocytes from allogeneic strains may reflect the effect of any of a number of variables in the system. One important question concerns whether the mere presence of a completely foreign histocompatibility antigen on the surface of the cell may in itself serve as a "block" of some sort to cell interactions. This question was approached in reciprocal experiments in which, on the one hand, CAF_1 BGG-primed cells were tested for their capacity to help T cell-depleted DNP-KLH-primed parental cells, and, on the other hand, parental helper cells were tested for their capacity to interact with CAF_1 DNP-primed B cells (58).

The first of these experiments is shown in Fig. 6. Groups I and II

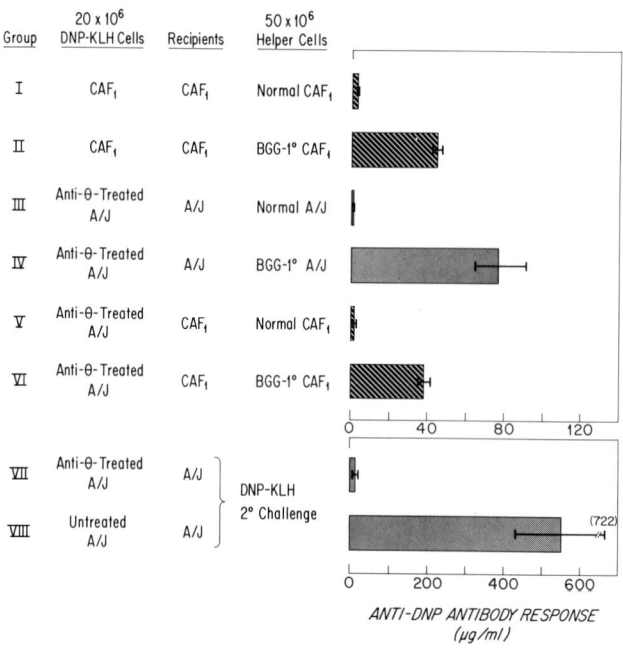

FIG. 6. Demonstration of physiologic cooperative interactions between T and B lymphocytes sharing one major histocompatibility specificity in common and differing by another: Using F_1 hybrid helper T cells with parental B cells. The scheme outlined in Fig. 4 was followed. The donor cell–recipient strain combinations are indicated. Recipients in groups I–VI were secondarily challenged with 50 μg of DNP-BGG (dinitrophenyl bovine γ-globulin). Groups VII and VIII received 20 μg of DNP-KLH. Mean serum anti-DNP antibody levels of groups of 6 mice on day 7 after secondary challenge are illustrated. Horizontal bars represent ranges of the standard errors. Statistical comparisons of the various groups gave the following results: groups I and II, $0.01 > P > 0.005$; groups III and IV, $0.001 > P$; groups V and VI, $0.005 > P > 0.001$; groups VII and VIII, $0.001 > P$. Taken from Katz et al. (58).

and groups III and IV demonstrate the positive control cooperative responses obtained with CAF_1 and A/J cell populations, respectively, in their totally syngeneic combination. Likewise, group VII illustrates the effectiveness of T cell depletion of the anti-θ-treated A/J population as compared to its untreated control (group VIII) in response to DNP-KLH. In the experimental groups, when anti-θ-treated A/J DNP-primed cells are adoptively transferred to irradiated CAF_1 recipients, a good cooperative response to DNP-BGG is obtained provided CAF_1 BGG-primed cells are present (group VI). The possibility of an allogeneic effect is ruled out by the lack of response in group V recipients. The reciprocal experiment (not shown) also demonstrated the capacity of parental BGG-primed helper T cells to physiologically cooperate with DNP-primed CAF_1 B cells in this system. This latter positive result is also most important, as will be discussed below, in providing further evidence against the possibility of nonspecific suppressive influences of an allogeneic effect being a viable alternative explanation for the failure of physiologic T–B cell cooperation to occur between mixtures of parental cells in these conditions, since if such suppressive effects were present in substantial amounts one might reasonably expect them to be manifested in mixtures of F_1 B cells with parental T cells.

B. Demonstration That the H-2 Histocompatibility Gene Complex Determines Successful Physiologic Lymphocyte Interactions

Since the strains employed in the above studies, i.e., BALB/c (H-2^d) and A/J (H-2^a), not only differed at the major histocompatibility locus but for many other polymorphisms as well, one could only speculate that the relevant area of the genome responsible for permitting (or preventing) "physiologic," i.e., antigen-specific, T–B cell cooperative interactions to occur was located in the gene complex coding for the major histocompatibility specificities. In the next series of experiments, we therefore utilized congenic-resistant mouse strains to answer questions concerning the respective roles of genes coding for the major histocompatibility specificities.

The protocol and results of one series of combinations of T and B cells in which the DNP-primed B cells were derived from A/J (H-2^a) donor mice are shown in Fig. 7 (59). For convenience, the relevant genetic similarities and/or differences are listed for each combination. Groups I and II demonstrate the intact cooperative functional capacities of the irradiated (*in situ*) bovine γ-globulin (BGG)-primed and the anti-θ-treated DNP-primed cells of syngeneic A/J origin

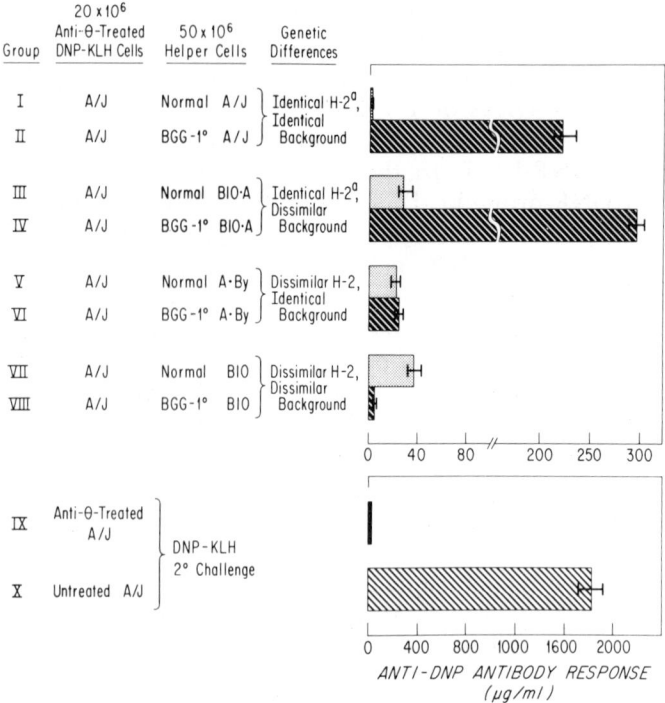

FIG. 7. Failure of physiologic cooperative interactions to occur between T and B lymphocytes differing at the major histocompatibility locus. The scheme followed is outlined in Fig. 4. Recipients for all cell combinations were $(A \times B10)F_1$ hybrids. Combinations and strain origins of T and B cells and the relevant genetic differences are indicated. Recipients in groups I–VIII were secondarily challenged with 50 μg of DNP-BGG; groups IX and X received 20 μg of DNP-KLH. Mean serum anti-DNP antibody levels of groups of 5 mice on day 7 after secondary challenge are illustrated. Vertical bars represent ranges of the standard errors. Statistical comparisons between the various groups gave the following results: groups I and II, groups III and IV, and groups IX and X, $0.001 > P$ in all cases; groups V and VI, $0.98 > P > 0.95$; groups VII and VIII, $0.80 > P > 0.70$. Taken from Katz et al. (59).

within the environs of $(A \times B10)F_1$ irradiated recipients (group II) as compared to control recipients of normal cells (group I). Similarly, BGG-primed T cells derived from congenic-resistant B10.A donors, which are identical with A/J at the major $H-2^a$ locus but dissimilar with respect to background genotypes, are capable of exerting a clear helper effect in cooperating with A/J B cells (groups III and IV). In sharp contrast, T cells from A.By or B10 donors, which are both $H-2^b$, fail to cooperatively interact with A/J B lymphocytes (groups V–VIII). This is true irrespective of whether or not the genetic background other than $H-2$ is identical, as in the case of A.By donor cells (group VI).

There are several possible explanations for the failure of physiologic T–B cell cooperation to occur across the major histocompatibility barrier. Certain of these possibilities which appear to be quite unlikely include the following:

1. Failure of transferred T and B cells to migrate to appropriate sites in the lymphoid organs *in vivo*, and/or rejection of one or the other cell type. These possibilities have been eliminated by using the F_1 recipient as a neutral host environment in which very good cooperative interactions could be obtained between H-2 identical cell mixtures and, moreover, by the corroboration of these data in a fully *in vitro* system (58).

2. A "block" of some sort to cell–cell interaction by the presence of a foreign major histocompatibility specificity on the cell surface of one or the other of the lymphocyte classes. This has been ruled out in our initial experiments which demonstrated highly effective cooperation between reciprocal combinations of parental F_1 hybrid T and B lymphocytes and provided that the carrier antigen employed is one to which both parental strains involved are genetic responders (Fig. 6). These findings demonstrate, moreover, that the existence of one common major *H-2* haplotype is sufficient for effective interaction to occur between two cell populations even though the F_1 cells also possess a set of foreign *H-2* specificities.

3. Ineffective or inefficient macrophage–lymphocyte interaction due to major histocompatibility differences. This possibility plays little, if any, significant role in these particular experiments since the major macrophage component is most likely provided by the irradiated F_1 host. The latter not only share a common haplotype with both parental *H-2* specificities but also support good cooperative responses between adoptively transferred isogeneic T and B cells. Furthermore, other studies from our laboratory have provided evidence that, in *in vitro* mouse spleen cell cultures, antigen-bearing macrophages from allogeneic donors are as effective as those from syngeneic donors in presenting DNP-KLH to T and B cells in the elicitation of secondary anti-DNP responses (60). The latter observations, although appearing on the surface to conflict with the observations of Rosenthal and Shevach (61) in guinea pigs, which show a clear preference for histocompatible antigen-bearing macrophages in the induction of *in vitro* proliferative responses of T lymphocytes, are not as contradictory as they seem. Hence, it must be recalled that elicitation of a helper cell function for antibody responses does not require proliferation of T cells as evidenced by the capacity of primed T cells to exert this function even after exposure to X-irradiation (48). It is possible, therefore, that histocompatibility require-

ments for macrophage–T cell interactions, such as those shown by Rosenthal and Shevach (61), are essential for proliferative but not for nonproliferative responses in T lymphocytes. Moreover, it is conceivable that the stringencies of such requirements for macrophage–T cell interactions differ in the guinea pig and the mouse, although we are not inclined to believe this to be the case.

4. Nonspecific suppressive influences exerted by the adoptively transferred allogeneic T cells on the DNP-specific B cells. This seems remote since as discussed above, nonspecific enhancement, rather than suppression, due to allogeneic effects was the major difficulty to overcome in developing the system (57). Moreover, primed parental T cells were shown to serve as effective helper cells for F_1 B cells under circumstances where comparable suppressive effects, had they existed, might be expected to manifest themselves (58). Finally, in an experiment designed to test this possibility directly,

TABLE III
FAILURE OF HISTOINCOMPATIBLE T CELLS TO INTERFERE WITH PHYSIOLOGIC COOPERATION BETWEEN SYNGENEIC T AND B LYMPHOCYTES

Group	Protocol[a]		Anti-DNP antibody response[b] (μg/ml)
	20×10^6 Anti-θ-treated DNP-KLH B cells	50×10^6 Irradiated helper cells	
I	BALB/c	Normal BALB/c	1.2
II	BALB/c	BGG-1° BALB/c	152.7
III	A/J	Normal A/J	5.8
IV	A/J	BGG-1° A/J	173.4
V	BALB/c	Normal A/J	7.3
VI	BALB/c	BGG-1° A/J	4.9
VII	BALB/c	BGG-1° BALB/c + BGG-1° A/J	189.4

[a] 50×10^6 normal or bovine γ-globulin (BGG)-primed spleen cells were transferred intravenously to nonirradiated CAF_1 recipients; 24 hours later, the recipients were irradiated and then given a second transfer consisting of 20×10^6 anti-θ-treated DNP-primed B lymphocytes from either syngeneic or allogeneic donors as indicated. Secondary challenge with 50 μg of DNP-BGG in saline was given intraperitoneally immediately thereafter.

[b] The data are expressed as geometric mean serum anti-DNP levels of groups of 5 mice on day 7 after secondary challenge. Statistical comparisons between the various groups yielded the following results: (1) groups I and II, $0.001 > P$; (2) groups III and IV, $0.001 > P$; (3) groups II and VII, $0.80 > P > 0.70$. Taken from Katz et al. (62).

proof has been obtained that no appreciable nonspecific suppressive influence exists to explain the absence of cooperative responses between histoincompatible T and B cells (62). Thus, as shown in Table III, concomitant transfer of histoincompatible carrier-primed T cells does not appreciably diminish the cooperative response between isogeneic T and B cells (group VII). Likewise, it should be pointed out that in a detailed analysis of the appropriate conditions to conduct these experiments, we were unable to obtain physiologic cooperation between histoincompatible T and B cells over a very wide range of cell doses.

This reasoning has led us to conclude, therefore, that the genetic restrictions for physiologic cooperation between T and B cells in the immune response concern the actual cooperative interaction between these cells. The studies described above as well as the observations of Kindred and Shreffler (54) provide clear evidence that the relevant gene or genes involved belong to the major histocompatibility complex. In the following section we will present the results of our experiments in which we have attempted to identify more precisely the genetic region concerned with H-2 primarily involved.

C. IDENTIFICATION OF HISTOCOMPATIBILITY GENES INVOLVED IN CONTROL OF T–B CELL INTERACTIONS

In our initial studies (58), no cooperation occurred with mixtures of T and B cells from BALB/c (H-2^d) and A/J (H-2^a) donors, respectively (Fig. 5). These particular strains are identical at S and the entire D end of the H-2 complex but possess major differences at the K end. Many differences are known to exist in the I region as well. What this tells us is that gene identities only at S and D are insufficient to permit optimal cooperative interactions to occur under these conditions. It is important, therefore, to determine precisely what gene or combination of gene differences are sufficient to either permit or restrict physiologic T–B cell cooperation.

In view of these findings, which indicate that differences at K and I gene regions prevent effective T–B cell cooperation, we asked whether identities at only K and I are sufficient to allow effective cooperation. In the following experiment (63), we have utilized the microculture system developed in our laboratory for eliciting cooperative T–B cell responses to soluble DNP-carrier conjugates as described elsewhere (58, 64, 65). As shown in Fig. 8, DNP-primed B cells from A/J (H-2^a) donors effectively interact with irradiated KLH-primed T cells from B10.BR donors which differ from A/J at genes in

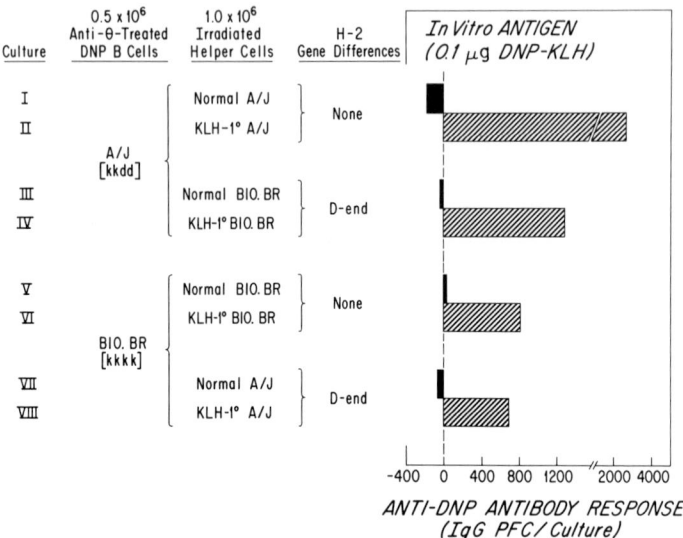

FIG. 8. DNP-ASC-primed spleen cells from A/J and B10.BR donors were depleted of T cells by *in vitro* treatment with anti-Θ serum plus complement and then cultured with either irradiated normal or KLH-primed spleen cells in the combinations indicated. Primed donors were immunized with either DNP-ASC in alum or KLH in CFA 6 months earlier and then boosted with 25 μg of the respective antigen in saline 1 month prior to culture. Cells were cultured with either no antigen (not shown) or DNP-KLH. The background responses of nonstimulated cultures have been subtracted from the numbers of DNP-specific PFC developed in cultures containing DNP-KLH—hence the negative values depicted here. IgG (indirect) DNP-specific PFC responses are shown. Responses in the IgM class (not shown) were parallel. Taken from Katz *et al.* (63).

the S and D regions (group IV). In the reciprocal mixed cell cultures, DNP-primed B cells from B10.BR interacted with KLH-primed T cells from A/J donors (group VIII) as well as isogeneic T cells (group VI) to develop secondary *in vitro* anti-DNP antibody responses to DNP-KLH. As shown in this figure, these data do not reflect nonspecific allogeneic effects as an explanation for successful cooperation between A and B10.BR lymphocytes since reciprocal controls using irradiated normal rather than KLH-primed cells failed to develop secondary responses to DNP-KLH (groups III and VII). These results are, in essence, the reciprocal situation of our initial combination of BALB/c and A/J, which failed to cooperate despite identities at S and D (58). The development of cooperative responses between A/J and B10.BR which differ for genes in S and D but are identical for K and I region genes indicate that the critical genes involved in T–B cell cooperation exist in the latter regions. It must be stated, however, that these results should be considered with some degree of caution until fully corroborated in an *in vivo* system.

The data described above raise the intriguing possibility that identities at the *I* gene region either alone or together with *K* or *D* end identities are critical determinants for T–B cell interaction. By taking advantage of our previous demonstration (Fig. 6) of highly effective cooperation between reciprocal combinations of parental and F_1 hybrid T and B lymphocytes when the carrier molecule employed is one to which both parental strains are genetic responders (58), we next asked the question of whether F_1 carrier-primed T cells can serve as helper cells for either or both parental B cells when: (a) the response to the carrier molecule employed is under genetic control such that one parental strain is a responder and the other is a nonresponder, and (b) the determinant specificity of the parental B cells being assessed is not under genetic control and bears no relationship to the specificity of the carrier molecule (37). The experimental system utilized an immune response gene controlling responses to the terpolymer L-glutamic acid-L-lysine-L-tyrosine (GLT) to which A strain mice (H-2^a) are nonresponders whereas BALB/c (H-2^d) and (BALB/c × A)F_1 hybrids (CAF$_1$) are responders (see Fig. 1). These studies demonstrated that GLT-primed T cells of CAF$_1$ donors can provide for responder BALB/c, but not for nonresponder A/J, the required stimulus for the anti DNP responses of DNP-specific B cells of these respective parental strains to the DNP conjugate of GLT.

The protocol and results of this adoptive transfer experiment is shown in Fig. 9. As an extension of our previously published data (37), the experiment illustrated here includes secondary antigen challenge with macrophage-bound DNP-GLT in addition to the routinely employed intraperitoneal challenge with soluble DNP-carriers (66). As shown in Fig. 9, BALB/c (group II) and A/J (group VIII) DNP-specific B cells are effectively "helped" by KLH-specific T cells of CAF$_1$ origin in developing secondary adoptive anti-DNP antibody responses to DNP-KLH. Similarly, GLT-primed CAF$_1$ T cells cooperate very well with B cells from BALB/c donors in response to either soluble or macrophage-bound DNP-GLT (groups IV and VI). In marked contrast, however, is the failure of these same GLT-specific F_1 T cells to serve as helper cells for DNP-specific B cells from A/J donor mice irrespective of whether soluble or macrophage-bound DNP-GLT is employed for secondary challenge (groups X and XII). There is no possibility that the different results obtained

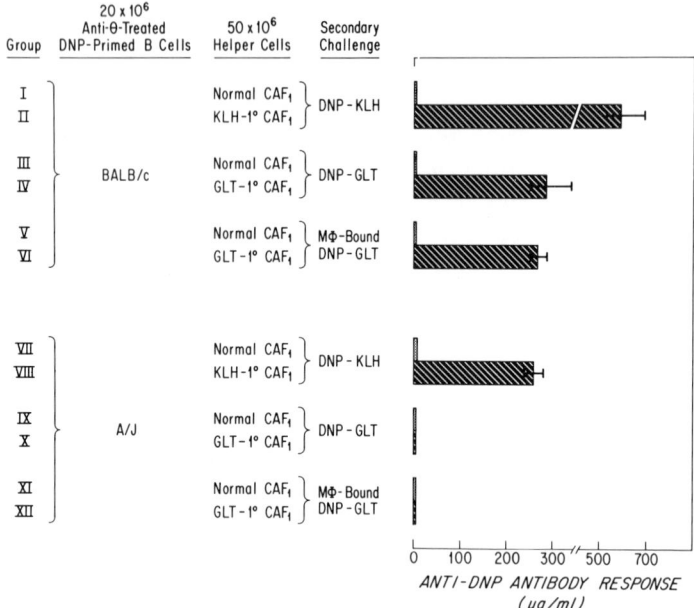

FIG. 9. Involvement of *I* gene in control of T and B lymphocyte interactions. Recipients for all cell combinations were CAF_1 hybrids. The transfer scheme is described in the text. Combinations, strain origins, and specificities of T and B cells are indicated. Secondary challenge was performed intraperitoneally with either 20 μg of soluble DNP-KLH or 100 μg of soluble DNP-GLT or intravenously with 10^7 F_1 macrophages (Mφ) containing 2.4 μg of DNP-GLT per mouse as indicated. Mean serum anti-DNP antibody levels of groups of 5 mice on day 7 after secondary challenge are illustrated. Horizontal bars represent ranges of the standard errors. Taken from Katz and Benacerraf (66).

with BALB/c and A/J B cells reflect marked functional disparities between them since the same pool of cells of respective origins were used in the cooperating mixtures in recipients of CAF_1 KLH-primed cells in which intact function was manifested in both cases (groups II and VIII). The same reasoning applies in the case of the GLT-primed CAF_1 cells, which functioned very well as helpers for BALB/c B cells (groups IV and VI), although failing to do so for A/J cells (groups X and XII).

The two experiments described above permit us to draw certain, albeit not definitive, conclusions concerning the histocompatibility genes involved in controlling optimal T-B cell interactions. Perhaps the most definite statement that can be made is that the genes involved are most likely located to the left of the *S* region, i.e., somewhere in the *K* and/or *I* region(s). It is really not possible to go any further than that with the possible exception of stating that differences in the *I-C* subregion of the *H-2* complex do not prevent effective physiological T-B interactions since the A and B10.BR combinations do, in fact, differ in this subregion (16). It is not possible to conclude, as yet, whether identity at the *I* region alone or identity at the *I* region together with genes coded for at the *K* end of *H-2* are sufficient for cooperation. The data obtained in the A/J ↔ B10.BR combinations (Fig. 8) should not be construed to mean that identities of genes in *both* the *K* and *I* regions are required for effective cell interaction. Thus, we know from the DNP-GLT studies that under certain circumstances a difference in *Ir* genes can prevent effective cooperation when the carrier antigen employed is the one to which the *Ir* gene control is directed (Fig. 9). Similarly, it must be stressed that the response to DNP-KLH employed in the A/J ↔ B10.BR experiment is not governed by known *Ir* gene differences among the A/J and B10.BR strains. The existence of identities of *K* region genes in this combination could well be insufficient for effective cooperation to occur under circumstances where the carrier used is one to which the response is controlled by an *Ir* gene that is present in one but not the other. Further definition of these possibilities requires additional experimentation of the type presented above using appropriate recombinant strains.

D. Relevance of Genetic Requirements for T-B Cell Interactions

Before speculating on the biological implications of the above data, it is essential to emphasize the point that these experiments demonstrate that certain identities of *H-2* genes are required for the *most effective* T-B cell interactions; such identities may not constitute an absolute requirement for T-B interactions to occur under certain circumstances. Thus, Bechtol *et al.* (33) have observed that tetraparental mice derived from responder and nonresponder strains may produce antibodies of nonresponder allotype under conditions of hyperimmunization. More recent studies from our own laboratories by Benacerraf *et al.* (38) have demonstrated that in a totally *in vitro* system (responder × nonresponder) F_1 T cells primed to the terpolymer L-glutamic acid, L-alanine, L-tyrosine (GAT), which fail to provide helper function for nonresponder B cells in response to GAT added to cultures in free soluble form, will "help" such B cells when the GAT is added to cultures in small quantities attached to macrophages. However, as presented above (Fig. 9), DNP-GLT on macrophages failed to elicit a cooperative anti-DNP response between F_1 responder T cells and parental nonresponder B cells *in vivo*. Finally, it should be reiterated that as seen in the allogeneic effect, activated allogeneic T cells provide the necessary stimulus for triggering antigen-activated B cells if the specificity of the T cell is directed against surface alloantigen differences on the B cell themselves (53).

Within this framework, and recognizing that clearly much additional work is needed to define precisely which gene(s) in the major histocompatibility complex are most critically involved in T-B cell interactions, we are able to evaluate the significance of the need for a common gene product on T and B cells for physiologic cooperation to be optimally effective in the development of humoral immune responses. The requirement for a common gene product on T and B cells for physiologic cooperation to occur clearly suggests something of critical importance relevant to the mechanism by which such interactions occur. On the basis of our observations, we have proposed that these genetic considerations provide evidence for the existence on the B lymphocyte surface membrane of a site closely related to the histocompatibility specificity that is critically involved in physiologic T-B cell interaction (37, 58, 59, 63). We envisage this relevant site as an "acceptor" molecule either for the active T cell product or the T cell itself. The necessity for the T and B cells to possess the same gene or genes for physiologic cooperation requires that the same gene product is expressed on both cells or, alternatively, if two gene products are expressed in the respective cell types, the genes concerned have remained closely linked.

As discussed at length in the preceding sections, the number of specific H-linked *Ir* genes that have been identified and the specific manner in which they permit immune responses to distinct antigens to take place, particularly at the T cell level, has suggested that they are somehow involved in either the specificity or the function of the T cell antigen receptors and may, therefore, be clonally expressed in this class of lymphocytes. Our experiments on the F_1-parent cooperative responses to DNP-GLT described above (Fig. 9) may be interpreted to indicate that *Ir* genes may also be expressed in B cells and demonstrate that their activity is concerned with successful T-B cell interactions in specific immune responses involving carrier recognition.

However, an alternative explanation for our results is that GLT-activated F_1 T cells, under control of the relevant *I* gene on one of its *H-2* alleles are limited to effective cooperation only with the B lymphocytes of the parent expressing the histocompatibility specificities coded for by the allele possessing the GLT *Ir* gene. According to this alternative, there would be no requirement for the functional expression of the *Ir* gene product in the B cell, but only a requirement for the *Ir* gene product or associated *I* region gene product(s) from the T cell to govern the interaction with the B cell at the histocompatibility site on the B cell surface.

The identity at the *I* region of the *H-2* complex required for physiologic T and B cell cooperation may be interpreted to indicate that the surface molecules on T and B cells responsible for this phenomenon are coded for in this region. The recent finding that alloantisera against lymphocytes prepared between congenic mice which differ at the *I* region react with B and T cells (67–69) is consistent with the hypothesis that these antisera are specific for surface molecules concerned with cooperative interactions between these cells.

To elaborate further, we envisage the following sequence involved in effective T–B cell interactions: The antigen-activated T lymphocyte, in close proximity to the appropriate B cell, either engages direct contact at the specific "acceptor" site (s) on the B cell surface and/or releases the active products that have specific complementarity for, and bind to, the specific "acceptor" sites on the B lymphocyte. The relevant surface molecules involved are conceivably products of the histocompatibility gene complex. It is likely that the antigen-binding event on the specific B cell surface Ig receptors has already taken place before the relevant interaction with the T cell or its product occurs. Perhaps one of the important consequences of the antigen-binding event followed by subsequent movement, capping, and endocytosis of the B cell surface immunoglobulin receptors (70) is either appropriately to expose greater numbers of "acceptor" sites or even to induce steric conformational changes in the acceptor molecule. Likewise, it is conceivable that the process of activation of the T cell results in a critical steric or structural alteration in the active moiety, which allows it then to interact with the B-cell acceptor. This mechanism would explain the discriminant regulation involved in normal immune responses since only those T and B lymphocytes whose surface sites have been either appropriately exposed or structurally altered by activation events would be capable of successful interaction.

VII. Identification of *I* Region Gene Products

The growing recognition of the biological significance of genes in the *I* region of the *H-2* complex stimulated pursuit of the possibility of producing alloantisera against these cell surface membrane determinants to use in studies designed to identify, assay, isolate, and biochemically define the *I* region gene products. This task has been successfully approached by several independent laboratories in the last two years and has been marked by the incredible pace at which progress has been made in this area. The history of developments along these lines has been recently reviewed in great detail by Shreffler and David (16) and will not be reiterated here. Instead, we will describe, in general terms, the nature of the antigen system defined by the alloantisera produced by various investigators and the possible relationship of this system to function in the development of immune responses.

This entire area of investigation was made possible only by the development and identification of pairs of recombinant strains of mice which differ only in the *I* and *S* gene regions of the *H-2* complex. Utilizing such recombinant pairs, reciprocal cross-immunizations with lymphoid tissues resulted in production of a variety of different antisera which react with cell membrane alloantigens shown to be controlled by genes located in the *I* region. The various recombinant strains used to prepare and the defined specificities of these various antisera are reviewed elsewhere (16). The antigen system defined by such antisera in the mouse has now been designated *Ia* (*I* region-associated antigens) and encompasses the entire set of serologically detected specificities controlled by genes in the *I* region of which ten such specificities have been identified to date by various investigators (16).

The anti-*Ia* antisera are generally multispecific and accordingly have been studied by direct testing and absorption analyses to assign the various *Ia* specificities to appropriate haplotypes (16). Studies of this type, which attempt to localize the *Ia* specificities on the *H-2* genetic map, have resulted in the proposed designation of three distinct *Ia* loci—*Ia-1*, *Ia-2*, and *Ia-3*—which fall into one of the three *I* subregions—*Ir-1A*, *Ir-1B*, and *I-C*, respectively. Further definition of additional *Ia* specificities and their assignment to the genetic map will undoubtedly be forthcoming in this rapidly moving field.

The biochemical studies performed thus far have only quite recently been reported by Cullen *et al.* (71) but are clearly definitive in establishing the distinction between *Ia* antigens and *H-2* antigens. These studies were performed utilizing an established assay system for detection of *H-2* antigens that have been radiolabeled on the cell surface membrane (72). The method involves dissociating the cell membrane in a nonionic detergent, separating the antigens of interest from the remainder of the membrane constituents by immunoprecipitation with specific antisera (i.e., either anti-*H-2* or anti-*Ia*), solubilization of the precipitates with sodium dodecyl sulfate (SDS), and then electrophoresis on SDS polyacrylamide gel. The resulting gels are then scanned for the presence of the radioactive label. Using this procedure, Cullen *et al.* (*71*) demonstrated the presence of a peak, after reduction, of molecular weight 30,000 in the specific immune precipitates developed with anti-*Ia* sera as contrasted with peaks of 45,000 daltons in immunoprecipitates developed with specific anti-*H-2K* or *H-2D* sera. The 30,000 MW antigen was shown to be a glycoprotein associated with cell membranes on normal lymph node and spleen lymphocytes, but not on various tumor cells (*71*). Moreover, it was shown that removal of *H-2K* and *H-2D* antigens from a radiolabeled detergent extract by appropriate anti-*H-2K* and anti-*H-2D* sera did not remove the 30,000 MW *Ia* antigen peak (*71*). Finally, in complete concordance with the aforementioned biochemical evidence, Unanue *et al.* (*73*) have very recently demonstrated the distinct existence of *Ia* molecules on the cell surface in studies on the movement of cell surface antigens. Thus, anti-*H-2 sera* directed against the *D* or *K* antigens, or anti-*Ia* sera were found to induce movement, capping, and aggregation of the respective specific determinants to which they are directed completely independently of one another. Thus, on both biochemical and cytological grounds, it is now firmly established that *Ia* antigens exist as molecular entities on the cell surface membrane distinct from other molecules coded for by genes in the *K* or *D* regions of *H-2*.

In terms of the tissue distribution of *Ia* antigens, however, the picture is not yet as ultimately conclusive. There is no doubt that the *Ia* antigens are present in greatest quantities on lymphocytes in the secondary lymphoid organs — i.e., lymph nodes and spleen — and are not present on cells of brain, liver, or kidneys or on erythrocytes (*74*). The confusion has centered about which cells of the lymphoid system possess these surface structures. Initially, it was thought that the anti-*Ia* sera reacted predominantly with T lymphocytes (*67, 74, 75*) whereas somewhat later the studies of Sachs and Cone (*68*) and Hämmerling *et al.* (*69*) provided compelling evidence that the *Ia* antigens were present exclusively on B cells. More recently, it has been shown that the antigens may exist on both cells, although in what appears to be different quantities (and perhaps distribution patterns), and that some anti-*Ia* sera may react exclusively with B cells whereas others may react with both B and T cells (*76*). The distribution of reaction with given antisera may vary depending on the strength of the antisera and/or sensitivity of the assay systems employed to detect reactivity. At any rate, there is general agreement that the strongest reactivity of these antisera is with antigens on B lymphocytes (60). Quite recently, cytological analyses have shown that by radioautography the highest level of labeling with anti-*Ia* sera is on B cells, most of which are labeled, whereas only a small proportion of T cells pick up label and in smaller amounts (77). Similarly, Unanue *et al.* have shown by fluorescence that certain anti-*Ia* sera react with peripheral B cells but not with T cells (73). The latter investigators have also shown that the same anti-*Ia* sera react with surface membrane components on macrophages (73), providing the first direct evidence for the existence of *Ia* antigens on such cells.

The key point worth emphasis here is that the discovery of this new and intriguing antigen system makes it very clear that the genes in the *I* region code for a number of antigenic specificities present on lymphoid cells which, although distinguishable upon genetic analysis, are not as yet easily, if at all, distinguishable on the basis of their roles in cell function(s). This will be discussed at greater length in the following section.

VIII. Relationship of Histocompatibility Gene Products to Each Other in Nature and Function

In order to develop a better understanding of the relationship of histocompatibility antigens, *Ir* genes, and immune recognition, studies have been carried out in several laboratories in the past several years on the functional effects of certain specific alloantisera on lymphocyte responses to antigen. The first studies of this type were made in guinea pigs by Shevach *et al.* (78), who examined the effect of specific alloantisera on lymphocyte stimulation induced by antigens under *Ir* gene control. Their experiments demonstrated that the *in vitro* proliferative response of lymphocytes from strain 2 or strain 13 animals both to antigens under *Ir* gene control (DNP-GL in strain 2 and GT in strain 13) and to PPD which is not known to be under genetic control were inhibited by the appropriate alloantiserum to a similar degree. However, when cells from $(2 \times 13)F_1$ animals were used, only the response linked to the histocompatibility antigens against which the serum was directed could be inhibited by a given alloantiserum. Thus, anti-2 serum inhibited the response of F_1 cells to DNP-GL but not to GT, whereas the anti-13 serum inhibited the response to GT but not to DNP-GL. The authors concluded from these data that the alloantisera were inhibiting T lymphocyte antigen recognition through interference with the activity of *Ir* gene products on the cell surface. Studies in the mouse by Lonai (47), which have demonstrated that anti-*H-2* sera block the induction of tritiated thymidine uptake from responder mice immunized with (H,G)-A—L and (Phe,G)-A—L, have been similarly interpreted.

Subsequent studies in the guinea pig performed more recently were designed to delineate whether the inhibitory antibodies in the alloantisera were directed against H antigens or against the products of the *Ir* genes (79, 80) by examining the capacity of anti-2 serum to inhibit the function of the Ir-GA gene, which in most outbred Hartley guinea pigs is linked to genes bearing strain 2 specificities, when the GA gene occurs in an outbred animal lacking strain 2 H genes. In this situation, anti-2 serum which effectively inhibited the *in vitro* proliferative response to GA of T cells derived from animals that were GA^+ and $2^\pm$, had little or no effect on such responses of T cells from GA^+2^- guinea pigs. Moreover, an antiserum prepared in strain 13 animals against lymphoid cells of a GA^+2^- outbred animal failed to exhibit any inhibitory activity whereas a strain 13 anti-GA^+2^+ antiserum specifically inhibited the response to GA of cells from $(2 \times 13)F_1$ guinea pigs. These data indicate that the inhibitory activity of anti-2 serum on GA responses is mediated via antibodies directed toward strain 2 H antigens rather than antibodies specific for the product of the GA *Ir* gene, leading the authors to speculate on the possible covalent linkage of *Ir* gene products with H antigens (79).

In a recent series of experiments, Pierce *et al.* (81, 82) have analyzed the effects of alloantisera on Mishell-Dutton *in vitro* primary antibody responses in the mouse. These studies have shown that antisera directed against *H-2* antigens markedly inhibit (up to 90%) the primary antibody response to sheep erythrocytes (SRBC); both IgM and IgG antibody classes are so affected with whole anti-*H-2* sera. The inhibitory activity can be absorbed with lymphoid cells bearing the appropriate haplotype but cannot be absorbed by mouse immunoglobulins. When F_1 cells are tested, anti-*H-2* sera directed against either parental haplotype will effectively inhibit the primary *in vitro* response.

The specificity characteristics of the inhibition of *in vitro* antibody responses can be summarized as follows (81, 82): (1) antisera directed against the entire *H-2* complex will block both IgM and IgG responses; (2) antisera tested in congenic strains against non-*H-2* gene products will also inhibit in certain cases, thus indicating the involvement of other specificities in these phenomena; (3) antisera directed against unique K specificities—i.e., private specificity H-2.19—will inhibit both IgM and IgG responses; (4) antisera directed against specificities in the K end of H-2 block the whole response, whereas anti-D sera fail to inhibit at all; and (5) finally, antisera directed against I specificities inhibit selectively responses of the IgG antibody class.

The cellular locus of action of these antisera is of particular interest in view of the discussion concerning histocompatibility requirements for cell interactions (Section VI). Thus, it appears that the antisera act at two levels: the first, on macrophages in exerting their inhibitory effects; when this occurs both IgM and IgG responses are blocked (82). Nonetheless, macrophages that have been exposed to the appropriate alloantiserum are not deficient in their capacity to bind and handle antigen. It is clear therefore that the mechanism of inhibition at the level of the macrophage involves events other than simple antigen uptake by these cells and probably indicates a block in macrophage–lymphocyte interactions. In addition, the alloantisera can also be shown to inhibit at the level of the lymphocyte populations; however, only IgG responses are inhibited in the latter circumstances implying the probable action of antibodies directed against I region antigens when inhibition is operative at the level of the lymphocytes.

Quite recently, radioautographic studies have been carried out independently in two laboratories on the effects of specific anti-H-2 sera on the binding of antigens under Ir gene control by thymocytes in the mouse. Hämmerling and McDevitt (45) analyzed the effects of anti-H-2 and anti-Ig sera on binding by thymocytes of (T,G)-A—L in responder and (responder × nonresponder)F_1 mice. Their observations were that: (1) thymocyte binding of (T,G)-A—L could be inhibited 50–70% (*but never completely*) by anti Ig sera containing antibodies directed against IgM and kappa specificities, but not by those directed against IgG determinants; (2) alloantisera directed against either the entire H-2 complex or against K or D end specificities *completely* inhibited thymocyte binding of (T,G)-A—L; (3) in the case of F_1 cells, antigen-binding could be inhibited by antisera directed against either responder or nonresponder parental haplotype. The latter observation is at first glance surprising in view of the functional observations in guinea pigs of Shevach *et al.* (78) discussed above, but consistent with the recent findings that thymocytes are capable of binding antigen in nonresponder mice both in the (T,G)-A—L system (83) and in the GAT system (46).

Studies in our own laboratories by Kennedy *et al.* (*46*) have been carried out on antigen-binding thymocytes in the Ir-GAT system in mice. These studies have shown that: (1) GAT-binding thymocytes are present, and in comparable numbers, in both responder and nonresponder animals; (2) the binding of GAT by these cells can be completely inhibited by alloantisera directed against the appropriate haplotype, in agreement with the observations of Hämmerling and McDevitt (*45*); (3) on the other hand, thymocyte binding of GAT was not inhibited by anti-Ig antisera directed against either IgM or IgG specificities. The reason for the difference in the capacity of anti-Ig to inhibit binding in Hämmerling and McDevitt's study and the failure of Kennedy *et al.* to observe such inhibition is not yet resolved but is perhaps explainable on the possible existence of antimembrane antibody activity known to be present in antimouse immunoglobulin sera.

IX. Function of Products of H-Linked *Ir* Genes and of Other *I* Region Gene Products: Relationship of These Products to Activation of Immunocompetent Cells

In this section, we will attempt to bring together in a résumé fashion what we have presented in the preceding sections in order to develop a cogent hypothesis concerning the functional relationships of *Ir* genes and other *I* region products in the development of immune responses. The products of H-linked *Ir* genes must be endowed with considerable specificity since different genes are required for the ability to respond to unrelated antigens and since in several cases these genes have been shown to map at different loci.

Considering that compelling evidence has been presented that virtually rules out the possibility that H-linked *Ir* genes are V-region genes of immunoglobulin (a role that belongs to the allotype-linked *Ir* genes), the very clear specificity involved in the function of H-linked *Ir* genes must therefore be explained by the existence of an additional recognition system in immunocompetent cells distinct from that of the immunoglobulin system. It is also apparent that the *Ir* system is more restricted than that represented by the immunoglobulin V-region dictionary, although the precise size of the *Ir* gene repertoire must remain conjectural until further knowledge is developed in this area.

As discussed in Section IV, perhaps the most intriguing aspect of our knowledge concerning *Ir* gene function is that the recognition function controlled by *Ir* genes is expressed in T cells, which are precisely those lymphocytes about which the least knowledge exists concerning the chemical nature of the antigen receptor. Based upon the data obtained in antihistocompatibility antisera–inhibition studies of antigen-induced *in vitro* blast transformation in guinea pigs (78) and mice (47), it has been proposed that the *Ir* gene product functions, indeed, as *the* or one of the antigen receptors on T cells. However, any hypothesis that assigns the role of antigen receptor to the H-linked *Ir* gene products must contend with two fundamental observations described herein. First, it is documented in two systems that thymocytes from nonresponder animals are able to bind the antigen under *Ir* gene control and in numbers comparable to those found in responder animals. Second, on the basis of functional studies with GAT, it has been shown that although nonresponder animals are unable to develop GAT-specific helper T cell function, they can nevertheless be stimulated by GAT to express suppressor T cell activity. In the absence of conclusive evidence concerning the relationship of helper versus suppressor T cells — i.e., whether these are indeed one and the same, or alternatively different cells with distinct receptors — the aforementioned data nevertheless indicate the existence of antigen-binding capacity by T cells in nonresponder animals, albeit that the binding results exclusively in suppressor activity. If, indeed, the hypothesis that *Ir* genes are antigen receptors on T cells is viable, then, as discussed in Section V, we must consider the following alternatives: (1) Helper and suppressor T cells are distinct and possess different receptors with analogous specificity. (2) Helper and suppressor T cells have identical receptors, which are, in fact, the *Ir* gene products, but in nonresponder animals these gene products are capable of binding antigen only inadequately (i.e., either due to lower avidity and/or in lower numbers). (3) The *Ir* gene products are not per se the primary antigen-receptor of the T cell, but rather are intimately associated with such receptors, and it is essential that they be present and interacted with, specifically, for the T cell to be differentiated into cells capable of exerting effector functions of helper cells and cells concerned with cellular immunity. The last hypothesis is also compatible with the possibility that *Ir* gene function is expressed only in a subpopulation of T cells, concerned with the positive regulation of both T cell and B cell activity, which have generally been identified as "helper" T cells (48).

Irrespective of which of these hypotheses is correct, the recognition controlled by the *Ir* gene system in immune responses in T cells bears directly on the pathway along which a given immune response will develop. In other words, the *Ir* gene products are positioned strategically at the crossroads between immunity and tolerance, particularly at the T cell level, and it is therefore not surprising that, as will be documented in the last section of this review, the *Ir* genes play a significant role in the pathogenesis of certain conditions where immune responses are involved.

Another major advance in cellular immunology in the last few years has been the recognition that cell interaction among T cells, B cells, and macrophages are conditioned by the presence of surface molecules coded for in the major histocompatibility gene complex in several species. As discussed in Section VI, it appears that the genes involved in these interactions are located in the mouse to the left of the *S* region, i.e., in the *K* and/or *I* region of the complex. In view of the identification of multiple *I* region specificities that exist in greatest quantities on B lymphocytes, and moreover, the distinction of these molecules from the *Ir* gene products themselves, it is very conceivable that one or more of these *I* region molecules are concerned with the mechanisms of such cell interactions. Indeed, the evidence obtained very recently in studies concerned with inhibition of *in vitro* immune responses by such anti-*I* reagents support this hypothesis. It is of considerable interest in this regard that the MLC reactions occur between T and B lymphocytes which differ genetically by surface molecules coded for predominantly in the *I* region, and likewise these reactions are inhibited by appropriate anti-*Ia* reagents.

It is clear to us that the proximal relationship of *Ir* gene products to other *I* region genes in the chromosome is not merely fortuitous. That is to say that this relationship has both evolutionary and functional connotations of great significance. We would like to develop the following hypothesis for the functional relationship between *Ir* gene products concerned with recognition of antigen and other products of the *I* region most probably concerned with cell interactions. Thus, it is conceivable that the interaction of antigen with the *Ir* gene product on the T cell is the essential prerequisite for the activation of the critical *I* region molecules on the T cell which control the subsequent interaction of such activated cells (or the release of active molecules from these cells) with either B lymphocytes or other T lymphocytes. According to this hypothesis, the *Ir* gene product would exhibit both recognition and regulatory functions. In order to perform such regulatory functions, the *Ir* genes would be expected to be spatially related on the T cell membrane in close proximity to other products of the histocompatibility complex concerned with cell interactions.

In favor of the above hypothesis, we can cite the following evidence. (1) In the guinea pig, as presented in Section VIII, it is clear that the alloantisera that inhibit the *Ir* gene-controlled antigen-induced blast transformation of F_1 lymphocytes do so not by reacting with the products of *Ir* genes themselves, but rather by reacting with histocompatibility molecules coded for in the major histocompatibility complex. It is significant that although they do not react with the *Ir* gene product, the alloantisera must interact on an F_1 T cell with the products coded for on the same haplotype as the *Ir* gene concerned if such antisera are to be suppressive. Antisera directed against products coded for on the opposite haplotype are ineffective in this regard. (2) The finding as detailed in Section VI that, for an antigen the response to which is under *Ir* gene control, the cooperation between (responder × nonresponder)F_1 T cells and parental B cells is restricted to the B cells bearing the responder parental haplotype can also be interpreted as indicating that an *Ir* gene on the same haplotype as the molecules concerned with T–B cell interactions must be activated if the latter are to take place successfully.

X. The Histocompatibility-Linked *Ir* Genes and Disease

The importance of H-linked immune response genes in the pathogenesis of diseases where the immune system plays a crucial role is becoming increasingly apparent, primarily in experimental laboratory models, but also in clinical medicine.

In the context of this volume, it is appropriate to consider first and foremost the role of H-linked *Ir* genes in the development of tumor immunity and tumor rejection. It is now well established that malignant neoplasms bear distinct tumor-specific antigens, among which some surface antigens are responsible for the stimulation of tumor immunity. The immune responses to tumor-specific antigens and particularly to tumor-specific transplantation antigens (TSTA) are recognized as being very complex, involving cellular immunity, cytotoxic and blocking antibodies and the development of suppressor cells. It is not the province of this review to consider in detail the various forms of immunity generated by tumor specific antigens nor the delicate balance of these responses as they affect tumor growth.

However, as we have been able to document in this review, all immune responses to thymus-dependent antigens, and particularly cellular immune responses, are probably under the control of one or more specific H-linked *Ir* genes, depending upon the complexity or degree of foreignness of the antigen. The immune response of tumor-bearing hosts to TSTAs and other tumor antigens could also be expected to be under control of H-linked *Ir* genes. This has indeed proved to be the case in selected tumor systems. For reasons unrelated to the study of tumor immunity, Lilly investigated the genetic factors controlling the susceptibility to Gross virus leukemogenesis in inbred mouse strains (84, 85). He was able to identify two major genes controlling this process. One of these genes, termed *RgV-1*, was found to be closely linked to *H-2* genotype and to map in the left side of the *H-2* complex, precisely where *Ir* genes are encoded (85). Similarly, susceptibility to Friend virus leukemia was also shown to be linked to *H-2*. At the time these findings were made, it appeared reasonable to propose that the relationship between tumor susceptibility and *H-2* genotype could be explained by the absence of the appropriate *Ir* gene in the susceptible strains rendering them incapable of developing an adequate immune response against the tumor-specific antigens. This interpretation received support from the findings by Lilly that resistance was dominant and that no relationship could be shown between susceptibility to leukemia and the presence of virus receptors on the cells (84). More recently this interpretation was verified by the experiments of Sato *et al.* (86), who described the following system:

Two BALB radiation leukemias are strongly rejected by hybrids of BALB with certain other mouse strains, although BALB mice themselves exhibit no detectable resistance whatever. Hybrids immunized with progressively larger inocula are resistant to 200×10^6 or more leukemia cells; their serum is cytotoxic for the leukemia cells *in vitro* and protects BALB mice against challenge with these BALB leukemias. The antigenic system thus identified has been named X.1.

In (BALB × B6) hybrids the major determinant of resistance was shown to be a B6 gene which maps in the left side of the *H-2* complex. This is likely to be the *Rgv-1* locus of Lilly, which may thus be identified in this case as an *Ir* allele conferring ability to respond to X.1 antigen on MuLV and leukemia cells, and therefore responsible for production of X.1 antibody and the rejection of X.1$^+$ leukemia cells by hybrid mice (see Fig. 1). Thus, H-linked immune response gene control of tumor immunity has been demonstrated in this experimental system.

These findings can be generalized to other tumor systems and may indeed explain the well known phenomenon that tumors which arose in parental hosts grow more slowly in certain selected F_1 hybrid recipients than in animals syngeneic with the parental host. This phenomenon, which was originally described by Hellstrom (87,

88) and studied in many laboratories by, among others, Sanford (89, 90), Fisher (91, 92), and Oth (93) [reviewed recently by Oth (94)], is probably best explained on the basis of a stronger immune response by the F_1 hybrid strains than by the syngeneic host. As expected, the ability to resist tumor growth better than the syngeneic host is only displayed by F_1 hybrid bearing selected H-2 haplotypes and was shown to be clearly determined by genes at the H-2 complex contributed by the allogeneic parent. Moreover, these differences between syngeneic hosts and F_1 hosts in their ability to resist the growth of implanted tumors are abolished by treatments which impair immune responsiveness such as antilymphocyte serum (91) or X-irradiation (95, 96).

Current studies in our laboratory (97) using DBA/2 P815 mastocytoma and a methylcholanthrene-induced sarcoma of C57Bl/6 origin are in agreement with this interpretation. Thus, the capacity to mount successful immune responses against tumor antigens depends upon the possession of appropriate Ir genes. Conversely, the most malignant tumors would be expected to develop in hosts which lack the Ir gene required for the development of tumor immunity.

The effect of H-linked Ir genes has also been recognized in other diseases, besides tumors, where the immune response plays a part. The development of autoimmune thyroiditis in the mouse was shown by Rose et al. to depend upon the presence of an H-linked Ir gene (98). The susceptibility of rats to develop experimental allergic encephalomyelitis after the injection of encephalitogenic protein was shown by Williams and Moore (99) to be controlled by an Ir gene linked to the major histocompatibility locus of the rat. The susceptibility of mice to the pathogenic effect of lymphocytic choriomeningitis virus was shown to be linked to H-2 genotype and to depend upon the ability to form a strong immune response against the virus (100). In this disease the animals which form the stronger immune response develop brain lesions and die. As would be expected, susceptibility to the lethal effect of the virus is dominant and linked to H-2.

There is also evidence of the activity of H-linked Ir genes in man and of their effect on the pathogenesis of allergic diseases. Levine et al. (101) have studied the inheritance in selected families of the susceptibility to develop hay fever and to synthesize reagents against ragweed antigens and found this response to be linked to HL-A in a highly significant number of cases.

Thus, within a relatively short time the importance of H-linked Ir genes in the pathogenesis of several diseases where immune responses play an important role has become recognized.

Acknowledgments

We are extremely grateful to our many colleagues and collaborators who participated in the studies performed in our laboratories cited here. These include Drs. Dieter Armerding, Hans Balner, Martin Dorf, Toshiyuki Hamaoka, James Kennedy, Frank Lilly, Paul Maurer, David Osborne, Jr., Carl Pierce, Donald Shreffler, Emil Unanue, R. Michael Williams, and Judith Kapp. We are particularly indebted to Dr. Martin Dorf for invaluable help in the gathering of materials to prepare Figs. 1 and 3 and this review and Dr. Dieter Armerding for help in preparing Fig. 2. The excellent secretarial assistance of Ms. Candace Maher in the preparation of the manuscript is greatly appreciated.

The studies performed in our laboratories were supported by Grants AI-10630 and AI-09920 from The National Institutes of Health.

References

1. McDevitt, H. O., and Benacerraf, B. (1969). *Advan. Immunol.* **11**, 31.
2. Benacerraf, B., and McDevitt, H. O. (1972). *Science* **175**, 273.
3. Benacerraf, B. (1974). *Ann. Immunol. (Inst. Pasteur)* **125C**, 143.
4. McDevitt, H. O., and Chinitz, A. (1969). *Science* **163**, 1207.
5. Ellman, L., Green, I., Martin, W. J., and Benacerraf, B. (1970). *Proc. Nat. Acad. Sci. U. S.* **66**, 322.
6. Armerding, D., and Rajewsky, K. (1970). *Protides Biol. Fluids, Proc. Colloq.* **17**, 185.
7. Günther, R., Rüde, E., and Stark, O. (1972). *Eur. J. Immunol.* **2**, 151.
8. Armerding, D., Katz, D. H., and Benacerraf, B. (1974). *Immunogenetics* **1**, 329.
9. Dorf, M. E., Balner, H., de Groot, L., and Benacerraf, B. (1974). *Transplant. Proc.* **6**, 119.
10. Balner, H., Dorf, M. E., de Groot, M. L., and Benacerraf, B. (1973). *Transplant. Proc.* **5**, 1555.
11. Levine, B. B., Ojeda, A., and Benacerraf, B. (1963). *J. Exp. Med.* **118**, 953.
12. McDevitt, H. O., and Sela, M. (1965). *J. Exp. Med.* **122**, 517.
13. McDevitt, H. O., Deak, B. D., Shreffler, D. C., Klein, J., Stimpfling, J. H., and Snell, G. D. (1972). *J. Exp. Med.* **135**, 1259.
14. Dorf, M. E., Plate, J. M. D., Stimpfling, J., and Benacerraf, B. (1975). *J. Immunol.*, in press.
15. Klein, J., and Shreffler, D. C. (1971). *Transplant. Rev.* **6**, 3.
16. Shreffler, D. C., and David, C. S. (1975). *Advan. Immunol.*, in press.
17. Lieberman, R., Paul, W. E., Humphrey, W., Jr., and Stimpfling, J. H. (1972). *J. Exp. Med.* **136**, 1231.
18. Dorf, M. E., Lilly, F., and Benacerraf, B. (1974). *J. Exp. Med.* **40**, 859.
19. Ellman, L., Green, I., and Benacerraf, B. (1971). *J. Immunol.* **107**, 382.
20. Bach, F. H., Widmer, M. B., Bach, M. L., and Klein, J. (1972). *J. Exp. Med.* **136**, 1430.
21. Blomberg, B., Geckeler, W. R., and Weigert, M. (1972). *Science* **177**, 178.
22. Eichmann, E. (1972). *Eur. J. Immunol.* **4**, 301.
23. Pawlak, L. L., and Nisonoff, A. (1973). *J. Exp. Med.* **137**, 855.
24. Landucci Tosi, S., Mage, R. G., and Dubiski, S. (1970). *J. Immunol.* **104**, 641.
25. McDevitt, H. O. Personal communication.
26. Ellman, L., Green, I., and Benacerraf, B. (1970). *Cell. Immunol.* **1**, 445.
27. Kapp, J. A., Pierce, C. W., and Benacerraf, B. (1973). *J. Exp. Med.* **138**, 1107.
28. Green, I., and Benacerraf, B. (1971). *J. Immunol.* **107**, 374.
29. Mitchell, G. F., Grumet, F. C., and McDevitt, H. O. (1972). *J. Exp. Med.* **135**, 126.

30. Green, I., Paul, W. E., and Benacerraf, B. (1969). *Proc. Nat. Acad. Sci. U. S.* **64**, 1095.
31. Dunham, E. K., Unanue, E. R., and Benacerraf, B. (1972). *J. Exp. Med.* **136**, 403.
32. Ordal, J. C., and Grumet, F. C. (1972). *J. Exp. Med.* **136**, 1195.
33. Bechtol, K. B., Herzenberg, L. A., and McDevitt, H. O. (1972). *Fed. Proc., Fed. Amer. Soc. Exp. Biol.* **31**, 777. (Abstr.)
34. Kapp, J. A., Pierce, C. W., and Benacerraf, B. (1973). *J. Exp. Med.* **138**, 1121.
35. Shearer, G. M., Mozes, E., and Sela, M. (1972). *J. Exp. Med.* **135**, 1109.
36. McDevitt, H. O., and Landy, M., eds. (1973). "Genetic Control of Immune Responsiveness: Relationship to Disease Susceptibility." Academic Press, New York.
37. Katz, D. H., Hamaoka, T., Dorf, M. E., Maurer, P. H., and Benacerraf, B. (1973). *J. Exp. Med.* **138**, 734.
38. Benacerraf, B., Kapp, J. A., Pierce, C. W., and Katz, D. H. (1974). *J. Exp. Med.* **140**, 185.
39. Gershon, R. K. (1974). *Contemp. Top. Immunobiol.* **3**, 1.
40. Basten, A. (1974). *In* "Immunological Tolerance: Mechanisms and Potential Therapeutic Applications" (D. H. Katz and B. Benacerraf, eds.), pp. 107. Academic Press, New York.
41. Claman, H. N., Phanuphak, P., and Moorehead, J. W. (1974). *In* "Immunological Tolerance: Mechanisms and Potential Therapeutic Applications" (D. H. Katz and B. Benacerraf, ed.), pp. 123. Academic Press, New York.
42. Gershon, R. K., Maurer, P. H., and Merryman, C. F. (1973). *Proc. Nat. Acad. Sci. U. S.* **70**, 250.
43. Kapp, J. A., Pierce, C. W., and Benacerraf, B. (1974). *J. Exp. Med.* **140**, 172.
44. Kapp, J. A., Pierce, C. W., Schlossman, S., and Benacerraf, B. (1974). *J. Exp. Med.* **140**, 648.
45. Hämmerling, G. J., and McDevitt, H. O. (1974). *J. Immunol.* **112**, 1734.
46. Kennedy, J., Unanue, E. R., and Benacerraf, B. (1975) (in press).
47. Lonai, P. (1973). *Fed. Proc., Fed. Amer. Soc. Exp. Biol.* **32**, 993. (Abstr.)
48. Katz, D. H., and Benacerraf, B. (1972). *Advan. Immunol.* **15**, 1.
49. Miller, J. F. A. P., and Mitchell, G. F. (1969). *Transplant Rev.* **1**, 3.
50. Claman, H. N., and Chaperon, E. A. (1969). *Transplant. Rev.* **1**, 92.
51. Leuchars, E., Cross, A. M., and Dukor, P. (1965). *Transplantation* **3**, 28.
52. Aisenberg, A. C. (1970). *J. Exp. Med.* **131**, 275.
53. Katz, D. H. (1972). *Transplant. Rev.* **12**, 141.
54. Kindred, B., and Shreffler, D. C. (1972). *J. Immunol.* **109**, 940.
55. Katz, D. H., Paul, W. E., Goidl, E. A., and Benacerraf, B. (1970). *Science* **170**, 462.
56. Hamaoka, T., Katz, D. H., and Benacerraf, B. (1972). *Proc. Nat. Acad. Sci. U. S.* **69** 3453.
57. Hamaoka, T., Osborne, D. P., Jr., and Katz, D. H. (1973). *J. Exp. Med.* **137**, 1393.
58. Katz, D. H., Hamaoka, T., and Benacerraf, B. (1973). *J. Exp. Med.* **137**, 1405.
59. Katz, D. H., Hamaoka, T., Dorf, M. E., and Benacerraf, B. (1973). *Proc. Nat. Acad. Sci. U. S.* **70**, 2624.
60. Katz, D. H., and Unanue, E. R. (1973). *J. Exp. Med.* **137**, 967.
61. Rosenthal, A. M., and Shevach, A. S. (1973). *J. Exp. Med.* **138**, 1213.
62. Katz, D. H., Hamaoka, T., Dorf, M. E., and Benacerraf, B. (1974). *J. Immunol.* **112**, 855.
63. Katz, D. H., Dorf, M. E., and Benacerraf, B. (1974). *J. Exp. Med.* **140**, 290.
64. Armerding, D., and Katz, D. H. (1974). *J. Exp. Med.* **139**, 24.
65. Armerding, D., and Katz, D. H. (1974). *J. Exp. Med.* **140**, 19.

66. Katz, D. H., and Benacerraf, B. (1974). In "The Immune System: Genes, Receptors, Signals" (C. F. Fox, ed.), p. 59. Academic Press, New York.
67. David, C. S., Shreffler, D. C., and Frelinger, J. A. (1973). Proc. Nat. Acad. Sci. U. S. 70, 2509.
68. Sachs, D. H., and Cone, J. L. (1973). J. Exp. Med. 138, 1289.
69. Hämmerling, G. J., Deak, B. D., Mauve, G., Hämmerling, U., and McDevitt, H. O. (1974). Immunogenetics 1, 68.
70. Ault, K. A., and Unanue, E. R. (1974). J. Exp. Med. 139, 1110.
71. Cullen, S. E., David, C. S., Shreffler, D. C., and Nathenson, S. G. (1974). Proc. Nat. Acad. Sci. U. S. 71, 648.
72. Schwartz, B. D., and Nathenson, S. G. (1971). J. Immunol. 107, 1363.
73. Unanue, E. R., David, C. S., Dorf, M. E., and Benacerraf, B. (1974). Proc. Nat. Acad. Sci. U. S. 71, 5014.
74. Götze, D., Reisfeld, R. A., and Klein, J. (1973). J. Exp. Med. 138, 1003.
75. Hauptfeld, V. D., Klein, D., and Klein, J. (1973). Science 181, 167.
76. Frelinger, J. A., Neiderhuber, J., David, C. S., and Shreffler, D. C. (1974). J. Exp. Med. 140, 1273.
77. Goding, J., Nossal, G. J. V., Shreffler, D. C., and Marchalonis, J. (1975). (in press).
78. Shevach, E. M., Paul, W. E., and Green, I. (1972). J. Exp. Med. 136, 1207.
79. Shevach, E. M., Green, I., and Paul, W. E. (1974). J. Exp. Med. 139, 679.
80. Bluestein, H. (1973). Fed. Proc., Fed. Amer. Soc. Exp. Biol. 32, 985.
81. Pierce, C. W., Kapp, J. A., Solliday, S. M., Dorf, M. E., and Benacerraf, B. (1974). J. Exp. Med. 140, 921.
82. Pierce, C. W., Kapp, J. A., Solliday, S. M., Dorf, M. E., and Benacerraf, B. (1975). J. Exp. Med. (in press).
83. Hämmerling, G. J., and McDevitt, H. O. (1974). J. Exp. Med. (in press).
84. Lilly, F. (1971). Proc. 2nd Convocation Immunol., (S. Cohen, G. Cudkowicz, and R. T. McCluskey, eds.), p. 103. Karger, Basel.
85. Lilly, F., and Pincus, T. (1973). Advan. Cancer Res. 17, 231.
86. Sato, H., Boyse, E. A., Aoki, T., Iritani, C., and Old, L. J. (1973). J. Exp. Med. 138, 593.
87. Hellstrom, K. E. (1966). Int. J. Cancer 1, 349.
88. Hellstrom, I., and Hellstrom, K. E. (1966). Ann. N. Y. Acad. Sci. 129, 724.
89. Sanford, B. H. (1967). Transplantation 5, 557.
90. Sanford, B. H., and Soo, S. F. (1971). J. Nat. Cancer Inst. 46, 95.
91. Fisher, B., Soliman, O., and Fisher, E. R. (1970). Cancer Res. 30, 66.
92. Fisher, B., Soliman, O., and Fisher, E. R. (1970). Cancer Res. 30, 2035.
93. Oth, D. (1971). Bull. Cancer 58, 363.
94. Oth, D. (1972). Thesis, Univ. of Nancy, Nancy, France.
95. Oth, D., and Burg, C. (1965). C. R. Soc. Biol. 159, 2231.
96. Oth, D., and Burg, C. (1967). Cong. Colloq. Univ. Liege 43, 31.
97. Williams, R. M., Dorf, M. E., Germain, R. N., and Benacerraf, B. Unpublished data.
98. Vladiatiu, A. O., and Rose, N. R. (1971). Science 174, 1137.
99. Williams, R. M., and Moore, M. J. (1973). J. Exp. Med. 138, 775.
100. Oldstone, M. B. A., Mitchell, G. F., and McDevitt, H. O. (1973). Fed. Proc., Fed. Amer. Soc. Exp. Biol. 32, 964.
101. Levine, B. B., Sternber, R. H., and Fotino, M. (1972). Science 178, 1201.

HORIZONTALLY AND VERTICALLY TRANSMITTED ONCORNAVIRUSES OF CATS

M. Essex

Department of Microbiology, School of Public Health, Harvard University, Boston, Massachusetts

I. Introduction	175
II. Characteristics of Feline Oncornaviruses	178
A. Morphology	178
B. Biochemical and Biophysical Characteristics	180
III. Antigenic Structure and Serologic Detection	181
A. Virus Core Antigens	181
B. Virus Envelope Antigens	184
IV. Virus–Host Cell Relationships	186
A. Replication of Feline Leukemia Virus in Cultured Cells	186
B. Transformation of Cultured Cells by Feline Sarcoma Viruses	188
C. Endogenous Oncornaviruses of Cats	189
V. Cell Surface Antigens Induced by Feline Oncornaviruses	191
VI. Experimental Induction of Tumors with Feline Oncornaviruses	194
A. Induction of Leukemia	194
B. Induction of Fibrosarcoma	197
VII. Immune Response to Experimental Infections	199
A. Immune Response to Feline Sarcoma Virus Infections	199
B. Immune Response to Experimental Infections with the Feline Leukemia Virus	203
VIII. Virus Transmission and Natural History of Feline Leukemia	205
A. The Pathology of Naturally Occurring Leukemia	205
B. Horizontal Virus Transmission under Laboratory Conditions	208
C. Horizontal Virus Transmission under Field Conditions	211
D. Vertical Transmission of Feline Oncornaviruses	216
E. Incidence of Virus Infection in Laboratory and Field Cat Populations	220
F. Serologic Studies of Cats with Naturally Occurring Leukemia	223
G. The Frequency of Feline Leukemia Virus Infection in Feline Diseases Other Than Leukemia and Sarcoma	226
IX. Comparison of Feline Oncornavirus Infectivity Patterns to Those of Other Oncogenic or Potentially Oncogenic Viruses	230
X. Public Health Significance of Feline Oncornaviruses	233
XI. Summary and Conclusions	235
References	237

I. Introduction

Although eight or more morphologically distinct groups of RNA viruses have been described, all RNA viruses thus far proved to have oncogenic potential fall into a single group with common characteristics. This group has been designated the oncornaviruses (Nowinski et al., 1970), leukoviruses (Fenner, 1968), or deoxyriboviruses (Temin, 1974). Not coincidentally, the oncornaviruses are also the only group of RNA viruses that possess reverse transcriptase (Baltimore, 1970; Temin and Mizutani, 1970), and thus the ability to form a DNA "provirus" (Temin, 1971; Temin and Baltimore, 1972) with the potential for stable interaction with cellular DNA.

As soon as it became apparent that the "filterable agents" originally described as the causes of leukemia and fibrosarcoma in chickens (Ellerman and Bang, 1908; Rous, 1910) and laboratory mice (Gross, 1951; Harvey, 1964) were oncornaviruses, optimism that similar agents would be isolated from mesodermal tumors of man and other outbred mammals was apparent. The primary technological approaches available were electron microscopy for the detection of morphologically similar particles, the concentration of biophysically similar particles by ultracentrifugation, and later, the serologic detection of oncornaviruses having the common "interspecies" virus core antigen (Geering et al., 1968). These approaches resulted in the description of C-type oncornavirus-like particles in many animal species, including man (Burger et al., 1964; Porter et al., 1964; Dmochowski et al., 1965; Levine et al., 1967), monkeys (Theilen et al., 1971; Wolfe et al., 1971), cattle (Miller et al., 1969; Kawakami et al., 1970), pigs (Howard et al., 1968), dogs (Chapman et al., 1967), cats (Jarrett et al., 1964a,b; Rickard et al., 1967; Kawakami et al., 1967), hamsters (Stenback et al., 1968; Kelloff et al., 1970), guinea pigs (Nadel et al., 1967; Hsiung, 1972), rats (Weinstein and Moloney, 1965; Klement et al., 1971), and snakes (Zeigel and Clark, 1969). The initial optimism was followed by pessimism, however, when the demonstration of infectivity for many of the "particles" seen in the electron microscope proved elusive, and the demonstration of oncogenicity even more so. A single exception was the existence of particles associated with leukemias, lymphomas, and fibrosarcomas of cats (Jarrett et al., 1964a,b; Rickard et al., 1967; Kawakami et al., 1967; Snyder and Theilen, 1969), and it was readily apparent that the feline agents were both infectious and oncogenic. The finding that oncornaviruses apparently caused naturally occurring leukemia and fibrosarcoma in cats was doubly significant because this represented the first such observation in an outbred mammalian species. Since laboratory mice were inbred for such things as a high leukemia incidence, it was possible that many murine oncornaviruses could be unnatural recombinants that were selected along with the given strain of mice.

Disappointment associated with the relative lack of success in finding oncornaviruses of men and other higher animals by means of these approaches was followed by increased efforts directed at the detection of subvirion viral components and unexpressed genomes. Cells that were thought to contain "turned off" oncornaviruses were exposed to chemical inducers, immunologic stimulation, and cocultivation with others presumed to be susceptible to productive infection.

Numerous new oncornavirus particles were activated using such procedures. Accordingly, a popular hypothesis proposed that such latent viruses were present in all individuals of higher animal species, and when appropriately activated, the cause of cancer (Huebner and Todaro, 1969; Todaro and Huebner, 1972). Success in activating latent viruses was, however, still most frequent with the same species—chickens, mice, and cats. Also, few, if any, of the "activated" particles proved to be oncogenic. Cells were also tested for the presence of nucleic acids that would hybridize with RNA or DNA probes prepared from oncornaviruses, and some success was again realized. Controversy then developed over the issue of whether such latent particles were present in all cells and individuals, or only in cancer cells (Baxt et al., 1972, 1973; Hehlmann et al., 1972, 1973).

The detection of so many latent and apparently nononcogenic agents suggested for the first time that frankly oncogenic oncornaviruses might represent the exception rather than the rule. Many, and possibly all, cat cells were found to have "turned-off" oncornaviruses (Fischinger et al., 1973; Livingston and Todaro, 1973; Sarma et al., 1973, 1974b), but these agents were easily distinguishable in several ways from the prototype feline oncornaviruses that cause leukemia and sarcoma. First, the latent viruses, unlike the prototype feline leukemia (FeLV) and sarcoma (FeSV) viruses, were primarily xenotropic; they did not grow in a permissive fashion in most cat cells, but did grow in cells from other species (Fischinger et al., 1973; Livingston and Todaro, 1973; Sarna et al., 1973). Second, the latent viruses were morphologically (Stephens et al., 1972), serologically (Oroszlan et al., 1972, 1973; Boone et al., 1973a; Gilden et al., 1974), and biophysically (Oroszlan et al., 1972; East et al., 1973), distinguishable from the leukemia (FeLV) and sarcoma (FeSV) viruses. Third, the latent viruses were apparently nononcogenic.

At the same time it became evident that endogenous, apparently nononcogenic RNA tumor viruses were present in cats, extensive evidence accumulated which indicated that the prototype leukemia and sarcoma viruses were horizontally transmitted (Jarrett, 1972; Essex and Snyder, 1973; Essex et al., 1973a; Hardy et al., 1973b; Jarrett et al., 1973b). Similarly convincing evidence for vertical chromosomal transmission of FeLV and FeSV was not available. As a result, the natural history of oncogenic feline oncornaviruses seemed to parallel the natural history of most cytopathic viruses of man and animals, rather than the transmission patterns seen for oncornaviruses of laboratory mice. FeLV and FeSV were not unique as horizontally transmitted oncogenic viruses, however, because the Herpesvirus that induces Marek's disease, a lymphoma of chickens, is also highly contagious (Nazerian, 1973). Furthermore, the Epstein–Barr virus associated with Burkitts' lymphoma of man is horizontally transmitted, and apparently not vertically transmitted (Klein, 1973). The feline leukemia–sarcoma system thus provides a valuable model for the study of naturally occurring virus induced tumors of mammals. The opportunity to study the pathogenesis of tumor development and tumor immunity in this system has been of particular interest to myself and several of my colleagues, and emphasis will be directed to these studies in this review.

The term leukemia will be used here in the broad sense to include lymphomas as well as blood and bone marrow tumors unless otherwise indicated. Several recent reviews on oncornavirus virology (Temin, 1971; Tooze, 1973; Bauer, 1974) and immunity (Essex, 1974; Lamon, 1974) have been published. Brief reviews on various aspects of feline leukemia are also available (O. Jarrett, 1970; W. F. H. Jarrett, 1972; Essex et al., 1973a; Hardy, 1974).

II. Characteristics of Feline Oncornaviruses

A. Morphology

Oncornaviruses associated with leukemia and sarcoma of chickens, mice, and cats are morphologically very similar. In addition, virtually all the latent endogenous activated oncornaviruses of these species are also similar, and frequently indistinguishable from the prototype viruses. They bud from cytoplasmic and vacuolar membranes in an "immature" form and are described as type C when "mature" as visualized in extracellular spaces.

In thin sections, type C FeLV has been described as 90–115 nm in diameter, which is slightly larger than the diameter for avian and murine leukemia viruses (Kawakami et al., 1967; Laird et al., 1968a,b; Rickard et al., 1969; Theilen et al., 1969; Burger and Noronha, 1970; Noronha et al., 1974). This diameter is increased to

120–140 nm when the 14–30 nm envelope spikes are included in the total diameter (Dougherty and Rickard, 1970). They may play an important role in adsorption to susceptible cells, and thus infectivity. The spikes are apparently difficult to preserve for visualization.

Mature "C"-type FeLV has a spherical electron dense central nucleoid or core of 60–90 nm and an electron lucent space between the core and envelope (Laird *et al.*, 1968a,b; Rickard *et al.*, 1969; Theilen *et al.*, 1970). Negative staining of the core shows coiled strands of 30 Å, which presumably represent the nucleoprotein (Nowinski *et al.*, 1970). Electron micrographs of the isolated RNA of FeLV (Whalley, 1973) and RD-114 (Kung *et al.*, 1974) have been published.

Immature FeLV buds from the cell by first forming in the cell membrane a dense thickening of about the same diameter as the virus particle. The buds then display a thickening below the cell membrane, which eventually condenses as an inner ring, associated with the formation of a short stalk and eventually pinching off from the cell. The immature particle contains a very thick ring below the bilayered envelope (Dalton, 1972), and a thicker electron-dense inner ring of about 65 nm with an electron-lucent center of about 45 nm (Theilen *et al.*, 1970). The morphology is not affected by the types or species of cells from which the virus replicated (Dalton, 1972; Essex *et al.*, 1972a). Reviews on oncornavirus morphology as interpreted from thin sections have been published (de Harven, 1968; Dalton and Haguenau, 1973).

FeSV has been described as essentially identical to FeLV by electron microscopy (Snyder and Theilen, 1969; Snyder, 1971), but such analyses are difficult to interpret because all pools of FeSV thus examined contain a great excess of helper FeLV (Sarma *et al.*, 1970c; Dougherty, 1971; Sarma *et al.*, 1971a,d; McDonald *et al.*, 1972; Sarma *et al.*, 1972).

The RD-114-type endogenous cat oncornaviruses have not been studied as thoroughly by thin-section electron microscopy, but in general characteristics they are very similar to FeLV (McAllister *et al.*, 1972; Sarma *et al.*, 1973). Noronha *et al.* (1974) found that the ratio between overall diameter of the particle and diameter of the central nucleoid was slightly wider (about 2:1) for RD-114 than for FeLV (about 3:2). Negative staining with phosphotungstic acid appears to allow easy differentiation because 60–70% of the RD-114 virus particles show multiple "tails" whereas these appear in less than 5% of the FeLV or murine leukemia virus particles (Stephens *et al.*, 1972).

B. Biochemical and Biophysical Characteristics

FeLV has a buoyant density of 1.14 to 1.16 gm/cm^3 in sucrose, which is similar to figures obtained for other oncornaviruses (O'Connor et al., 1964; Kawakami et al., 1967). The envelope is composed of at least two glycoproteins of approximate molecular weights 70,000 and 100,000 (Nowinski et al., 1972; Graves and Velicer, 1974; Pal et al., 1974; Strand and August, 1974), which are slightly larger than the figures given for avian and murine oncornavirus envelope glycoproteins (Bauer, 1974). Inside the envelope are five smaller polypeptides of molecular weight 30,000 (p 30), 21,000 (p 21), 15,000 (p 15), 11,000 (p 11), and 10,000 (p 10) (Schafer et al., 1971; Green et al., 1973; Jarrett, 1973; August et al., 1974; Graves and Velicer, 1974; Strand and August, 1974; Pal et al., 1975).

These proteins are somewhat similar for the FeLV and RD-114 groups (McAllister et al., 1972, 1973; Gilden et al., 1974), but qualitative differences have been reported. The major internal protein of RD-114, for example, was described as having a slightly higher molecular weight (33,500) and a higher isoelectric point (9.1) than FeLV (25,000 and 8.3) using the same procedures (Oroszlan et al., 1971, 1972). This protein has also been sequenced, and distinct differences were observed between FeLV and RD-114 (Oroszlan et al., 1973; Gilden et al., 1974). These differences were just as great when RD-114 was compared to FeLV as when either RD-114 or FeLV was compared to the murine oncornaviruses. Since pools of FeSV free of FeLV are not available, detailed knowledge of proteins or nucleic acids of FeSV has obviously been unattainable.

The RNA of FeLV and RD-114 is 65–75 S (O. Jarrett et al., 1971; Roy-Burman and Kaplan, 1972). A 4 S component, presumably transfer RNA, has also been found (O. Jarrett et al., 1971) and the 70 S component apparently becomes about 37 S when denatured (O. Jarrett et al., 1971; Roy-Burman and Kaplan, 1972; Whalley, 1973). The RNA of RD-114 has been described as 70 S by two groups (McAllister et al., 1972, 1973; Roy-Burman and Kaplan, 1972; Kung et al., 1974), and 50 S by another (East et al., 1973).

A difference in the average base composition for the RNA's of FeLV and RD-114 has been observed (Roy-Burman and Kaplan, 1972). The RNAs of FeLV and RD-114 have also been compared by hybridizing synthetic DNA templates made with reverse transcriptase from viral RNA with the heterologous and homologous virion RNA's. Distinct differences are seen between the FeLV–FeSV group when compared to the RD-114-endogenous virus group (Baluda and Roy-Burman, 1973; Benveniste and Todaro, 1973; East et al., 1973;

TABLE I

MORPHOLOGICAL AND BIOCHEMICAL PROPERTIES OF FELINE LEUKEMIA-SARCOMA VIRUSES (FeLV–FeSV) AND RD-114-ENDOGENOUS GROUPS OF FELINE ONCORNAVIRUSES

Property	FeLV–FeSV group	RD-114 group
Morphology by thin section technique		
Size	90–115 nm	90–110 nm
Percentage of particles with envelope spikes	Greater than 75%	Less than 10%
Arrangement	Type C	Type C
Particle to nucleoid ratio	3:2	2:1
Morphology by negative stain technique	5% or less have multiple "tails"	60–70% have multiple "tails"
Density in sucrose	1.14–1.17 gm/cm^3	1.16 gm/cm^3
P 30 core antigen		
Size	25,000 Daltons	33,500 Daltons
Isoelectric point	8.3	9.1
RNA		
Sedimentation coefficient	60–75 S	50–70 S
Estimated molecular weight	1.1×10^7	5×10^6
Homology with other oncornavirus RNAs (hybridization)	Less than 5% with RD-114 and all others tested	10–20% with M7 baboon virus; less than 5% with others tested

Quintrell et al., 1974). Nucleic acids from both groups show some degree of homology with normal feline cells (Baluda and Roy-Burman, 1973; Fujinaga et al., 1973; Gillespie et al., 1973; Neiman, 1973; Ruprecht et al., 1973) but the extent of homology is considerably greater for the endogenous-RD-114 group (Gilden et al., 1974). Both groups have reverse transcriptase in the virion (Spiegelman et al., 1970a,b; Fujinga and Green, 1971; Roy-Burman, 1971; McAllister et al., 1972), however the enzymes are readily distinguishable (Livingston and Todaro, 1973; McAllister et al., 1973).

Table I summarizes the biochemical and morphological properties of the FeLV–FeSV and RD-114-endogenous virus groups.

III. Antigenic Structure and Serologic Detection

A. VIRUS CORE ANTIGENS

The designation "group-specific antigen," or gs, has become the most widely used term for describing oncornavirus core reactivity.

The term seemed appropriate because core antigens detected for all "strains" of oncornaviruses found within a given animal species appeared to show complete cross-reactivity. This was not true for the envelope antigens, which show predominantly subgroup specific activity by virus neutralization. The intraspecies cross-reactivity is primarily due to reactions directed at the gs 1 or p 30, which also has group reactivity (Green et al., 1973; August et al., 1974) and is the major structural protein in the virus core (Geering et al., 1968, 1970; Gilden and Oroszlan, 1971; Gilden et al., 1971; Schafer and Noronha, 1971). We now know, however, that at least one species, the cat, has two distinct groups of oncornaviruses.

These are the RD-114 endogenous group and the oncogenic FeLV–FeSV group (Bauer, 1974; Essex, 1974; Gilden et al., 1974). Each feline group shows no more cross-reactivity between their respective gs antigens than they do, for example, with mouse oncornaviruses (Oroszlan et al., 1972; Schafer et al., 1973; Gilden et al., 1974). It now appears that several interspecies determinants may be present on the same molecule (Oroszlan et al., 1971; Gilden et al., 1971; Strand and August, 1974). Oncornavirus-induced cell membrane antigens also often give strong intraspecies "group-specific" reactions (Bauer, 1974; Essex, 1974). Unless otherwise specified, the gs term will be used here in the traditional manner, to describe the reaction directed to either purified or unpurified gs 1 or p 30.

The gs is most readily detected in virions after treatment with ether and/or detergents to rupture the envelope and release the core. This antigen is also present in reasonably large quantities in the cytoplasm of virus producer cells and sometimes in nonproducer cells as well. Identification of gs provided a valuable way to detect FeLV and FeSV in tissues of cats with laboratory induced or naturally occurring tumors. In early studies, immunodiffusion was extensively used (Hardy et al., 1969; Sibal et al., 1970; Fink et al., 1971; Hardy, 1971; Schafer and Noronha, 1971). Tumor tissues and/or plasma were homogenized and concentrated by ultracentrifugation, treated with ether, and allowed to react with antiserum prepared in rabbits to purified ether-treated virus. This procedure was cumbersome and impractical for testing large numbers of samples as in the clinical or seroepidemiological situation, but still reliable, and useful in many experimental situations. Complement fixation (Sarma et al., 1970b, 1971b,c; Essex et al., 1972a), passive hemagglutination inhibition (Sibal et al., 1970; Fink et al., 1971), and radioimmunoassay (Parks and Scolnick, 1972; Scolnick et al., 1972) have been used in a similar manner to detect core antigens. The development of antisera specific to FeLV reverse transcriptase also allows the serologic detection of this virus-associated enzyme in appropriate materials by inhibition of its activity on synthetic templates (Aaronson *et al.*, 1971; Aaronson, 1973).

A substantial improvement from the standpoint of economy and efficiency was the adaptation of fixed-cell immunofluorescence to the detection of FeLV gs (Ubertini *et al.*, 1971; Hilgers *et al.*, 1972; Hardy *et al.*, 1973a) in the cytoplasm of infected cells. In addition to the obvious value of such a test to detect virus proteins in cells infected *in vitro*, the modification by Hardy and co-workers (Hardy *et al.*, 1973a,b; Hardy, 1974) to detect FeLV gs in blood smears has provided a valuable tool for seroepidemiologic and clinical studies. A fixed-cell immunofluorescence test for RD-114 has also been described (Riggs *et al.*, 1974).

Gs expression in the absence of virus production was shown to occur under certain circumstances with oncornaviruses of mice and chickens (Huebner and Todaro, 1969; Huebner *et al.*, 1970, 1971; Gilden and Oroszlan, 1972; Todaro and Huebner, 1972). The same subvirion expression of gs can also occur in the FeLV–FeSV system, but in this case it has only been demonstrated in heterologous species. Dog and monkey tumors induced with FeSV or FeLV, for example, often fit this criterion (Gardner *et al.*, 1970, Deinhardt *et al.*, 1972, 1973; Wolfe *et al.*, 1972; Rickard *et al.*, 1973a). The virus genes for gs synthesis can also be completely repressed, and this appears to occur in a minority of tumors induced with FeLV or FeSV in nonfeline species (Rickard *et al.*, 1973a). In the RD-114 group, the relationship of virus proliferation and production of structural proteins to species infected appears opposite to FeLV–FeSV (McAllister *et al.*, 1972, 1973; Fischinger *et al.*, 1973; Livingston and Todaro, 1973; Todaro *et al.*, 1973a,b). RD-114 is xenotropic, and the genome is completely repressed in cells from most cats, but virus production occurs readily in most nonfeline species (Fischinger *et al.*, 1973; Livingston and Todaro, 1973). When endogenous feline gs is present it can be detected using the same types of procedures with antisera specifically prepared to the RD-114 virus (McAllister *et al.*, 1973; Sarma *et al.*, 1973; Fischinger *et al.*, 1973; Livingston and Todaro, 1973; Filbert *et al.*, 1974; Riggs *et al.*, 1974).

A surprising cross-reactivity has been observed between the p 30's of RD-114 and the endogenous baboon virus designated M7 (Sherr *et al.*, 1974; McAllister, personal communication). The degree of cross reactivity seen between these two, is greater than that seen between either RD-114 or M7 and any other virus studied, including

TABLE II
RELATIONSHIPS BETWEEN MAJOR ANTIGENS OF FELINE LEUKEMIA VIRUS (FeLV),
FELINE SARCOMA VIRUS (FeSV), AND RD-114

Antigen	FeLV–FeSV	RD-114
P 30 (core)		
Interspecies	Common for all mammalian viruses including FeLV–FeSV and RD-114 groups	
Species	Distinct for FeLV–FeSV	Distinct from FeLV–FeSV, similar to M7 baboon virus
Envelope	At least three subgroups, each distinct from RD-114 and other oncornavirus groups	Overlap with M7 virus, distinct from others, including FeLV–FeSV
Reverse transcriptase	Distinct for FeLV–FeSV	Overlap with M7 virus, distinct from others, including FeLV–FeSV
Cell membrane	Distinct for FeLV–FeSV	Distinct from FeLV–FeSV group

the exogenous primate oncornaviruses. Table II summarizes antigenic activities observed for the FeLV–FeSV and RD-114-endogenous groups of feline oncornaviruses.

B. VIRUS ENVELOPE ANTIGENS

An efficient immune response to virion envelope antigens results in neutralization of the virus and termination of infection under ideal conditions. The glycoprotein envelope antigens of oncornaviruses are probably concentrated in the spike areas (Bauer, 1974; Essex 1974). Envelope antigens, as detected by virus neutralization, allow us to categorize oncornaviruses into subgroups. Since this classification corresponds perfectly with the same subgroup classification seen for virus–host cell attachment site interference, it is likely that antibody neutralization functions by tying up the antigens needed for infectivity. Avian oncornaviruses were the first to be characterized by the use of these antigens, and all that were isolated from either natural or laboratory sources fell into several distinct subgroups (Vogt, 1970).

The naturally occurring FeLV–FeSV group has been categorized in a similar fashion using A, B, and C subgroups (Sarma and Log, 1971, 1973a,b). All naturally occurring isolates of B or C subgroup viruses were found to contain A subgroup virus as well, but isolates of subgroup A alone have been found (Sarma and Log, 1973a,b), and at least one isolate containing all three subgroups has been found

(Fl 74 strain). Most natural isolates of FeLV and all isolates of FeSV thus far described are mixtures of subgroups A and B (Sarma and Log, 1973b). It is possible that additional virus envelope antigens specific for individual members of each subgroup, but with weaker immunogenicity, might also be present, as in the avian system (Ishizaki and Vogt, 1966).

Virus neutralization can be measured by many procedures that allow blocking of infectivity. Those used most successfully include the blocking of induction of virus core antigens as measured by complement fixation (Sarma and Log, 1971, 1973a,b; Post *et al.*, 1971), or fixed cell immunofluorescence (Hardy, 1974 and personal communication) and the blocking of focus formation using either cell transformation by FeSV (Post *et al.*, 1971; Sarma *et al.*, 1974b; Schaller *et al.*, 1974) or FeLV pseudotypes of murine sarcoma viruses (Fischinger *et al.*, 1973; Jarrett *et al.*, 1973b).

Early studies comparing FeLV to FeSV by virus neutralization showed an incomplete cross-reactivity (Post *et al.*, 1971). In retrospect, this appears to have been due to the fact that the strain of FeLV used consisted of subgroup A virus only while the FeSV used contained subgroups A and B rather than any distinct differences between all FeLV's and all FeSV's. The subgroups present in the commonly used "strains" of FeLV and FeSV are listed in Table III. The envelope antigens of all subgroups of FeLV–FeSV are completely distinct from those of the RD-114 group (Fischinger *et al.*,

TABLE III
SUBGROUPS OF FELINE ONCORNAVIRUSES PRESENT IN VARIOUS STANDARD STRAINS OF FELINE LEUKEMIA VIRUS (FeLV) AND FELINE SARCOMA VIRUS (FeSV)

Strain	Virus subgroup		
	A	B	C
FeLV			
Jarrett 5	+	+	−
Jarrett 9	+	+	−
F174 (Kawakami-Theilen)	+	+	+
F-161 (Rickard)	+	−	−
F-422 (Rickard)	+	−	−
FeSV			
ST (Snyder-Theilen)	+	+	−
GA (Gardner-Arnstein)	+	+	−
SM (McDonough)	+	+	−

1973; Sarma and Log, 1973b), but RD-114 envelope antigens can be assayed in a similar manner. Some cross-neutralization is observed between the endogenous baboon M7 agent and RD-114 (McAllister, personal communication).

In addition to the serologic procedures based on detection of virus core and envelope antigens, other biophysical and biochemical procedures are extremely valuable for detecting feline oncornaviruses. The most commonly used are incorporation of uridine-^{3}H into particles of the appropriate size and shape, electron microscopy, and detection of reverse transcriptase activity. Since these procedures are essentially identical whether feline or other oncornaviruses are the target, they will not be dealt with here.

IV. Virus–Host Cell Relationships

A. Replication of Feline Leukemia Virus in Cultured Cells

With the exception of a few atypical strains developed in the laboratory (Wright and Korol, 1969; Aaronson and Todaro, 1970) murine oncornaviruses will normally not grow in cells from nonmurine species. Field isolates of FeLV and FeSV, in addition to growing productively in feline cells (Jarrett et al., 1968b; Rickard et al., 1969; Theilen et al., 1969), also replicate in cultures from most other species tested. These include such diverse species as the dog (O. Jarrett et al., 1970, 1971; Sarma et al., 1970c; Lee, 1971; Essex et al., 1972a); hamster (Sarma et al., 1970c; Gilden et al., 1972; Monti-Bragadin and Ulrich, 1972), pig (O. Jarrett et al., 1970, 1971; Lee, 1971), monkey (Deinhardt et al., 1970; McDonald et al., 1972), ox (Lee, 1971; Chan et al., 1974a), and man (Jarrett et al., 1969a, 1970; Chang et al., 1970; Hampar et al., 1970; Sarma et al., 1970c; Essex et al., 1972b; McAllister et al., 1973; Chan et al., 1974a). Rat and mouse cells appear to be resistant (O. Jarrett, 1971; Laird et al., 1973).

The primary restrictive mechanism thought to be responsible for regulating infection is the presence or the absence of host cell membrane receptors for FeLV envelope subgroup antigens. The situation is somewhat confused, however, as illustrated by the following observations. (a) Fibroblasts from certain human individuals were sensitive to infection with one strain of subgroup AB virus, while cells from other individuals were resistant (Chang et al., 1970). We have confirmed this observation using lymphoblasts from different human individuals and a different virus strain (Essex, unpublished observations). Since the same virus strain was used under identical conditions, this observation would be easiest to explain on the basis of a lack of receptors on human cells of certain genetic types. This occurs with different strains of chicken cells exposed to the same subgroup of avian oncornaviruses (Vogt, 1970), but has not been described previously for infection of cells of heterologous species. (b) Subgroup A FeLV's (but not B and C) were observed to be incapable of infecting human and canine cells by one group (Jarrett et al., 1972, 1973), but this observation was disputed by another (Sarma, 1973, personal communication). One explanation for this could be the use of different human cell lines, as suggested by the Chang observations above. Related experiments suggest that B or C subgroup FeLV replicates as well in human cells as in cat cells in some circumstances (O. Jarrett, 1971), but not in others (Sarma et al., 1970c). Numerous other explanations could be offered to explain minor differences in relative susceptibility when seen in different laboratories, such as an increased or decreased sensitivity for established cell lines as opposed to primary or secondary cultures (Lee et al., 1972), different levels of interferon production, and different degrees of sensitivity to interferon (Rodgers et al., 1972).

Leukemogenic oncornaviruses, unlike sarcomagenic RNA viruses, are generally thought of as existing in a noncytocidal steady-state fashion with infected cells. It should be stressed, however, that most in vitro studies with FeLV are done with fibroblastic or epithelial cells which are apparently not transformed by the virus in vivo either, since all tumors induced with FeLV are leukemias or lymphomas. The few reported studies that have involved infection of lymphoid cells have used established human cultures (Hampar et al., 1970, 1973; Essex et al., 1972b). These lines are already "transformed" in the sense that they contain Epstein–Barr virus genomes (Zur Hausen and Schulte-Holthausen, 1970; Nonoyama and Pagano, 1971) and have characteristics of infinite growth potential, unlike cord blood lymphocytes, or those from Epstein–Barr virus negative healthy individuals (Pope et al., 1969; Chang et al., 1971; Nilsson et al., 1971). It might be unrealistic to expect substantial additional physiologic changes in such cells following exposure to a second virus, and experiments involving infection of fetal or cord blood lymphocytes of several species with FeLV and other nonsarcomagenic oncornaviruses, such as those done with the Epstein–Barr virus might be worthwhile. Two observations have suggested that feline oncornaviruses might induce at least minimal metabolic changes in established lines. Hampar et al. (1973) found that infection of human lymphoblast lines with either FeLV or RD-114 resulted in transient syncytial cell formation, and we reported an early increase in glucose uptake and lactic acid production in human and feline monolayer cells infected with FeLV (Bardell and Essex, 1974). Increased glycolysis has been regularly associated with transformation by avian and murine sarcoma viruses (Morgan and Ganapathy, 1963; Temin, 1968; Hatanaka et al., 1969; Hatanaka and Gilden, 1970; Hatanaka and Hanafusa, 1970), but not by their leukemogenic counterparts. The replication of FeLV in cat cells has been shown to be inhibited by pretreatment with homologous interferon (Rodgers et al., 1972). A mixed cell cytopathogenicity test, similar to the test used for murine leukemia viruses (Klement et al., 1969; Rowe et al., 1970) and employing the same XC indicator line, has recently been described as an assay for FeLV (Rangan et al., 1972a,b, 1973).

B. Transformation of Cultured Cells by Feline Sarcoma Viruses

Feline sarcoma viruses, like avian, murine, and simian RNA sarcoma viruses, are apparently "defective" or "incomplete" in that they will not function in the absence of competent helper oncornaviruses. Although FeSV can be isolated from many cats with naturally occurring fibrosarcomas (Snyder, 1971; Essex and Snyder, 1973), characterization studies have concentrated on the first three isolates. These are the Snyder-Theilen (ST) FeSV first described in 1969 in northern California (Snyder and Theilen, 1969; Snyder et al., 1970), the Gardner-Arnstein strain isolated in southern California (Gardner et al., 1970), and the McDonough strain (McDonough et al., 1971) isolated on the east coast of the United States.

FeSV will transform cells from a wide range of species similar to the number productively infected by various subgroups of FeLV. Species that have been shown to be susceptible to FeSV transformation include the cat (Sarma et al., 1971a,d, 1972; McDonald et al., 1972), dog (Sarma et al., 1970c), marmoset (Deinhardt et al., 1970; McDonald et al., 1972), baboon (Melnick et al., 1973), sheep (Theilen et al., 1974), pig (Sarma et al., 1971a,d), ox (Chan et al., 1974a,b), and man (Chang et al., 1970; Sarma et al., 1970c; McAllister et al., 1971a). Although entry into the cell is presumably related to the same envelope subgroup antigen receptors, the process of transformation itself is not dependent on completion of the virus replication cycle. This is illustrated by observations that FeSV can infect and transform but apparently not replicate in rat cells (Laird et al., 1973; Maruyama et al., 1974). Additionally, certain individual cell lines within a susceptible species, such as man, show transformation without virus production, while others show both transformation and release of active FeSV (Chang et al., 1970).

Comparisons of the three major strains of FeSV have been done by Sarma and his co-workers (Sarma et al., 1971a,d, 1972). All showed "one-hit" focus titration kinetics indicating a substantial excess of "helper" virus in the pools, and all showed essentially the same species host range for transforming activity. Some differences were observed; for example, the GA strain had a larger excess of helper virus, and induced foci in feline embryo fibroblasts that were morphologically distinguishable from those induced by the ST strain (Sarma et al., 1971a,d).

Due to the relative biochemical and biophysical similarities between mammalian oncornaviruses, "hybrids" containing the core proteins and genome of a virus from one species can be "coated" with and thus assume the host range specificities for the virus from another species. Furthermore, cosedimentation of two separate groups of viruses results in a spectrum of infectivity encompassing the limits of both. Murine sarcoma viruses, for example, will not grow in or transform human cells when accompanied only by murine oncornavirus "helpers." When cosedimented with FeLV the resulting pseudotype designated MuSV(FeLV) will infect and transform human cells (Fischinger and O'Connor, 1970; Fischinger and Moore, 1971).

These observations led to optimism that helper FeLV might be a useful tool to activate undetectable sarcoma and leukemia virus genomes suspected to be present in species such as man and the dog (Fischinger and O'Connor, 1970; Chapman et al., 1970; McAllister et al., 1971b). The passage of FeLV or FeSV through cells of nonfeline species did not visibly alter the biological properties (Sarma et al., 1970c; McAllister et al., 1971a), so identification of progeny virus was not expected to be a problem. These procedures proved to be successful for the activation of "turned-off" sarcoma viruses artificially introduced into hamster cells (Sarma et al., 1970a; Gilden et al., 1972; Monti-Bragadin and Ulrich, 1972), but success with naturally occurring tumors of nonproducer species has yet to be realized.

C. Endogenous Oncornaviruses of Cats

The RD-114-endogenous group of feline oncornaviruses was discovered unintentionally (McAllister et al., 1972). Observations that unexpressed mammalian oncornavirus genomes could, in certain instances, be activated by interaction with feline oncornaviruses resulted in experiments designed to activate human viruses. The injection of human sarcoma cells into the brains of fetal cats resulted in the detection of RD-114, a previously undescribed virus. Since all FeLV and FeSV strains had distinctly different serologic characteristics (Klement and McAllister, 1972; McAllister *et al.*, 1972, 1973), the possibility that RD-114 was a new human virus had to be considered. Neither the principal virus core antigen (Oroszlan *et al.*, 1971) nor the virus envelope antigens (Klement and McAllister, 1972), nor the virus-induced cell membrane antigens (Boone *et al.*, 1973a; Oshiro *et al.*, 1974) cross-reacted with those of the FeLV–FeSV group. What actually occurred in the initial isolation is unclear because the recipient cat fetal tissues were subsequently shown to harbor both FeLV and RD-114 (Sarma *et al.*, 1974a) and renewed attempts to repeat the same isolation by injecting the RD human rhabdomyosarcoma cell into other fetal kittens were unsuccessful (Gardner *et al.*, 1973).

Subsequent studies revealed that many, if not all, primary and established cultures from cats contained repressed viruses, designated CCC, RDV, or the endogenous feline oncornaviruses (Fischinger *et al.*, 1973; Livingston and Todaro, 1973; Noronha *et al.*, 1974; Sarma *et al.*, 1973, 1974a). These viruses were normally completely repressed, but occasionally spontaneous release occurred, and activation was facilitated by treating the cells with chemicals, such as iododeoxyuridine. The endogenous viruses were described as "xenotropic," because they readily infected cells from those nonfeline species tested, but normally did not grow productively in feline cells. When high input doses are used, however, some replication in feline cells can occur (Sarma *et al.*, 1973). A mixed-cell cytopathogenicity type of assay has also been described for use with the RD-114 group (Klement and McAllister, 1972; Rand and Long, 1973).

Expression of virus production does not seem to be related to tumor development, since all of 100 feline tumors tested for RD-114 virus core antigens were negative, and 20 of 20 cats with tumors were negative for RD-114 neutralizing antibody (Sarma *et al.*, 1973).

Although one set of experiments indicated specific homology between RD-114 RNA and a specific site on human D-group chromosomes (Price *et al.*, 1973), numerous other studies using various methods of nucleic acid hybridization indicated extensive homology with cat cells but little or no homology with human cells (Fujinaga *et al.*, 1973; Baluda and Roy-Burman, 1973; Neiman, 1973; Okabe *et al.*, 1973b; Ruprecht *et al.*, 1973). Molecular hybridization procedures were also used to compare the relatedness of the RD-114

TABLE IV
CELL CULTURE PROPERTIES OF FELINE ONCORNAVIRUSES

Activity	FeLV[a]	FeSV[a]	RD-114
Replication in cells from:			
Cat	+	+	−[b]
Dog	+	+	+
Human	+	+	+
Transformation of fibroblasts:			
Cat	−	+	−
Human	−	+	−
Formation of syncytia	+	+	+
Genome detected by nucleic acid homology in normal feline embryo cells	±[c]	±[c]	+
Activation from normal feline embryo cells	±[d]	±[d]	+

[a] FeLV, feline leukemia virus; FeSV, feline sarcoma virus.
[b] Limited replication in a few feline cultures.
[c] Limited homology (20–30%) in some lines (Quintrell et al., 1974).
[d] Occasional activation from normal cultures (Sarma et al., 1974a).

virion nucleic acids to those of the FeLV–FeSV group (Baluda and Roy-Burman, 1973; Benveniste and Todaro, 1973; East et al., 1973). As expected from the serologic studies, the two groups were not found to be closely related.

Since the endogenous feline oncornaviruses appear to be present in repressed form in all cats, and activation is not seen in individuals with tumors, the role of such viruses in oncogenesis, if any, is difficult to assess. Conversely, a role for the FeLV–FeSV group as endogenous viruses regularly transmitted in a vertical fashion is difficult to predict. Although FeLV is found in a minority of healthy cats, most appear free, and the number of positive cats increases dramatically following exposure to virus-excreting leukemic cats (Hardy et al., 1973b; Cotter et al., 1974; Essex, 1974; Essex et al., 1975c,d Sarma et al., 1974b). Furthermore, the development of leukemia and sarcoma is regularly associated with the presence of the FeLV–FeSV group (Hardy et al., 1973b, 1974). It is therefore possible that the RD-114 group plays no role at all in tumor development.

Various characteristics of *in vitro* growth and replication for RD-114 as well as FeLV and FeSV are listed in Table IV.

V. Cell Surface Antigens Induced by Feline Oncornaviruses

Cancer cells generally have altered cell membranes, characterized by the presence of new antigenic determinants that are recognized as such by the host immune defense mechanisms. The primary antigens of tumors induced by chemicals are individually distinct, but those induced by viruses are common and specific for the virus involved. The identification of embryonic antigens that are similarly cross-reacting confuses the issue of molecular mechanisms. Yet, the same tumor antigens are induced in all individuals of all species susceptible to tumor induction by a given virus, and they are not induced by other viruses or other carcinogens in postembryonic life. As a result, it is difficult to say whether viral nucleic acids are coding directly for the expression of such antigens, or merely derepressing host gene functions in a specific manner resulting in the expression of embryonic antigens common for all species. In a functional sense, this is probably not significant for virus-induced tumors because such cell surface antigens are recognized as foreign, and serve as reliable markers.

Cell surface antigens have been characterized for tumors induced by the avian and murine oncornaviruses. In the case of the avian viruses the predominant antigens are group specific, or common for all viruses in all subgroups. In the case of the murine oncornaviruses the cell membrane antigens are subgroup specific, but the subgroups are larger and different from those subgroups based on virion envelope antigens (Bauer, 1974; Essex, 1974). The cell membrane antigens described for avian and murine oncornaviruses appear to be expressed independently from the virus envelope proteins.

We described feline oncornavirus-associated cell membrane antigens (FOCMA) on the surface of cultured feline lymphoblastoid cells (Essex *et al.*, 1971a,b). Observations related to this were also made by others (Oshiro *et al.*, 1971; Riggs, 1971; Boone *et al.*, 1973b). We used the indirect membrane immunofluorescence test, with serum samples from cats injected with FeSV, and fluorescein-conjugated antisera to feline globulins. The target cell used as a standard, designated Fl 74 (Theilen *et al.*, 1969), was a culture established from a cat with lymphoma. It produces leukemogenic (but not sarcomagenic) virus of all three subgroups (Sarma and Log, 1973b). Subsequently we found that FOCMA could be induced in lymphoblastoid cells by infecting with FeLV *in vitro* (Essex *et al.*, 1972b) and in fibroblastic cells transformed by FeSV *in vitro* (Essex, unpublished observations).

FOCMA does not cross-react with similar cell membrane antigens induced by avian oncornaviruses, murine oncornaviruses, simian oncornaviruses, or the Epstein–Barr Herpesvirus. It also does not cross-react with the comparable cell membrane antigens induced by the feline endogenous-RD-114 oncornavirus group (Boone *et al.*, 1973a,b; Oshiro *et al.*, 1974). It has yet to be determined whether FOCMA is transformation specific as the counterpart antigens in the avian system seem to be (Kurth and Bauer, 1972; Gelderblom *et al.*, 1972). Our preliminary results suggest that the *in vivo* expression of FOCMA in cats appears to be strongest on malignant cells, and weaker or negative on nonmalignant virus producing lymphocytes in the same animals.

In addition to cat cells, FOCMA is expressed in human, dog, and monkey cells infected with FeSV or FeLV *in vitro* (Essex *et al.*, 1972b, 1973b; Essex, 1974). The kinetics of FOCMA expression in cultured cells infected with FeLV is related to the duration of time (or number of subcultures) that has elapsed since virus exposure. At 7-10 days post infection, for example, only 5-10% of the cells in susceptible cultures are FOCMA positive. This percentage gradually increases to 80-90% FOCMA-positive cells after several months, and remains at that level indefinitely. Whether this reflects a selection advantage for FOCMA-positive cells, an increased infectivity for "adapted" virus, or other mechanisms is unknown.

The high titers of FOCMA antibody found in dogs, monkeys, sheep, pigs, and cattle following exposure to FeSV indicates immunogenicity for the *de novo* synthesized antigen in heterologous species (Essex *et al.*, 1972b, 1973b; Essex, 1974). FOCMA can be induced by infection of cells with pure viruses representing each of the subgroups based on virion envelope classification, as well as all of the major "field" strains of FeLV and FeSV. Other indirect evidence also suggests that it is group specific as in the avian oncornavirus system, and distinct from the predominant virion envelope antigens. Antibody titers to FOCMA, for example, do not appear to correlate with virus neutralizing antibody titers directed to the virus envelope (see below), and adsorption of FOCMA antiserum with pelleted virus does not result in a significant reduction of FOCMA antibody titer. Although antisera from "regressor" cats and dogs was observed to label both the virus envelope and cell membrane using immunoelectron microscopy (Oshiro *et al.*, 1971), it is to be expected that regressor sera would contain both anti-FOCMA and virus-neutralizing antibodies. Antibodies directed to two different antigens would of course not be distinguished by antiglobulin reagents. Although the RD-114-endogenous group of viruses induces a cell surface antigen, the observation that RD cells infected with FeLV did not cross-react with RD-114 indicates the distinctiveness of the two systems.

Studies by Maruyama and Dmochowski (1969) using mixed hemadsorption indicated a reaction between monkey anti-Rauscher murine leukemia virus serum and cells infected with both murine and feline oncornaviruses. This type of reactivity was apparently confirmed using membrane immunofluorescence, rabbit anti-FeLV serum, and target cells infected with murine and feline leukemia viruses (Yoshiki et al., 1973, 1974). This has been interpreted as deposition of one or more of the virion core interspecies group-specific antigens on the cell membrane. The reaction seems to be detected only when using heterologous sera from animals hyperimmunized with pure virus. The failure to detect such a reaction using homologous anti-FOCMA sera may be due to a relative immunodepression of the homologous species for production of such antibodies. This observation, as well as observations of different cell membrane antigen systems induced by the avian and murine oncornaviruses, suggest that multiple determinants are probably present in the feline system.

VI. Experimental Induction of Tumors with Feline Oncornaviruses

A. INDUCTION OF LEUKEMIA

The first clue that feline leukemia might be caused by a virus was provided by Jarrett's group in 1964 (Jarrett et al., 1964a,b). They prepared suspensions from mediastinal lymphoma tissue and injected the resultant supernatant into each of 4 newborn kittens within a day of birth. The kittens developed disease after periods ranging from 9 to 18 months. Three of the four had pathologically confirmed leukemia, and one was questionable. Tissues from one of the cats that developed lymphoma were examined using an electron microscope, and "viruslike" particles similar to those associated with murine leukemia were described. An etiological role for the observed particles could not be established on the original passage, however, because the inoculum was not certified to be free of living cells.

Soon after these experiments were repeated, and the cell-free induction of the disease through several passages was confirmed by W. Jarrett et al. (1966) and others (Kawakami et al., 1967; O. Jarrett et al., 1968a, 1969b; Rickard et al., 1968; Theilen et al., 1968). Virtually all pathologic forms of leukemia–lymphoma have been induced, including myeloid leukemia (W. F. H. Jarrett et al., 1971, 1973c). The virulence of some virus strains seemed to increase following laboratory inoculation because the Cornell group observed an incubation period of 9–12 months for the first passage, but reduced latent periods of 30–139 days in subsequent passages with a mean of 53 days. In that series lymphoid neoplasia was induced in 56 of 68 (82%) newborn kittens (Rickard, 1968, 1969; Rickard et al., 1968, 1969). Experiments by the University of California group indicated a similarly brief latent period on the first passage, and leukemia induction using FeLV concentrated from plasma (Kawakami et al., 1967; Theilen et al., 1968, 1970). In all the studies FeLV was detected by electron microscopy in tumor tissue.

One group also separated and concentrated FeLV from plasma using density gradient centrifugation (Kawakami et al., 1967) in the same manner previously described for murine oncornavirus isolation (O'Connor et al., 1964). Cell-free FeLV was shown to be more efficient for tumor induction than whole cells. This was attributed to a relative inefficiency of the immune response to the virus itself as opposed to tumor cells (Theilen et al., 1970). Our subsequent studies on the role of immunity to tumor cell membrane antigens (see below) suggest that this explanation may be correct.

Further studies done by the Glasgow group involved 37 neonatal kittens inoculated with FeLV (O. Jarrett et al., 1970; W. F. H. Jarrett, 1971; Mackey et al., 1972). Although a few cats developed leukemia at only 1 or 2 months post-infection, most had an incubation period of 11 months or more, and 11 were still alive 3.5 years later. One-third of the cats died from causes other than hematopoietic neoplasms. The experimental induction of tumors with FeLV in this and other studies resulted in the induction of a wide range of pathologic forms, many being quite different from the tumor used to prepare inocula (Mackey et al., 1972; Jarrett et al., 1973c; Rickard et al., 1973b).

The incubation period for induced leukemia appeared shortest for the Rickard and Kawakami-Theilen strains, and longest in the Jarrett studies. Our current studies with naturally occurring cases suggest that the longer latent periods probably more accurately reflect the natural situation (Essex et al., 1975c,d).

The observation that many cats injected with FeLV died with unrelated infectious diseases was important, since it subsequently proved to be associated with FeLV-induced atrophy of the thymus and immunosuppression (Anderson et al., 1971; Mackey et al., 1972; Perryman et al., 1972; Hoover et al., 1973). Thymic atrophy was due to extensive depletion of cortical thymocytes, while the medullary components persisted (Hoover et al., 1973).

Most studies concerning the induction of leukemia involved the administration of concentrated FeLV by parenteral injection. Studies by Hoover et al. (1972), have indicated that administration of FeLV by instillation of droplets into the nose was also an effective way to induce leukemia in cats. The Rickard strain was used, and 3 of 7 kittens developed leukemia within latent periods of 170–330 days. Seven of 8 controls inoculated with the same virus suspension developed leukemia within 82–120 days. This suggests that prolonged incubation periods and resistance to leukemia development are more representative of the natural exposure situation.

Electron microscopic and gradient centrifugation studies established that viremia occurs in at least some cases of feline leukemia (Kawakami et al., 1967; Laird et al., 1968a). Our recent studies indicate that viremia occurs in most cats with both induced and naturally occurring leukemia (Hardy et al., 1973b, 1974; Jarrett et al., 1973b). FeLV apparently also replicates from many other tissues in most cats with induced leukemia, and is seen budding from cells of bone marrow, spleen, lymph node, tracheal, nasal, and oral epithelium, salivary gland, and intestinal epithelium (Jarrett et al., 1973b).

FeLV also induces leukemia in dogs (Rickard, 1969; Rickard et al., 1973a). This is of interest in the sense that the dog, like man, is a species from which RNA tumor viruses have not been isolated despite many attempts. Using cell-free FeLV of the Rickard strain, 12 of 19 (63%) puppies inoculated either *in utero* or on the day of birth developed leukemia. By contrast, none of the six inoculated 2 or 3 days after birth developed disease within a one-year observation period. The pathology of the tumors was not unlike that seen with spontaneous lymphoma of dogs. It included generalized lymphadenopathy and involvement of the spleen and thymus.

The dependence on immaturity for tumor development appeared to be related to virus replication. The incubation period for tumor development was much shorter for dogs inoculated *in utero* than for those inoculated after birth. Dogs inoculated before birth were virus producers as judged by both electron microscopy and subsequent induction of tumors in other dogs and cats with cell-free inocula. Cells from tumors established from prebirth inoculations also had high positive titers of virus core antigens. The tumors induced following postparturition injections were "nonproducers" or FeLV negative, and either negative or very weakly positive for virus core antigens in tumor cell cytoplasm. This "nonproducer" type of tumor cell infection is not unusual for RNA virus-induced sarcomas, but the situation of nonproducer leukemias is unusual if not unique. The fact that virus expression is clearly related to host development in this system and that both producer and "nonproducer" tumors can be induced in the same species makes this an ideal model for the study of "nonproducer" human leukemias assumed by many to be associated with the presence of "turned-off" oncornaviruses.

B. INDUCTION OF FIBROSARCOMA

The discovery of leukemogenic oncornaviruses of chickens and mice was rapidly followed by the isolation of sarcomagenic oncornaviruses in the same species. It was therefore quite logical that Jarrett's discovery of FeLV would stimulate investigators to search for comparable sarcomagenic variants in cats. The first description of a feline sarcoma virus was by Snyder and Theilen (1969), and this was soon followed by other similar reports (Gardner et al., 1970; McDonough et al., 1971).

In the experiments by Snyder and Theilen (1969), multiple subcutaneous fibrosarcomas were collected from a cat, homogenized, and injected into five 2-day-old kittens. All developed fibrosarcomas at the site of inoculation, and one had multiple metastases. The incubation period was 20–61 days. On the second passage, cell-free filtrates were administered to 3 kittens, and all again developed tumors. In the latter case the incubation period was much shorter— 10 to 15 days. The relatively prolonged incubation period for those given cellular material appears to have been related to both the nature of the inoculum and increased oncogenicity due to passage. Studies with cell-free preparations of the original tissue also resulted in short incubation periods, as did subsequent passages (Snyder et al., 1970; Snyder, 1971; Essex and Snyder, 1973). The induced tumors, like the original spontaneous neoplasm, were composed of highly vascular masses of whorls and interwoven bundles of fusiform and polygonal cells. Many mitosis were present. Electron microscopy of tumor tissue revealed particles similar or identical to FeLV.

In the experiments by Gardner et al. (1970), a recurrent subcutaneous fibrosarcoma in a 5-year-old cat was the original source of inoculum. The tumor used in the studies had been irradiated 2 months before and was present at the site of previous surgery for the primary tumor. The cell homogenate was injected into fetuses in utero, and tumors developed in 2 of 3 within 67–93 days. Subsequent transplants of induced tumors resulted in tumor development in 14 of 16 inoculated kittens. The latent period varied from 20 to 77 days. Cell-free concentrates were also administered to 24 young kittens in 2 passages, and 15 developed tumors with latent periods that varied from 14 to 30 days. As with the ST strain, the latent period was shorter when cell-free inocula were given. Virtually all the tumors had identifiable C-type virus particles replicating from bone marrow, lymph nodes, thymus, spleen, and tumor tissue. Most tumors also contain virus core antigens as detected by complement fixation. Similar studies were done with the third isolate (McDonough et al., 1971), which seemed to be very similar to the first two.

Electron microscopic examination of spontaneous fibrosarcomas indicated that 2 of 2 young cats (2 years of age or less) had tumors with many virus particles (Snyder, 1971). Only 1 of 5 tumors from older cats (7–14 years) had virus by electron microscopy and very few particles were observed in this tumor. All three tumors with identifiable particles were transmissible using cell-free inocula. Cell-free passage of only one "virus free" tumor was attempted, but that was also successful. Comparative studies of these and GA-FeSV indicated that ST had the shortest latent period (Essex and Snyder, 1973). The latent period for tumor induction with two additional isolates was somewhat longer, and it was longest with GA-FeSV.

Age and dose response curves were also determined for the ST strain (Essex et al., 1971a,b; Snyder and Dungworth, 1973). The results obtained were similar to those cited in previous studies with avian and murine sarcoma viruses (Bryan, 1946; Blumenschein and Moloney, 1969). Kittens receiving smaller virus doses tended to have longer incubation periods and were likely to develop tumors that subsequently regressed when compared to those receiving high doses. The development of detectable metastasis was most common in cats given intermediate doses that developed progressive primary tumors with latent periods of moderate duration. Kittens given high virus doses apparently died before metastases had a chance to develop. The effect of increasing age was similar to the effect of decreasing virus dose. Older animals had longer latent periods, tended to develop slower growing tumors that subsequently regressed, and had fewer detectable virus particles in the tumors.

In the original experiments with ST-FeSV (Snyder and Theilen, 1969), cell-free filtrates were also injected into two newborn puppies. Both developed multiple subcutaneous fibrosarcomas at the inoculation site within 10–15 days. Histopathologically the tumors were similar to those induced in cats. The GA-FeSV was also highly oncogenic for dogs when fetuses were injected in utero (Gardner et al., 1970). When tumors were induced in postnatal puppies with either strain, regression usually occurred (Gardner et al., 1970; Theilen et al., 1970; Essex et al., 1973b) even though some developed to a very large size. Regressing tumors of both dogs and older cats contained neutrophils, lymphocytes, fibroblasts, mast cells, and macrophage-like cells (Snyder et al., 1970; Slauson, 1973).

ST-FeSV was also used to induce tumors in rabbits (Theilen *et al.*, 1970), pigs (Pearson *et al.*, 1973), sheep (Theilen, 1971; Theilen *et al.*, 1974), rats (Maruyama *et al.*, 1974), and several species of monkeys (Deinhardt *et al.*, 1970, 1973; Theilen *et al.*, 1970; Essex *et al.*, 1972b; Rabin *et al.*, 1972, 1973; Wolfe *et al.*, 1972). The tumors induced with cell-free FeSV in rabbits, pigs, sheep, and large breeds of monkeys regressed in the same manner as dog tumors induced with FeSV. Tumors induced in young squirrel or marmoset monkeys did not regress, but went on to kill the host (Deinhardt *et al.*, 1970, 1973; Rabin, 1971; Essex *et al.*, 1972b; Rabin *et al.*, 1972, 1973; Wolfe *et al.*, 1972). Tumors induced in rats and sheep with transformed cells also did not regress (Maruyama *et al.*, 1974; Theilen *et al.*, 1974). The tumors induced in monkeys often contain virus core intracytoplasmic antigens, and the host sera often contained antibodies to such antigens, but tumors induced with cell-free inocula did not contain budding virus particles (Rabin *et al.*, 1972; Wolfe *et al.*, 1972; Deinhardt *et al.*, 1973). FeSV could be "rescued" from nonproducer tumors by *in vitro* manipulations of cultured tumor cells (Deinhardt, personal communication), and the induction of tumors with cultured or passaged marmoset cells often resulted in the induction of tumors that did produce FeSV *in vivo* (Essex *et al.*, 1972b; Wolfe *et al.*, 1972).

VII. Immune Response to Experimental Infections

A. Immune Response to Feline Sarcoma Virus Infections

As described above, the ST-FeSV induces malignant fibrosarcomas that usually regress in older animals given low virus doses. We collected serum samples from FeSV-injected cats before and after virus administration and tested the samples (as described above) for antibody to the feline oncornavirus associated cell membrane antigen (FOCMA) (Essex *et al.*, 1971a,b, 1973b; Essex and Snyder, 1973; Essex, 1974). In the first experiment 21 cats injected with ST-FeSV were studied. Of twelve that developed tumors that subsequently regressed, the FOCMA antibody titers ranged from 4 to 256 at 3–7 weeks post-infection. Antibody was assayed by determining the terminal 2-fold dilution where 50% or more of the cells were labeled. Most cats that developed regressing sarcomas or no tumors were 6 months or older at the time of inoculation, and cats which developed progressing tumors were usually 3 months of age or younger. Antibody titer showed a greater relationship to tumor status than to age at time of exposure. Those few older cats that

TABLE V
Feline Oncornavirus-Associated Cell Membrane Antigen (FOCMA) Antibody Titers in Serum Samples Taken from Cats Injected with Oncogenic Doses of the Snyder-Theilen Strain of Feline Sarcoma Virus (FeSV)

Group	Titer[a]										Total	Geometric mean
	0	1	2	4	8	16	32	64	128	256		
Progressors												
Number	22	9	6	5	—	—	—	—	—	—	42	0.6
Percentage	52	21	15	12	0	0	0	0	0	0	100	
Regressors												
Number	—	—	—	7	2	6	3	4	2	1	25	19.2
Percentage	0	0	0	28	8	24	12	16	8	4	100	
No tumor developed												
Number	—	—	—	—	1	4	—	1	2	—	8	29.8
Percentage	0	0	0	0	12	50	0	12	25	0	100	

[a] Reciprocal of highest serum dilution giving positive test.

developed progressive tumors also had low or negative antibody titers, while those of younger ages that did not develop tumors had moderate or high antibody titers (Essex et al., 1971a, 1973b).

We have now examined FOCMA antibody titers of 75 cats injected with ST-FeSV (see Table V). Of 42 that developed progressing lethal tumors, none had antibody titers higher than 4, and most had no detectable antibody at all. Of 33 that either developed no tumors or developed tumors that subsequently regressed, all had antibody titers in the range of 4 to 256. Less than 10% developed tumors that did not undergo either rapid progression or complete and permanent regression. They were not included in the analysis.

We also performed similar studies with cats given GA-FeSV (Schaller et al., 1974). The GA-FeSV is somewhat less virulent (Essex and Snyder, 1973). Of 23 cats inoculated with this strain, 7 developed tumors that were classified as either "slow progressors" or "temporary regressors" with subsequent remission. The rapid progressors given GA-FeSV had a mean survival time of 21 weeks, which is several times longer than for kittens given ST-FeSV. Those undergoing temporary remission or "slow" tumor progression had a mean survival time of more than 40 weeks. Seven of 9 rapid progressors had no detectable FOCMA antibody, and 2 had very low titers. As expected, all 7 with complete regression or no detectable tumor development also had high titers. These two groups thus had humoral antibody responses that were similar to those found in cats given ST-FeSV that had undergone the same type of pathologic response. The two less dramatic groups designated "slow progressors" and "temporary regressors" had FOCMA antibody titers that fell between the extremes observed for rapid progressors and permanent regressors in both degree of elevation and duration of titer.

The same samples that were collected from cats injected with GA-FeSV were tested for the presence of virus-neutralizing antibodies using an ST-FeSV focus reduction assay. No correlation was found between the presence of significant virus-neutralizing antibody titer and tumor progression. Cats with progressing tumors were just as likely to have significant virus-neutralizing antibody titers as cats with regressing tumors or those that developed no tumors at all. Thus no correlation between FOCMA antibody titer and virus-neutralizing antibody titer was observed. A lack of correlation between antibodies to virus core antigens and FOCMA was also present. Both progressors and regressors had significant responses to virus core antigens.

Antibodies to FOCMA were found in newborn kittens whose mothers were exposed to FeSV or FeLV (Essex et al., 1971a, 1973a,b; Essex and Snyder, 1973). Although only low to moderate titers of antibodies (2–16) were present, the kittens resisted the development of progressive tumors when given 100 to 1000 times the lethal dose of ST-FeSV. In this experiment it was not possible to say whether the tumor resistance was due to an anti-FOCMA tumor cell cytotoxic response, or to neutralization of the virus inoculum with antibodies also present in the same sera, or both.

The detection of various antibody activities in cats injected with FeSV conflicted with the expected lack of such a response as predicted by the oncogene hypothesis (Huebner and Todaro, 1969). The detection of antibody to virus core antigens also conflicted directly with a previous report claiming that no such activity was found in cats (Gardner et al., 1970). This discrepancy was apparently due to the use of tests that would detect complement-fixing antibodies in only one case (Gardner et al., 1970), and the detection of reactive non-complement-fixing antibodies by the other group (Olsen and Yohn, 1972; Yohn and Olsen, 1973). Feline antibodies that do not fix guinea pig complement have been characterized (Olsen et al., 1974a,b,c). The tests used to detect non-complement-fixing antibodies were the paired radioiodine labeling technique and complement-fixation inhibition (Olsen and Yohn, 1972; Yohn and Olsen,

1973). These procedures had been used previously to demonstrate similar non-complement-fixing antibody activity in chickens, a species also thought to be immunotolerant to oncornavirus core antigens (Rabotti and Blackham, 1970, Roth et al., 1971).

Although increases in antibody titers were observed in cats after inoculation of FeSV, background titers were present in most cats that were tested prior to virus injection (Yohn and Olsen, 1973). The background titers to the virus core antigens were present in most conventional or specific-pathogen-free cats, but not in germ-free cats. Since the antibody activity was directed to a cross-reactive interspecies-type antigen, it is quite possible that the antibody activity was directed to endogenous RD-114 type antigens. The RD-114 genome is apparently present in all cats, but FeLV-FeSV type viruses are not. Expression of the RD-114 gs antigen and/or antibody production could be activated by exposure to nonspecific immunostimulants not present in the germ-free environment. This possibility is suggested because our studies to detect anti-FOCMA activity in uninoculated "specific-pathogen-free" cats from the same colony indicated that most had no evidence of previous exposure to FeLV-FeSV (Essex et al., 1975b).

Dogs injected with FeSV were also examined for their immunologic response to FOCMA and other antigens. We checked antibody titers to FOCMA in 7 dogs that developed regressing tumors (Essex et al., 1973b). All developed titers at 3–6 weeks that ranged from 8 to 32. Only 1 dog with a "progressing" tumor was available for analysis. This animal developed a titer of 2. Slauson (1973) has checked dogs with regressing FeSV-induced tumors using a cytotoxic test directed against FOCMA antigens on cultured autologous cells. Antibody titers peaked when regression began, declined slightly during regression, and rose again as regression was completed. The lymphocyte-mediated cytotoxicity response was also studied, but it did not parallel regression as the humoral antibody response did. Antibodies produced in dogs to the cell membrane antigen were also identified by immunoelectron microscopy (Oshiro et al., 1971). Virus-neutralizing antibodies (Slauson, 1973) and complement-fixing antibodies directed to virus core antigens were also identified in dogs injected with FeSV.

Marmoset monkeys injected with FeSV have been examined for evidence of an immune response to virus core antigens and FOCMA. Most monkeys that survive for 6 weeks or longer have antibodies to virus core antigens (Wolfe et al., 1972; Deinhardt et al., 1973). We studied the FOCMA antibody responses of 7 marmosets given transplants of FeSV-induced marmoset tumors (Essex et al., 1972b). Despite the development of progressive malignant tumors in all but one animal, all developed significant titers of FOCMA antibodies. The titers ranged from 4 to 1024, and in 5 of the 7 animals, the titers were 128 or higher. The observation that animals with progressive tumors produced high antibody titers was in marked contrast to the situation in cats, where only the animals that resisted progressive tumor development had high antibody titers. The variation seen in marmosets could have been related to the fact that they received tumor transplants rather than cell-free FeSV. The fact that they represent a heterologous unnatural host for FeSV should also be considered.

Antibodies to the FOCMA-type antigen have also been identified in other species exposed to FeSV, including pigs (Pearson et al., 1973) and sheep (Essex and Theilen, unpublished).

B. Immune Response to Experimental Infections with the Feline Leukemia Virus

The first studies to detect an immune response in cats to FeLV or related antigens such as FOCMA involved the detection of complement-fixing antibodies to virus core antigens (Gardner et al., 1970; Huebner et al., 1971; Sarma et al., 1970d, 1971b). All cats that were tested were negative. This led to the proposal that cats were immunologically tolerant to the virus core antigens owing to regular vertical transmission of the virus in all individuals (Huebner et al., 1970). This position was also supported by observations that direct injection of pure FeLV in lymph nodes gave no evidence for stimulation of immune cells (Anderson and McKeating, 1970).

Studies by several groups have demonstrated that parenterally injected cats can produce antibodies to core antigens that are detectable by both immunodiffusion and complement-fixation tests (Sibal et al., 1970; Noronha et al., 1972; Olsen and Yohn, 1972). Other studies showed that cats have significant titers of non-complement-fixing antibody that is regularly detectable by tests that are not dependent on the fixation of guinea pig complement (Olsen and Yohn, 1972; Yohn and Olsen, 1973). The interpretation of these data is confused by the possible reactivity with RD-114-endogenous virus interspecies antigens, but regardless of which antigen is being detected it illustrates that an immune response to feline oncornavirus core antigens does occur in cats. Whichever type of antibody is produced to virus core antigens, this response probably has little or no effect on FeLV replication, and the non-complement-fixing antibody appears to have no significant effect on tumor development or progression (Schaller et al., 1974). Antibodies directed to virus core proteins do not give virus neutralization. The discovery that such antigens are also deposited on the cell membrane (Yoshiki et al., 1973, 1974) raises the theoretical possibility that tumor cells could be attacked at such sites, but further studies are needed to clarify this issue.

We checked the FOCMA antibody responses of 10 cats that were inoculated with FeLV (Essex, 1974; Essex et al., 1975a) (see Table VI). Each was checked for antibody titers at monthly intervals. None of the 7 that developed leukemia or lymphoma had significant titers of antibody. Although only 3 cats failed to develop clinical leukemia following injection of virus, each had a higher antibody titer than any of those that developed leukemia.

Vaccination experiments using FeLV-producing, FOCMA-positive feline cells were recently described (Jarrett, 1974; Jarrett et al., 1974). Various doses of cells were administered to determine whether high titers of FOCMA antibody could be induced. Very high titers were induced, and the antibody persisted at high levels for more than a year. The cats given high cell doses still harbored FeLV. These results are reminiscent of those obtained with the Marek's disease vaccine (Nazerian, 1973). Cellular inocula were

TABLE VI
RELATIONSHIP BETWEEN DEVELOPMENT OF LEUKEMIA AFTER FELINE LEUKEMIA VIRUS INOCULATION AND DEVELOPMENT OF ANTIBODY TO FELINE ONCORNAVIRUS-ASSOCIATED CELL MEMBRANE ANTIGEN (FOCMA)

Cat No.	FOCMA antibody titers, weeks post-inoculation					Development of leukemia[a]
	4	8	12	16	20	
301	0	0	0	Died	Died	Yes
302	0	0	1	0	Died	Yes
303	0	0	0	Died	—	Yes
304	0	0	Died	—	—	Yes
305	0	0	1	1	Died	Yes
306	0	0	0	Died	—	Yes
307	0	0	0	0	Died	Yes
308	16	32	256	64	—	No
309	0	0	2	8	—	No
310	32		32	64	—	No

[a] By 130 days postvirus injection which was last observation.

highly efficient for inducing anti-FOCMA antibodies, but pure cell-free FeLV of all subtypes was relatively inefficient.

The inoculation of FeLV and other leukemogenic RNA tumor viruses induces thymic atrophy and immunosuppression (Notkins et al., 1970; Anderson et al., 1971; Dent, 1972; Perryman et al., 1972; Hoover et al., 1973). Almost all newborn kittens injected with FeLV had significantly prolonged allograft rejection times when compared to age-matched control cats (Perryman et al., 1972). In the same study the humoral antibody response to sheep red blood cells was not depressed. In mice, oncornavirus-mediated humoral antibody immunosuppression is related to the class of antigen and the time of antigen exposure in relation to virus exposure (Cerny et al., 1971). It is therefore difficult to conclude that the humoral response might not also be affected by FeLV until more extensive studies on the subject are concluded.

VIII. Virus Transmission and Natural History of Feline Leukemia

A. THE PATHOLOGY OF NATURALLY OCCURRING LEUKEMIA

The term "leukemia" is used in this review, and in much of the other literature on the subject, in the broad, rather than the narrow, sense to describe the leukemia–lymphoma complex in general. This is done not only because of the etiologic relationship between the two, but also because no evident histologic differences are seen between the malignant cells involved, whether they are restricted to the blood and bone marrow, as in true lymphocytic leukemia, or deposited in solid tissue sites, as in lymphoma. The term lymphosarcoma is used synonymously with the term lymphoma. In addition to the lymphoid neoplasms, FeLV has also been associated with different forms of myeloproliferative leukemias (Herz et al., 1970; Schalm and Theilen, 1970; W. Jarrett, 1971; W. Jarrett et al., 1971, 1973c), but they are much less frequently seen than the lymphoid neoplasms under both natural and experimental conditions.

Numerous reports have been written on the clinical signs, hematology, and pathologic lesions associated with feline leukemia (Holzworth, 1960a,b; Squire, 1966b; Anderson et al., 1969; Crighton, 1968a,b, 1969a,b; Nielsen, 1969; Gilmore and Holzworth, 1971; Jarrett, 1971). Except in a very brief and selective manner, this information will not be reviewed here.

The most commonly used classification for the lymphoid tumors is that proposed by the Glasgow group (Anderson et al., 1969; Crighton, 1968a, 1969b; W. Jarrett, 1971). Five types, based on anatomical location, are recognized. (a) In the *multicentric* form most lymphoid organs are involved, including bilateral involvement of lymph nodes. Other organs, such as liver, kidney, lungs, and bone marrow may be secondarily involved. (b) The *alimentary* form appears to start in the Peyer's patches, with major involvement being restricted to the gut wall and regional lymph nodes. (c) The *thymic* or *anterior mediastinal* form represents a large mass that replaces the thoracic thymus and involves local lymph nodes. (d) True *lymphoid leukemia* is characterized by the presence of either absolute peripheral blood lymphocytosis or the presence of large numbers of immature lymphoid cells in the blood, or both. The bone marrow is also massively involved. (e) The last category is only a representation to describe those cases that do not fit into one of the above four. These are primarily unusual instances, where local involvement occurs in such areas as the central nervous system and kidney. The clinical signs are usually a reflection of the organ systems that are involved. Diagnosis is often difficult without hematologic or histopathologic support. The most frequent hematologic findings in the lymphoid forms are normocytic normachromic anemia and absolute lymphocytopenia (Crighton, 1968b).

The histopathology of feline lymphoma is similar to that of rapidly growing lymphomas of many species, such as the Burkitt tumor of children (Squire, 1966a). The principal cell types seen in feline lymphoma are the stem cell, the lymphoblast, the prolymphocyte, the histiocyte, and the lymphohistiocyte (Mackey and Jarrett, 1972; Jarrett *et al.*, 1973c). The origin, sites of multiplication, and routes of migration of the malignant cells are distinct for each morbid anatomic form (Mackey and Jarrett, 1972). It is possible that the degree of lymphopenia and the degree and nature of the immunosuppression are also somewhat characteristic in each form (whether the T-cell-mediated immune functions or the B-cell-mediated functions are involved).

We checked clinically healthy cats naturally infected with FeLV to determine whether alterations in the hemogram were present. No evidence for subclinical anemia was found in infected cats, and total leukocyte counts were also the same for FeLV-infected cats and uninfected household controls. FeLV-infected healthy cats did, however, have lower mean absolute lymphocyte counts.

Significant geographical differences are observed between the comparative incidences of the various forms (Essex *et al.*, 1975a). We observed that about half of the cases collected in Boston between 1972 and 1974 were true lymphocytic leukemia, while 5% or less of the cases collected in Glasgow and New York during the same time period were this form. Similarly, the multicentric form was much more common in the New York cases, and the alimentary form was most common in the Glasgow cases. The differences were apparently too great to be due to either chance or biased selection. Different incidences of certain virus strains is one possible explanation, but this theory is confused by observations that single (but uncloned) isolates of FeLV induce a variety of forms in laboratory studies (Jarrett et al., 1973b).

The true age, sex, and breed incidence of feline leukemia-lymphoma is very difficult to establish because accurate population background data on healthy cats are almost nonexistent. Additionally, the accuracy of diagnosis is very variable when populations apart from those observed at large academic-associated veterinary clinics are considered. The only feline leukemia incidence figure determined using a population-based animal registry as background was the figure of 41.6 cases per 100,000 cats in the population at risk (Dorn et al., 1967, 1968). This incidence is considerably higher than that for man or other domestic animals (Priester and Mantel, 1971). Even in the Dorn et al. (1968) study, some cases could have been missed, and the incidence may be even higher. There is general agreement that leukemia is the most common cat tumor, accounting for at least one-third of the malignant tumors in this species. Because of the variation in frequency of different morbid anatomic forms observed for different cities, it is very likely that variations in the total incidence in the Alameda County, California, survey (Dorn et al., 1968) may be quite different in other geographical locations.

The true age incidence also varies for each form and therefore for different locations as well. Leukemia is not a tumor characteristic of old cats as are most tumors of domestic animals. A biphasic age curve probably occurs, with peaks at about 2 and 8 years (W. Jarrett, 1971). The mean age for feline leukemia has been estimated at 5–6 years. Of 106 cases we collected in Boston, the mean age at time of detection was 3.9 years (Essex et al., 1975a), and 78 (74%) were 5 years of age or younger. Background data on ages for healthy cats in this area were not available, however. Lymphoma is thought to be slightly more common in male cats, and slightly higher incidences have been reported for purebred cats, such as Siamese, as compared to the crossbred domestic "breed" (Dorn et al., 1968; Hardy et al., 1969; Schneider, 1971). The suggestion has been made that an observed increase in incidence in certain purebred cats may be simply a reflection of selective attention to serious health problems by the owners (Gilmore and Holzworth, 1971). Our results with cats in leukemia cluster households support this explanation (Essex et al., 1974, 1975c,d). We found no appreciable differences in incidences of either clinical leukemia, FeLV infection, or geometric mean FOCMA antibody titers for cats of the Abyssinian, Burmese, and domestic breeds living in the same house.

B. Horizontal Virus Transmission under Laboratory Conditions

The first hint that oncogenic feline oncornaviruses might be transmitted horizontally in an infectious manner was when "clusters" of naturally occurring leukemia were reported (Schneider et al., 1967; Brodey et al., 1970; Brodey, 1971). The second clue came when investigators in different laboratories found that a higher than expected number of uninoculated contact control cats developed either leukemia (Rickard, 1969; Rickard et al., 1969, 1973b), fibrosarcoma (Snyder, personal communication), or antibody titers to FOCMA (Essex et al., 1971a,b). Convincing evidence for horizontal virus transmission under laboratory conditions came when serologic studies showed antibody development in almost all exposed controls (Jarrett, 1972; Essex and Snyder, 1973; Essex et al., 1973a; Jarrett et al., 1973b; Essex, 1974), and experiments designed to expose kittens by contact to FeLV excretor cats resulted in a significant frequency of leukemia development (Jarrett, 1972; Essex et al., 1973a; Jarrett et al., 1973b).

Five of 26 contact control kittens developed leukemia in the experiments described by Rickard, and similar observations were to be reported later by Hoover et al. (1972).

These results came at a time when a seemingly contradictory hypothesis (Huebner and Todaro, 1969) had just become popular, and the Rickard observation was received with little enthusiasm. The oncogene theory, based primarily on observations made with laboratory mice and chickens, proposed that vertical chromosomal transmission of oncornaviruses represented the only important transmission route in mammalian species.

In an experiment describing the induction of antibody to FOCMA (Essex et al., 1971b), we found that 3 of 13 kittens that were 3–12 months old had moderate antibody titers at the time the experiment began. We postulated that contact exposure to FeLV or FeSV could account for the antibody titers because the cats had been housed in an experimental barn with other cats that were previously involved in FeSV experiments.

In another study we found an unexpected resistance to oncogenesis in newborn kittens given up to 1000 times the lethal oncogenic dose of FeSV (Essex et al., 1971a). Since almost all the kittens that resisted tumor development had FOCMA antibody, we concluded that the antibody was protective. Retrospective examination of breeding histories for all kittens and mothers indicated that all kittens that had antibody titers as neonates were from litters whose mothers were known to be previously exposed to FeLV. None of the 19 kittens in any of 5 litters whose mothers had not been exposed to FeLV showed unusual resistance, and none had detectable antibodies. All 9 kittens in 2 of 4 litters whose dams had been previously exposed to FeLV were resistant to tumor induction and positive for FOCMA antibodies (Essex et al., 1971a). We suspected that passive transmission of antibodies had occurred because (a) all kittens within each litter had approximately the same antibody titers, (b) the antibody was present as IgG within a few days of birth, (c) antibody levels rapidly deteriorated in the kittens as would be expected for passively acquired globulins, and (d) the passive colostral transmission of IgG was known to be efficient in cats (Scott et al., 1970). The mothers involved had not themselves been inoculated with feline oncornaviruses, but had been exposed because they nursed previous litters that were injected with FeLV. Because of this we postulated that the mothers had become infected by horizontal transmission, developed protective antibody titers, and transmitted the antibodies to subsequent litters (Essex et al., 1973b). The transmission of protective antibodies in a similar manner had also been demonstrated for newborn rats exposed to murine leukemia viruses (Ioachim, 1970).

Recently we followed a series of 17 contact control "tracer" kittens and 6 mothers that nursed inoculated litters for the development of detectable FOCMA antibody (Essex and Snyder, 1973; Essex et al., 1974) (see Table VII). None had detectable antibody at the time of exposure to their infected cagemates. Of 17 contact-exposed kittens, 14 (82%) developed detectable antibody within 3 months of exposure. All 6 nursing mothers became positive during the same time interval. The geometric mean antibody titer at 10–15 weeks post-exposure was 5.0 for the kittens and 23.1 for the queens. These results thus supported our previous hypotheses of horizontal virus transmission and the protection of neonates by passively transmitted maternal antibody. They suggested that horizontal virus transmission not only occurred, but appeared highly efficient under conditions of laboratory contact.

TABLE VII
DEVELOPMENT OF FELINE ONCORNAVIRUS-ASSOCIATED CELL MEMBRANE ANTIGEN (FOCMA) ANTIBODY IN CONTACT CONTROL CATS EXPOSED TO CAGE-MATES WHICH WERE INOCULATED WITH FELINE LEUKEMIA VIRUS (FeLV) OR FELINE SARCOMA VIRUS (FeSV)

Cat No.	FOCMA antibody titers weeks post-inoculation[a]		
	0	5–7	10–15
Kittens[b]			
401	0	0	16
402	0	2	16
403	0	0	8
404	0	4	ND[c]
405	0	4	4
406	0	32	16
407	0	0	0
408	0	0	2
409	0	ND	64
410	0	ND	4
411	0	ND	4
412	0	2	ND
413	0	0	ND
414	0	1	4
415	0	1	4
416	0	0	2
417	0	0	0
Incidence	0/17	7/14	12/14
Geometric mean	0	1.1	5.0
Nursing mothers			
501	0	0	32
502	0	4	8
503	0	0	8
504	0	ND	16
505	0	8	128
506	0	4	32
Incidence	0/6	3/5	6/6
Geometric mean	0	2.0	23.1

[a] After cage-mates were inoculated with FeLV or FeSV.
[b] One week to 12 weeks old.
[c] ND, not done.

At about the same time we reported similar experiments, done in collaboration with the Glasgow group (Jarrett, 1972; Essex et al., 1973a; Jarrett et al., 1973b), where other criteria, in addition to the development of FOCMA antibody, were used to monitor FeLV infection in contact-exposed "tracer" cats. In addition to FOCMA antibody, we checked for (a) the development of virus neutralizing antibodies, (b) the presence of virus core group specific antigens (gs) in peripheral blood leukocytes, (c) the detection of virus by electron microscopy in blood platelets and bone marrow, and (d) the development of clinical leukemia. In one experiment, each of 2 contact control kittens and the nursing mother became positive for FOCMA antibody, gs, and electron microscopically detectable virus within 3 months after two littermates were injected with FeLV. Both inoculated kittens and one contact control developed leukemia. In a second experiment 6 contact-exposed kittens and 4 inoculated littermates were observed. Five of 6 controls developed FOCMA antibody titers, and 5 of 6 also developed neutralizing antibodies. All 6 developed gs and virus particles detectable by electron microscopy. Two of the 6 "tracer" controls developed leukemia. The controls converted to positive for each test about 2–4 weeks after their FeLV injected littermates. These experiments also supported the existence of a highly efficient mechanism for horizontal transmission under the close contact conditions in laboratory cages.

Since all the experiments mentioned above involved exposure to kittens that were given inoculations, an experiment was done to expose kittens to a field case of lymphosarcoma (Jarrett et al., 1973b). Each of four 6-month-old kittens were exposed to the terminally ill leukemic cat in a $4 \times 6 \times 8$-foot room for 8 days. Before the experiment began each exposed cat was confirmed to be negative for FOCMA antibody and virus. All four became positive for antibody, or virus, or both, within 2 months.

The report by Hoover et al. (1972) that leukemia could be induced by instillation of FeLV droplets in the nasal cavity suggested a reasonable mechanism for horizontal infection to occur. Cats frequently groom each other, especially when a mother nurses her progeny. Budding C-type virus particles had previously been observed in many cat tissues, including salivary gland (Gardner et al., 1971). Our examination of different tissues from both experimentally induced and naturally occurring cases of leukemia indicated that virus was usually present in salivary glands as well as tracheal, nasal, and oral epithelium (Jarrett et al., 1973b). The infiltration of salivary gland tissue with malignant lymphocytes had been reported previously (Oksanen et al., 1971).

C. Horizontal Virus Transmission under Field Conditions

In 1967 Schneider et al. reported a cluster of 6 cases of leukemia over a 5-year period in a household containing 34 cats. Because 5 of the 6 cats that developed leukemia were related, and because evidence for vertical transmission of oncornaviruses in mice was overwhelming, a role for horizontal FeLV transmission was not considered likely by the author (Schneider, 1971). The reports by Brodey and his colleagues thus became the first stimulus for serious consideration of the role of horizontal transmission in the natural history of feline leukemia (Brodey et al., 1970; Brodey, 1971). They described 15 household clusters that involved 38 leukemic cats, and case clustering accounted for 21% of all leukemic cases. Other clusters of feline leukemia were also described (Hardy, 1971; Hardy et al., 1973a; W. Jarrett, 1971; Cotter et al., 1973).

In one particular cluster (Cotter et al., 1973, 1974) the evidence for horizontal transmission was very strong. This involved an instance where 11 cases of leukemia occurred in a population of 35 largely unrelated cats during a period of 39 months. In addition to the incidence itself, which was about 1600 times higher than that to be expected due to chance alone, several other observations suggested that horizontal transmission of FeLV was responsible. First, the high incidence of leukemia continued to occur at a predictable rate after the first few cases were identified. Second, all 11 cases were the same histopathologic form. These two observations essentially eliminated the possibility that the cluster was due only to chance. Third, less than half of the 35 cats were related to other cats in the house, and the leukemia case animals were no more likely to be related to other leukemic cats or to have other relatives in the house than the healthy controls. Fourth, a much higher number of healthy cats in the cluster house were viremic as compared to healthy control cats from outside the house. Finally, the geometric mean FOCMA antibody titer for healthy cats in the house was higher than that to be expected. In the study by Hardy et al. (1973b), 38 household clusters were studied. The clusters included 117 cats with leukemia and an average of 3.1 cases per household. Two-thirds of the cases were in unrelated cats.

Owing to cooperation by the staffs of the Angell Memorial Animal Hospital in Boston and the Animal Medical Center and Henry Bergh ASPCA Hospitals in New York we were able to conduct seroepidemiologic studies on more than 3000 cats from these areas that received no unnatural exposure (i.e., laboratory inoculation or contact with FeLV-injected littermates) to feline oncornaviruses. These studies were done in collaboration with Hardy and others (Essex et al., 1973b, 1974, 1975a,b,c,d; Cotter et al., 1974; Essex, 1974; Hardy et al., 1973b, 1974; Hardy, 1974). In addition to the FOCMA antibody test, extensive use was made of the fixed cell immunofluorescence test for detecting virus core gs in peripheral blood leukocytes and platelets (Hardy *et al.*, 1973a,b). The test for gs using peripheral blood smears was also shown to be an accurate index for the presence of infectious FeLV in the blood, or viremia (Hardy *et al.*, 1973b).

In households where a case of feline leukemia had been confirmed, the normal healthy cats were checked for FeLV using the gs test (Hardy *et al.*, 1973a,b). Of 543 healthy cats from such households, 33% were gs positive. Furthermore, healthy cats from cluster households (defined as those with two or more cases of leukemia) were twice as likely to be FeLV positive as healthy cats in households with only 1 leukemia case. As controls, 1462 healthy cats with no known exposure to leukemia were checked. Only 2 were FeLV positive, and these were both stray cats with unknown histories. None of 627 cats from isolated pet households confirmed as having no history of leukemia were positive. A positive correlation between FeLV infection of exposed healthy cats and the subsequent development of leukemia was also established (see below). FeLV positive healthy cats were at approximately a 900-fold greater risk for leukemia development.

Our studies were then concentrated on healthy cats in multiple case "cluster" households, and particularly on the cats in two houses (Cotter *et al.*, 1973, 1974; Essex *et al.*, 1974, 1975c,d; Essex, 1974). The first house, where 11 cases of leukemia had been observed, was described above. In the second house 10 cases of leukemia were observed in a population of about 150 over an 18-month period. In this case only about half of the sick or dead cats were available for diagnosis of disease or autopsy, so the rate of leukemia might have been considerably higher. Three different breeds were present in the house, and the leukemia incidence was about the same for each breed.

In the first house, 3 cats died of leukemia and 3 of other diseases before the serologic study began. Of the remaining 29, 14 were persistently gs positive. Of these, 2 were first tested and shown to be gs positive at the time a diagnosis of leukemia was made. Five developed leukemia after being confirmed as FeLV positive while still healthy. Three more died during the course of study from nonleukemic diseases. When all the healthy cats in the house were first tested, 8 of 21 (38%) were FeLV positive. None of the age, sex, and geographically matched controls from outside the house were positive. At the same time the geometric mean FOCMA antibody titer for the healthy cats was 4.7, a figure several times higher than that obtained for the age, sex, and geographically matched controls. These data supported our previous observations concerning a positive correlation between FeLV infection in healthy contact controls and exposure to leukemia cases, as well as the correlation between FeLV positivity in healthy cats and subsequent development of disease. Additionally, our use of the FOCMA antibody test on the same population also showed an infection rate for the healthy exposed cats that was significantly higher than that for unexposed controls.

In cluster house number 2, the results were equally dramatic. Of 125 healthy cats exposed to FeLV-excreting leukemic cats, 64 (51%) were gs positive. The geometric mean antibody titer for the healthy animals in this house was 5.9—more than 5 times as high as the figure for controls from outside the cluster. More than 93% of the healthy cats in this house were positive for gs antigen or FOCMA antibody, or both. In this house an analysis of FeLV positivity and FOCMA antibody titer was also done by breed (in the first house all cats except 1 were of the domestic breed). No evidence was found for a significantly higher infection rate in any of the 3 breeds. Two families that also had sufficient numbers of progeny were compared. One represented the progeny of an FeLV-positive mother with a low antibody titer. The other involved the progeny of a virus-free mother with a high FOCMA antibody titer. For the 12 progeny in one family and 13 in another, the incidence of gs positivity and the mean FOCMA antibody titer was essentially the same. Several other leukemia exposure households containing fewer cats were studied using the same tests, and similar results were obtained (Essex et al., 1975d).

The only obvious interpretation of these findings is that leukemia of cats is horizontally transmitted under natural conditions and that FeLV, as the cause, is spread as a highly contagious virus. As with most infectious diseases, however, leukemia apparently occurs only in a minority of the exposed individuals. Except for the information supporting a very different natural history for oncornaviruses of the two more thoroughly studied but very different species, laboratory mice and chickens, it is likely that the evidence of horizontal transmission for FeLV would be accepted without further questioning. It is beyond reason to expect that the overwhelming seroepidemiologic evidence could have occurred due to chance alone. This is stated not only because of the very wide differences seen between healthy cluster and noncluster control cats in both tests, but also because of the prospective predictability of the cluster microenvironments as established endemic foci for new cases of clinical leukemia. Criticism of the approach of studying cats in such cluster environments frequently includes the comment that "many other diseases of cats also occur more frequently under such crowded conditions." This is of course true, but it must be realized that the "other diseases" (primarily enteritis, pneumonitis, rhinotracheitis, and infectious peritonitis) are caused by highly contagious viruses and bacteria.

The data obtained in one epidemiologic survey, interpreted as failing to support the horizontal transmission of FeLV (Schneider, 1970, 1972a), thus requires close scrutiny. In that case horizontal transmission was thought to be unlikely because of three observations. First, leukemic cats were not observed to have a significantly higher degree of association with other cats. Second, neutered male leukemic cats were not found to have been castrated at older ages than were control males. Third, the leukemic case animals were not found to have a greater tendency for predatory dietary habits. The latter two criteria were considered to be related to the degree of mobility, and thus increased contact with other cats as measured directly in the first case. The problems involved in a study such as this are very great, and several possible points of criticism can be made. It is unfortunate that the behavioral parameters incorporated in the study were not confirmed as accurate reflections of horizontal transmissibility using as a "positive control" one of the other common infectious diseases of cats. Proof of an association between mobility and neutering for the ages considered has not been demonstrated in cats. Regarding the "predatory habits," the leukemic cats were 1.4–2.1 times as likely to be included in each of four such categories. The failure to establish statistical significance in this case could be simply because of insufficient numbers available for analysis. Aside from these details, two major limitations exist concerning the sensitivity of such an approach for confirming or disproving horizontal transmissibility. These are the very long incubation periods that must be expected for the development of leukemia under natural conditions (Hardy et al., 1973b; Essex et al., 1975c,d) and the likelihood that most cats exposed to FeLV do not develop leukemia, but resist owing to an active immune response (Essex et al., 1973a, 1974, 1975b,d; Essex, 1974).

The most logical route for horizontal transmission is oral. Tracheal, nasal, and oral epithelium as well as salivary gland tissue are sites where FeLV readily replicates (Gardner et al., 1971; Jarrett, 1972; Jarrett et al., 1973b). This would facilitate both excretion of large quantities of virus in oral secretions and ready access to susceptible target tissue after virus exposure. Other possibilities, that seem less likely, include exposure to FeLV excreted in urine and feces, transmission by blood-sucking ectoparasites that feed on viremic cats (Hardy *et al.*, 1974) or vaccination with infected vaccines (Gardner, personal communication). FeLV has been observed by electron microscopy to replicate from intestinal and kidney epithelium (Dougherty *et al.*, 1969; Dougherty, 1971; Hardy *et al.*, 1969, 1973a,b), but it seems unlikely that much viable virus would be dispersed by this route.

D. VERTICAL TRANSMISSION OF FELINE ONCORNAVIRUSES

The possible routes for transmission of oncornaviruses can be arbitrarily divided into three categories, and all appear to play a significant role in the cat. The first, horizontal transmission, as described above, appears to be the most important route for distribution of the FeLV–FeSV group. The second, true vertical chromosomal transmission, is where virus genes are permanently integrated into the cell nucleic acid component of all cells in all individuals of the species. The virus genome is then regularly transmitted through the germ cells. This type of transmission appears to be the most important, if not exclusive mechanism for the RD-114-endogenous virus group. The third category, vertical extrachromosomal or epigenetic transmission is somewhat more difficult to define, and it is equally difficult to assess the role of this route for the FeLV-FeSV group. This category includes transplacental infection of the fetus from an infected mother, as well as infection of neonates with milk-borne virus. The infection of young kittens by oral contact with an infected mother (grooming) should probably be considered as horizontal.

Horizontal transmission appears to play little or no role for distribution of the RD-114 group of viruses among cats. All cats appear to have these agents in an unexpressed form, so little or no purpose would be served by superinfection. A few cat fetuses express gs antigen or infectious virus, but postnatal cat tumors or normal tissues are almost always negative for genome expression (Gardner *et al.*, 1974; Sarma *et al.*, 1974a).

True chromosomal vertical transmission is extremely difficult to prove, especially as it concerns all individuals within an outbred species, as opposed to all clones of a given cell line or all individuals in a highly inbred strain. All oncornaviruses presumably have the potential for forming DNA proviruses which can interact in a stable unexpressed fashion with the DNA of susceptible somatic cells (Temin, 1971; Temin and Baltimore, 1972). This property does not necessarily imply vertical transmission, however. In Herpesvirus systems such as the Epstein–Barr virus of man, for example, the viral genome exists in a stable "turned-off" association with the nucleic acid of susceptible target cells (Zur Hausen and Schulte-Holthausen, 1970; Nonoyama and Pagano, 1971). It is then regularly transmitted through mitosis to all progeny cells in the same line, but the virus is apparently never vertically transmitted. This may be because the germ cells are more resistant to infection (Koprowski, 1972), or because the meiotic division step is more selective concerning integration or excision of exogenous DNA. The regular association of oncornavirus functions with unrelated phenotypic characteristics of the cell implies a regular site on somatic cell chromosomes for integration, but not necessarily vertical chromosomal transmission. Again, in analogy with Herpesviruses, negative evidence for a lack of virus production in certain selected tissues of most individuals does not of itself eliminate the possibility for horizontal transmission. With the Marek's disease and Epstein–Barr viruses, unexpressed genomes are characteristically found in most target cells, but virus is only produced in certain "privileged" sites and then efficiently spread to most individuals of the species by such materials as feather follicle debris (Nazerian, 1973) and oral secretions (Chang, 1971).

Despite these difficulties, the regularity of finding RD-114 nucleic acids in all feline embryos (Baluda and Roy-Burman, 1973; Fujinaga *et al.*, 1973; Neiman, 1973; Gillespie *et al.*, 1973; Okabe *et al.*, 1973a,b) and the success reported by Sarma *et al.* (1974a) for inducing RD-114 in 16 of 16 different feline cultures (from 9 cats) with iododeoxyuridine makes a very strong case for vertical genetic transmission. The total absence of neutralizing antibodies to RD-114 in normal and cancerous cats also indicates either a complete lack of production of virus proteins during immunosusceptible stages or complete tolerance due to regular expression at very early stages of embryogenesis. The RD-114 case is in fact probably the best evidence for regular transmission of oncornavirus genomes in an outbred mammalian species.

Vertical epigenetic or extrachromosomal transmission cannot yet be ruled out for the RD-114 group, but if it exists it must occur at very early postzygotic stages of embryogenesis. The chances for transplacental or neonatal transmission seem, like the horizontal route, very unlikely.

In marked contrast to the RD-114 group, little or no evidence exists for regular vertical chromosomal transmission of viruses of the FeLV groups. It appears that FeLV can, like other oncornaviruses, exist in somatic cells in a "nonproducer" or "turned-off" manner

(Baluda and Roy-Burman, 1973; Gillespie et al., 1973; Sarma et al., 1974a). As explained above, this does not imply vertical genetic transmission through the germ cells. The fact that FeLV-specific nucleic acid sequences are found only in a minority of the specimens studied by itself suggests exogenous entry rather than regular genetic transmission. Studies with virus free "clean" cat cultures indicated an absence of FeLV-specific RNA sequences (Okabe et al., 1973b). The lack of success for activating FeLV from virus-free cloned cat embryo cells also appears to be significant (Todaro et al., 1973b).

It is likely that true vertical genetic transmission and horizontal transmission are, at least to some degree, mutually exclusive. It is also possible that true regular vertical genetic transmission is incompatible with pathogenicity or oncogenicity in the evolutionary sense of survival, at least for diseases such as feline leukemia that most often kill before the reproductive years are over.

Vertical extrachromosomal transmission of the FeLV–FeSV group probably does occur, at least occasionally. When pregnant queens become viremic it is logical that they might infect unborn fetuses by the transplacental route, and neonates by nursing. This feature would not be unusual for oncornaviruses, but probably occurs to some extent with most pantropic animal viruses. Several groups have examined fetal and embryonic tissues for viruslike particles by electron microscopy, and virus core antigens using serological tests. The electron microscopic examination of tissues from normal fetal and adult cats gave results varying from a small percentage positive for C-type particles (Rickard et al., 1973b; Gardner et al., 1974) to a complete lack of success for finding such particles (Laird et al., 1968a; Jarrett, 1972; Riggs et al., 1973). The finding of C-type particles in fetal tissues does not necessarily indicate vertical transmission of FeLV. RD-114 is morphologically similar to FeLV when observed in thin sections, and many of the C-type particles seen in fetal tissues by Gardner et al. (1974) were found in tissues free of FeLV and RD-114 virus core antigens or infectious virus. The latter observation was interpreted as indicating the possibility of the existence of a third as yet undescribed class of feline oncornaviruses (Gardner et al., 1974).

Antigenic studies also indicate that fetal or adult tissues from some normal healthy cats also contain FeLV viral core proteins (Hardy et al., 1969, 1973a,b, 1974; Sarma et al., 1974a; Essex et al., 1974, 1975b,c,d). Our studies indicate that the percentage of positive normal cats varies from zero to more than 50% depending on degree of environmental exposure to FeLV. For this reason, attempts to demonstrate vertical transmission or the presence of C-type particles or antigens in normal adult or fetal tissues should be expected to produce variable results, especially when healthy cats of unknown histories are studied. The identification of FeLV in placental or fetal tissues from germ-free or specific-pathogen-free cats has not been reported.

We have observed that a high percentage of female cats with naturally occurring breeding problems such as abortion and fetal resorption are FeLV positive (Essex et al., 1975a). It is therefore tempting to postulate that the adverse effects on the fetus observed in these instances were due to transplacental transmission of FeLV from the viremic mother. It is well established that the leukemogenicity of FeLV is greatest when virus is administered to the very young. Horizontal transmission of virus appears to be common among adults, but it is quite possible that neonatal exposure would more frequently result in leukemia development. Adults not confined to close quarters in cluster households would probably receive only low exposure doses, and mount an effective immune response. Neonates, on the other hand, would receive large doses when being constantly groomed with infected saliva from viremic mothers. This exposure would also come at a time of relative immunologic immaturity.

In summary, the role for extrachromosomal vertical transmission in the natural history of FeLV is unclear at this time. It is likely that such transmission is infrequent. Yet it is also possible that this type of exposure might be the type that most frequently results in clinical leukemia. Following the same thesis that regular genetic vertical transmission would eliminate a need for horizontal transmission, the highly lethal effect seen with occasional extrachromosomal vertical transmission would appear to eliminate a role for regular vertical transmission because of adverse effects on survival of the species.

Another possible mechanism that has been suggested is that horizontally transmitted viruses (FeLV–FeSV) might act by activating or "turning-on" an oncogenic endogenous virus (Hardy et al., 1973b). No support for this exists at the present time, and a considerable amount of evidence argues against it. The only known endogenous virus of cats, RD-114, does not become expressed or activated when leukemia or other tumors occur (Gardner et al., 1974). Additionally, extensive in vivo testing of the RD-114 virus has failed to demonstrate any oncogenicity, at least during a 10–20-month observation period (McAllister, personal communication). FeLV, in contrast, is both oncogenic and regularly found in tumor-bearing animals. Even if the exogenous FeLV did act by turning on an endogenous agent that was present in all cells, it would require considerable stretching of the definition of cause to imply that the endogenous agent actually caused the tumor. The endogenous agent would not be able to operate alone, but the exogenous virus would—in the sense that all cats would contain the required endogenous genome sequences, but only those specifically activated by FeLV could be oncogenic.

E. Incidence of Virus Infection in Laboratory and Field Cat Populations

In Sections VIII,B and VIII,C above, evidence was presented for a very high frequency of FeLV infection in laboratory-exposed control cats housed with injected littermates, as well as healthy cats from naturally occurring leukemia cluster environmer.ts. Although several criteria were employed, the gs antigen blood smear test and the FOCMA antibody test were most extensively used. The former was taken as an indication of current FeLV infection; the latter as an index of previous exposure. In this section the infection status and serologic picture of cats from different environments with no known exposure to FeLV will be considered. Cats exposed to FeLV or FeSV were first thought to be immunologically tolerant and unable to produce antibody to virus core proteins (Gardner et al., 1970; Huebner et al., 1970, 1971). Extensive testing using different procedures demonstrated that this was not so (Sibal et al., 1970; Fink et al., 1971; Noronha et·al., 1972; Olsen and Yohn, 1972; Yohn and Olsen, 1973).

Tests for virus antigens using serologic procedures that specifically detect FeLV have indicated that very few healthy cats are positive outside of those in household environments where heavy exposure is known to have occurred. Those that react positively using the blood smear gs test are probably persistently viremic, with few exceptions. The incubation period for leukemia is long under natural conditions, and FeLV viremia persists for many months before the development of clinical disease (Hardy et al., 1973b; Cotter et al., 1974; Essex et al., 1975c). Healthy cats with short transient FeLV infections are rarely detected except by antibody seroconversion in a retrospective sense. The presence of viruslike particles by electron microscopy in normal cats is not specific for FeLV (Gardner et al., 1974), so data on this subject will not be reconsidered here. Likewise, the complement-fixation inhibition and paired radioiodine labeling serologic procedures as employed (Olsen and Yohn, 1972; Yohn and Olsen, 1973) might also detect RD-114 as well as FeLV.

The study by Hardy et al. (1973b, 1974) using the gs test on cats not known to be from leukemia exposure environments indicates only 2 of 638 healthy stray cats as positive, and no positives at all among 627 healthy cats from pet household environments where negative histories for leukemia and related diseases were first confirmed. The cats involved in this study were primarily from the New York City area. One hundred ninety-seven healthy cats from a colony where chronic administration of ^{90}Sr was practiced were also negative. One hundred fourteen healthy cats from urban and suburban Boston were also tested, and only 2 were positive (Essex et al., 1975b). In this case, histories on the cats were not obtained, and no attempt was made to screen for and eliminate those from households with histories of leukemia or related diseases.

Various tests have been used to detect FeLV-specific antibodies in healthy cats. Using passive hemagglutination, 8 of 15 cats in one instance (Fink et al., 1971) and 8 of 10 in another were found to have detectable antibody. A considerable range was found in antibody titers. Histories on the cats were not available. With virus neutralization, 13 of 59 (22%) cats without neoplasia (all but 7 were healthy) had detectable antibody (Sarma et al., 1974b). Three had antibody to subgroup A virus only, 6 to subgroup B only, 3 to subgroup C only, and 1 to both A and B virus subgroups. As in the previous case, detailed histories on either geographical location or possible leukemia exposure status were not available. Using indirect membrane immunofluorescence in a manner similar to that used to detect FOCMA antibody, Riggs et al. (1973) found 5 normal cats of 100 tested that reacted positively at a 1:4 serum dilution. The cats involved were from an SPCA shelter in the San Francisco area, but of unknown exposure status.

Using the FOCMA antibody test as an index for exposure to viruses of the FeLV–FeSV group, we determined antibody titers for 477 normal healthy cats from various cities (Essex et al., 1973a; Jarrett et al., 1973a; Essex, 1974; Essex et al., 1975a). Table VIII lists the results obtained for healthy cats from laboratory colony and pet household environments. None of the 50 cats from a specific-pathogen-free colony had detectable antibody, and 6.5% or less of the cats from 3 other laboratory colonies were positive. All the cats in each of the colonies were watched very closely for signs of illness, and no case of leukemia had ever been observed in any of the colonies. Two of the colonies were maintained as breeding facilities to provide kittens for oncornavirus experiments, but any kittens or dams used for experiments were maintained in a geographically dis-

TABLE VIII
FELINE ONCORNAVIRUS-ASSOCIATED CELL MEMBRANE ANTIGEN (FOCMA)
ANTIBODY TITERS IN HEALTHY CATS FROM VARIOUS ENVIRONMENTS

Source	No. tested	No. positive	Percent positive	Titer Range	Geometric mean
Laboratory colonies					
Specific-pathogen free	120	3	2.5	0–16	0.0
Other	101	3	3.0	0–4	0.0
Pet environments					
Suburban and urban Boston	163	102	62.6	0–256	1.2
Suburban and urban Detroit	32	15	46.9	0–32	0.7
Suburban and urban Glasgow	28	11	39.3	0–8	0.6
Urban New York	33	1	3.0	0–1	0.0
Leukemia cluster households					
House No. 1	121	100	82.7	0–256	5.9
House No. 2	17	13	76.5	0–64	4.7

tant facility and were never returned to the breeding colony. Our results indicate that FeLV infection is infrequent or rare under such conditions.

Samples collected from healthy cats residing in 4 major suburban and urban areas were also tested. Of 28 cats from the Glasgow area, 11 (39.3%) had antibody. For cats in the Detroit area, 15 of 32 (46.9%) were positive and of 33 cats from urban New York City only 1 was positive. Of 163 cats from suburban and urban Boston, 102 (62.6%) had some detectable FOCMA antibody. A few cats had titers ranging from 8 to 256, but most were very low, and the geometric mean in each case was about 1.0 or less. In all cases but those from New York City, the cats were not screened to eliminate those from households with a previous history of leukemia. Cats known to be from leukemia households were not included in any of the series. Except for those cats from several known leukemia households, no attempt was made to determine environmental histories. The only exception to this rule was the New York City cats, where all were confirmed to be from leukemia-free households. This was probably partially responsible for the low number of FOCMA-positive cats seen in the New York series. The urban New York cats, however, were also from high rise apartments where roaming does not occur and exposure to other cats is infrequent. The Boston, Glasgow, and Detroit samples were primarily from suburban cats where roaming is frequently practiced.

Since 163 samples were available for testing from healthy Boston cats, the results were also analyzed for different age categories (Essex *et al.*, 1975b). Young adults were most frequently positive, and had the highest geometric mean antibody titers. Cats over 5 years of age were less likely to be positive for detectable antibody, and the geometric mean titer was also lower. This suggests that young adults, presumably the most mobile group, may be more frequently exposed to FeLV. The same age group would be the most likely to resist leukemia due to an active immune response, which could account for the failure to correlate a significant increase in leukemia detection with increased mobility (Schneider, 1972a).

The results of serologic testing indicate that many more cats become infected with FeLV than the number that actually develop leukemia. A comparison of these results with those for healthy cats from leukemia cluster households suggests that exposure to larger doses in the cluster environments results in: (a) a much higher frequency of persistent rather than transient infections, (b) a higher frequency of development of detectable FOCMA antibody, and (c) higher titers in those cats with detectable antibody.

F. Serologic Studies of Cats with Naturally Occurring Leukemia

The electron microscopic examination of tissues has resulted in observations of C-type particles in approximately 55–90% of the cases of naturally occurring feline leukemia (Laird *et al.*, 1968a; Hardy *et al.*, 1969; Dougherty, 1971; Gardner *et al.*, 1971, 1974; Jarrett *et al.*, 1973a; Riggs *et al.*, 1973; Rickard *et al.*, 1973b; Essex *et al.*, 1975a). Considering the largely unavoidable variability in procedures used for selection of cases, tissues, blocks, grids, and sections, the degree of success has been quite constant. As with induced cases, bone marrow, lymph nodes, tracheal epithelium, and salivary gland tissues are most frequently positive. Almost all tissues and cell types examined were occasionally positive, including even erythrocytes (Oshiro *et al.*, 1972).

The serologic examination of tissues for FeLV–FeSV virus core antigens is more specific than electron microscopic examination. It is probably also more sensitive, at least when procedures such as fixed cell immunofluorescence are employed (Hardy *et al.*, 1969, 1973a,b; Jarrett *et al.*, 1973b; Essex *et al.*, 1975a). Using immunodiffusion with high-titered reference antisera prepared in rabbits, Hardy (1971) found 42 of 59 (71%) cases of leukemia positive. Others obtained similar results with a limited number of cases (Sibal *et al.*,

1970; Fink et al., 1971). Complement fixation has also been used (Sarma et al., 1970b, 1971b; Gardner et al., 1974). Twenty-nine of 64 cases were found to be positive using this procedure.

Fixed-cell immunofluorescence using peripheral blood smears is probably the most economical and convenient procedure, and it is at least as sensitive as the other tests (Hardy et al., 1973a,b). With this technique, more than 200 cats with leukemia have been tested. From 69% to 91% were positive (Hardy et al., 1973b, 1974; Hardy, 1974; Essex, 1974; Essex et al., 1975a).

Regardless of the procedure used to detect FeLV, differences in the proportion of positive cases have been observed for leukemic cats of different ages and from different geographical locations. Perhaps the most dramatic variation was the report by Gardner et al. (1974) that only 1 of 20 leukemic cats older than 10 years at the time of leukemic development were positive for FeLV while 28 of 44 cats less than 10 years of age were positive. Concerning geographical location, we found that only 70% of the Boston leukemic cats were positive for FeLV gs antigen in blood smears, while 85 to 90% of the cats from New York City were positive (Essex et al., 1975a). Some pathologic forms of leukemia–lymphoma are also more frequently virus positive than others (Hardy, 1971; Jarrett et al., 1973a; Essex et al., 1975a). We found a variation of positive percentages that ranged from 37% for the alimentary form to 92% for the multicentric form (Essex et al., 1975a). The frequency of different pathologic forms of leukemia–lymphoma varies considerably for different geographical areas, so the geographic, pathologic, and individual laboratory variations in positivity may have the same explanation. The explanation is unclear, but a likely possibility is the existence of different strains of FeLV, each endemic to or more common in certain areas, and each tending to induce certain types of the disease. Assuming that oncogenic potential also varies among FeLV strains, the differences between the ratio of virus positive (persistently viremic) cats to the number of antibody-positive, virus-negative cats in the same environment may be due to virus strain as well as age and dose.

Several procedures have also been used to detect antibody to virus core, envelope, and cell membrane antigens in cats with naturally occurring leukemia. Either all or most cats tested for antibody by either immunodiffusion (Hardy et al., 1969; Sibal et al., 1970; Fink et al., 1971; Hardy, 1971) or complement fixation (Gardner et al., 1970; Sarma et al., 1971b; Olsen and Yohn, 1972) were negative. A few were found to be positive by passive hemagglutination (Sibal et al., 1970; Fink et al., 1971). Nine of 38 cats with neoplasia (all but 2 had lymphoma) had detectable virus-neutralizing antibodies (Sarma *et al.*, 1974b). All but one had low titers, and all but two had antibodies to only one virus subgroup. Simultaneous FeLV antigen studies were not done, so it was not known if the leukemic cats with detectable antibody were virus positive or negative. Although another study indicated that viremic cats were invariably negative for virus-neutralizing antibodies at serum dilutions of 1:10 or above (Hardy, 1974; Hardy and Essex, unpublished), it is at least theoretically possible that infection with one subgroup might persist in the presence of high titers of antibody to a different virus subgroup.

We have determined the FOCMA antibody titers for cats with naturally occurring leukemia (Jarrett *et al.*, 1973a; Cotter *et al.*, 1974; Essex, 1974; Essex *et al.*, 1974, 1975a). As is the case with induced leukemia (see Section VII,B) either no detectable FOCMA antibody or very low titers were observed. Sixty-seven of 145 cats with naturally occurring leukemia had some detectable antibody, but the titers were very low (Essex *et al.*, 1975a). The geometric mean titer was only 0.8. Slight but not dramatic differences were seen in the frequency of detectable antibody, and/or the geometric mean titers for cats from different geographical areas or having different pathologic forms of leukemia. Riggs *et al.* (1973) found 17 of 52 (33%) cats with leukemia to be positive for antibody to the cell membrane antigen when a 1:4 dilution of serum was tested.

More extensive studies were done with healthy and leukemic cats in the large leukemia cluster household described in Section VIII,C above (Essex, 1974; Essex *et al.*, 1975c,d; Essex, Jakowski, Hardy, and Cotter, unpublished). Serial bleedings were taken from all cats in the environment at 3–5-month intervals for a 2-year period. During this time 9% of the cats converted from virus negative to positive and 2% went from FeLV positive to negative. The vast majority remained either virus positive or negative throughout the course of study, and about equal numbers of positive and negative cats were present in the house.

FeLV positive (viremic) cats were less likely to have high FOCMA antibody titers than uninfected cats (Essex *et al.*, 1975d). The geometric mean antibody titer for FeLV-infected cats was 3.4; for uninfected cats it was 10.0. Forty of 60 (67%) of the virus negative cats had a FOCMA antibody titer of 8 or higher, the range that is associated with resistance under laboratory conditions. Twenty of 61 (33%) of the viremic cats had antibody titers of 8 or higher. Of the healthy viremic cats followed for two years in this and a second cluster house (as described above in Section VIII,C), 31 of 69 (44.9%) developed lethal diseases (Essex *et al.*, 1975c). Only 5 of 59 (8.5%) of the cats that remained FeLV negative developed disease and died.

All but one of the cats that developed leukemia were virus positive. All cats that developed leukemia, and 29 of 34 (86%) that developed lethal diseases had low or negative FOCMA antibody titers.

A somewhat unexpected observation in these studies was the increase in the incidence of nonneoplastic diseases (4–5 times) in FeLV-positive cats when compared to virus-negative cats from the same environments. This suggested that the immunosuppression and thymic atrophy previously described in laboratory studies may also play a very important role under field conditions. Leukemia has a very long incubation period, and the incubation period for most of the other diseases observed is short. Persistently viremic nonleukemic cats thus appear to have long periods of increased susceptibility to other disease processes. A high incidence of FeLV infection has been observed previously by ourselves and others in cats with certain nonneoplastic diseases (Hardy et al., 1969; Hardy, 1971; Gardner et al., 1971; Cotter et al., 1973, 1974; Essex and Snyder, 1973; Essex et al., 1973a, 1975c). This had previously been explained as an activation of vertically transmitted latent FeLV by the nonneoplastic disease agent (Hardy, 1971). In view of the current seroepidemiological information and the observation that persistent FeLV infection often precedes the development of nonneoplastic diseases by many months, the FeLV immunosuppression-predisposition explanation appears more realistic.

The serologic picture presented by cats naturally exposed to FeLV appears similar to the picture seen in laboratory cats deliberately exposed to the virus. We can thus postulate that the immune response to both virion envelope and cell membrane antigens plays a very important role in disease outcome. Cats that mount an efficient virus neutralizing antibody response do not become viremic, and cats that mount an efficient anti-FOCMA response do not develop leukemia or sarcoma. If the virus-neutralizing antibody response is ineffective and persistent viremia occurs, cats still appear resistant to leukemia if FOCMA antibody titers are high. These cats can remain viremic and excrete FeLV as healthy carriers for several years. Such individuals may develop leukemia later in life if the immune response deteriorates, but they probably play a very important epidemiologic role in the distribution of virus to susceptible contacts.

G. The Frequency of Feline Leukemia Virus Infection in Feline Diseases Other Than Leukemia and Sarcoma

Feline oncornaviruses have been detected in, and associated with, certain disease syndromes other than leukemia–lymphoma and fibrosarcoma. As discussed in the previous section, FeLV infection is associated with both immunosuppression and a predisposition to the development of infectious diseases in general, so caution should be exercised before assigning an etiologic role for FeLV in many of the syndromes. Although cats with some diseases, such as infectious peritonitis, are frequently FeLV positive, very little is known about the immune response or the etiologic agents involved in this disease. It is possible, for example, that those aspects of the immune response that are most necessary to combat certain disease agents are the same elements most affected by FeLV. In addition to infectious peritonitis (Hardy et al., 1969, 1973a,b; Hardy, 1971; Hardy and Hurvitz, 1971; Cotter et al., 1973, 1974; Essex et al., 1975a), those syndromes reported to be associated with feline oncornaviruses include mammary carcinoma (Feldman and Gross, 1971; Riggs et al., 1973; Weijer et al., 1974), anemia (Gardner et al., 1972, 1974; Hardy et al., 1973b; Jarrett et al., 1973a; Priester and Hayes, 1973; Essex et al., 1975c,d), and glomerulonephritis (Anderson and Jarrett, 1971; Jarrett et al., 1973c; Essex et al., 1975c,d).

Probably the best case for FeLV acting as a cause of a nonneoplastic disease can be made for the nonregenerative anemias. Gardner et al. (1974) found that spleen tissues from 17 of 23 (74%) anemic cats were positive for virus core antigens by the complement-fixation test, and 11 of 13 (85%) were positive for C-type particles by electron microscopy. We also found that 53 of 76 (70%) of the cats with naturally occurring anemia in the absence of leukemia were FeLV positive by fixed cell immunofluorescence (Essex et al., 1975a). Both studies revealed as many anemic cats that were positive for FeLV as leukemic cats that were FeLV positive. In the prospective sense, we observed that 7.5% of 177 FeLV-positive cats subsequently developed lethal anemia during a 5.3-month observation period (Hardy et al., 1973b). In the same study 16.2% of the cats developed leukemia.

Anemia is the most frequent sign in clinical leukemia or lymphoma, and it is possible that some animals die in a preleukemic stage due to severe anemia before a diagnosis of leukemia can be made. To determine whether anemia was a regular occurrence following FeLV infection, we checked packed cell volumes for healthy cats with persistent viremia of 1–2 years' duration and control virus-negative associates in the same cluster households (Essex et al., 1975d). No evidence for subclinical anemia was found in the virus-positive group. This neither proves nor disproves the hypothesis that FeLV causes anemia either as an end in itself or as a preleukemic sign. It does indicate that a slowly degenerating anemia does not necessarily occur either concurrently with or soon after FeLV infection. The possibility that only certain strains of FeLV cause anemia as a specific entity has also been considered (Essex *et al.*, 1975c; O. Jarrett, personal communication).

Feldman and Gross (1971) reported that 5 of 11 spontaneous mammary tumors contained viruslike particles. The particles were somewhat similar to typical C-type FeLV. C-type particles have not been shown to cause carcinomas in any species, but B-type oncornaviruses are associated with mammary cancer of mice. Riggs *et al.* (1973) found 2 of 2 mammary tumors positive by electron microscopy, and Weijer *et al.* (1974) found 6 of 24 positive. Gardner *et al.* (1974) found 8 of 38 carcinomas positive, but no breakdown for the various types was presented. Regarding serologic studies, 2 of 5 tumor cell cultures were positive by membrane fluorescence (Riggs *et al.*, 1973), and 11 of 51 were positive by fixed cell immunofluorescence (Weijer *et al.*, 1974). Of 15 mammary carcinomas tested, Hardy (1971) found none positive by immunodiffusion. Gardner *et al.* (1974), using complement fixation, found no reactors among 44 cat tumors, including all types of carcinomas. One of 29 spleens from cats with unspecified carcinoma was positive.

Infectious peritonitis is a severe and invariably fatal disease characterized by fibrinous and granulomatous serositis in the abdominal or pleural cavities. Hepatic necrosis and meningitis are also often present (Robison *et al.*, 1971; Wolfe and Griesemer, 1971). The disease was not recognized until recently (Wolfe and Griesemer, 1966). It can be induced experimentally with cell-free filtrates (Wolfe and Griesemer, 1966; Zook *et al.*, 1968; Hardy and Hurvitz, 1971) and is believed to be caused by a virus that is considerably smaller than FeLV (Zook *et al.*, 1968; Ward, 1970).

Immunodiffusion tests for core antigens detected FeLV in 9 of 20 naturally occurring cases and 2 of 15 induced cases of feline infectious peritonitis (Hardy and Hurvitz, 1971). FeLV virus core antigens were also found in 5 of 25 cases by complement fixation (Gardner *et al.*, 1974), and 4 of 7 (Hardy *et al.*, 1973a) and 26 of 42 by fixed-cell immunofluorescence (Essex *et al.*, 1975a). The disease was also found in a significant number of cats in two large leukemia cluster households (see Section VIII,C) (Cotter *et al.*, 1973, 1974; Essex *et al.*, 1975c). In both households infectious peritonitis was observed to develop in both FeLV-positive and negative cats.

Numerous other infectious diseases of cats are frequently found in cats that are viremic with FeLV. In acute diseases, such as septicemia, pneumonia, and viral enteritis (panleukopenia), the etiological agents can be identified with certainty. It is very unlikely that

FeLV plays more than a secondary immunosuppressive type of role in these diseases.

In two other syndromes, the possibility that FeLV acts in a more direct role should be considered. The first is abortion and/or fetal resorption of unknown cause where we found 9 of 12 cases positive for FeLV by fixed-cell immunofluorescence (Essex et al., 1975a). As described in Section VII,D, this situation deserves more study to determine whether it may be related to infection of the embryo or fetus during early gestation by the viremic mother. It should also be noted that Chapman et al. (1974) found that FeLV caused abnormal embryogenesis when hamster fetuses were artificially exposed. The second syndrome where FeLV may play a more direct role is glomerulonephritis. This has been noted as a pathologic lesion in clinical leukemia (Anderson and Jarrett, 1971; Jarrett et al., 1973c) and immune complex deposits containing FeLV core antigens have been identified in diseased kidneys (Hardy, personal communication). We found 3 of 4 cases of naturally occurring glomerulonephritis to be

TABLE IX
Reported Incidences of Infection with Feline Leukemia-Sarcoma Viruses (FeLV–FeSV) in Disease Syndromes Other Than Leukemia and Sarcoma

Disease	No. positive/No. tested (% positive)			References
	Virus core antigens in tissues	Virus core antigens in blood	Particles by electron microscopy	
Nonregenerative anemias	17/23 (74%)	53/76 (70%)	11/13 (85%)	Gardner et al. (1974); Essex et al. (1975a)
Infectious peritonitis	9/20 (45%)	26/42 (62%) 5/25 (20%)	6/7 (86%)	Hardy and Hurvitz, (1971); Essex et al. (1975a); Gardner et al. (1974)
Hemobartonellosis	—	10/17 (59%)	—	Essex et al. (1975a)
Mammary carcinoma	11/51 (22%)	—	6/24 (25%)	Weijer et al. (1974)
Glomerulonephritis	—	3/4 (75%)	—	Essex et al. (1975a)
Abortion and fetal resorption	—	9/12 (75%)	—	Essex et al. (1975a)
Bacterial infections (systemic)	—	28/51 (55%)	—	Essex et al. (1975a)

FeLV positive (Essex et al., 1975a), and also observed the development of the disease in some cats in the leukemia cluster households with very high FOCMA antibody titers. A list of the diseases of cats (other than leukemia and sarcoma) that have been associated with the presence of FeLV is given in Table IX.

Brief mention should also be made of the feline syncytial virus because it is very frequently found in cats with clinical leukemia. Morphologically it is a myxovirus-like particle (Riggs et al., 1969; Hackett et al., 1970) that is often isolated from cats with many unrelated infectious and noninfectious diseases (Hackett and Manning, 1971; Scott, 1971). It also causes destruction of many cell cultures derived from infected cats. Partly because of this and because a similar syncytial virus has been found in lymphocytes from leukemic cattle (Malmquist et al., 1969), the agent is being studied in several laboratories.

IX. Comparison of Feline Oncornavirus Infectivity Patterns to Those of Other Oncogenic or Potentially Oncogenic Viruses

Feline oncornaviruses have many characteristics in common with oncogenic viruses of other avian and mammalian species. The FeLV–FeSV and RD-114-endogenous virus groups each have at least as many characteristics in common with certain oncornavirus groups of other species as they do with each other.

Biochemically, the murine oncornaviruses appear to be the closest relatives of the FeLV–FeSV group (Gilden et al., 1974), and the endogenous baboon oncornavirus is very similar to RD-114 (Sherr et al., 1974).

All avian oncornaviruses thus far described have similar or identical virus core antigens. Several subgroups, based on virion envelope antigens, have been described (Vogt, 1970; Bauer, 1974). Endogenous avian oncornaviruses have also been detected in all normal chicken and jungle fowl cells (Baluda and Nayak, 1970; Rosenthal et al., 1971; Weiss et al., 1971). Horizontal transmission of avian oncornaviruses also occurs (Rubin et al., 1961; Burmester and Purchase, 1970). Recent evidence (Weiss and Biggs, 1972) suggests that the endogenous viruses present in the genetic makeup of all chickens and jungle fowl are characterized by the apparently nononcogenic subgroup E agents. These viruses thus have a natural history that is similar to that of the RD-114 group. The field strains of oncogenic avian viruses identified in the United States have been subgroup A or B, and these appear to be primarily transmitted in a horizontal fashion, as are the FeLV–FeSV group. The presence of related endogenous and exogenous viruses is therefore characteristic for an avian and a mammalian species. The principal difference is the unrelatedness of the endogenous and exogenous feline viruses when compared to the avian agents. Another apparent difference is the xenotropic replication properties of RD-114, which are not apparent for the group E avian oncornaviruses. Knowledge of the avian E subgroup, however, indicates the theoretical possibility that endogenous vertically transmitted (and presumably nononcogenic) viruses with FeLV-FeSV type virus core antigens might exist in some feline species.

The situation with murine oncornaviruses is more difficult to interpret. All murine oncornaviruses thus far found, including the recent xenotropic isolates (Aaronson and Stephenson, 1973; Benveniste *et al.*, 1974), appear to have the same virus core antigens. This is similar to the avian situation, but unlike that in the cat. The murine viruses do not appear to fit a simplified virion-envelope subgroup classification system, however, as do the avian and feline agents. Many endogenous viruses have been "rescued" from nonproducer mouse cells (Todaro and Huebner, 1972; Rowe, 1973), including cloned lines, and most appear to be nononcogenic. The L-cell particle appears to represent a fully expressed nononcogenic agent.

The rather artificial selection of many inbred mouse strains, based on such properties as a high or low frequency of leukemia or mammary tumors, almost certainly resulted in the development of recombinant strains that display properties not seen in field isolates. Extensive studies with oncornaviruses of wild mice will obviously be very important to an understanding of the true natural history of the murine agents. Gardner and his associates (personal communication) have observed that most feral mice have indigenous oncornaviruses, and that many isolates have neuropathic as well as oncogenic properties.

Of the several monkey oncornaviruses recently described, one appears to resemble the exogenous FeLV–FeSV type of infectivity pattern involving horizontal transmission (Kawakami *et al.*, 1973), while another, the RD-114-like baboon agent, appears to be endogenous (Melnick *et al.*, 1973; Sherr *et al.*, 1974).

In addition to the very different biochemical-biophysical properties, the Herpesviruses, unlike the oncornaviruses, exhibit cytopathic characteristics. Despite this, the natural history of such agents as the Marek's disease virus of chickens and the Epstein–Barr virus associated with Burkitt's lymphoma appears to be relatively similar to that for exogenous oncornaviruses such as the FeLV–FeSV group. Both groups are efficiently transmitted in a horizontal fashion. Both also exist in a nonproducer "turned-off" association with certain somatic cells, and can be detected by nucleic acid hybridization or rescued with such agents as iododeoxyuridine (Hampar et al., 1972; Klein and Dombos, 1973). Seroepidemiologic studies indicate that both also infect many more individuals than the number that actually develop tumors. This presumably reflects, at least in part, a common evolutionary adaptation of the immune response in a capacity of surveillance directed at virus-altered cells. The same general picture is seen with polyoma in wild mice, where horizontal exposure to the

TABLE X
Oncogenicity and Mode of Transmission for Feline Oncornavirus and Other Selected Oncogenic Viruses

Virus	Oncogenicity		Mode(s) of transmission		
	In homologous species	In heterologous species	True vertical (chromosomal)	Extra-chromosomal vertical	Horizontal
Feline leukemia virus	+	+	−	+	+
Feline sarcoma virus	+	+	−	+	+
RD-114	−	−	+	−	−
Avian oncornaviruses subgroups A, B, C, D	+	±[a]	−	+	+
Avian oncornaviruses subgroup E	−	−	+	−	−
Murine oncornaviruses (general)	+	−	+	+	−
Marek's disease virus	+	−	−	−	+
Epstein–Barr virus	?	+	−	−	+
Polyoma virus	+	+	−	?	+
Gibbon lymphoma and simian sarcoma viruses	?	?	−	?	+
Herpes saimiri	−	+	−	?	+

[a] Positive for avian sarcoma viruses, negative for leukemia viruses.

virus is very frequent, but immune resistance highly efficient (Klein, 1973). Table X lists those characteristics relating to mode of transmission and oncogenicity for selected oncogenic and potentially oncogenic viruses.

X. Public Health Significance of Feline Oncornaviruses

Three early observations concerning the pathobiology of the FeLV–FeSV group resulted in concern regarding a possible role for these viruses in human tumors (Bross and Gibson, 1970; Hanes et al., 1970; Schneider, 1970, 1971, 1972b; Gardner, 1971; Bross et al., 1972; Essex, 1972). The observations were: (a) the FeLV group replicates in human cells, including lymphocytes (Jarrett et al., 1969a, 1970; Chang et al., 1970; Hampar et al., 1970; Sarma et al., 1970c; Essex et al., 1972b; Chan et al., 1974a); (b) FeSV transforms human fibroblasts (Chang et al., 1970; Sarma et al., 1970c, 1971a,d; McAllister et al., 1971b); and (c) FeSV will induce malignant tumors in monkeys (Deinhardt et al., 1970, 1972, 1973; Theilen et al., 1970; Essex et al., 1972b; Rabin et al., 1972, 1973; Wolfe et al., 1972). These properties were not characteristic for field isolates of other tumor viruses, with the exception of the primate Herpesviruses (Melendez et al., 1972). Accompanying the realization that many people are intimately exposed to cats, was the implication that transmission of the viruses to man should be investigated. Enthusiasm for such studies was restrained, however, primarily because observations based on the related murine and avian oncornavirus systems suggested that horizontal transmission of such agents either did not occur at all, or occurred only in a limited and unimportant way (Huebner and Todaro, 1969; Huebner et al., 1970, 1971). Observations that FeLV was frequently excreted by infected cats and highly contagious for contact-exposed cats (Sections VIII,B and C) rejuvenated interest for studying a possible cat–human link (Levy, 1974).

A few epidemiological studies have addressed the question of possible cat–human transmission (Dorn and Schneider, 1972). Two California-based studies concluded that no association was present between feline and human cancer (Hanes et al., 1970; Schneider, 1970, 1972b). Another group, studying data from New York, Minnesota, and Maryland, concluded that household contacts of "sick" cats had a slightly increased risk for development of both childhood (Bross and Gibson, 1970) and adulthood (Bross et al., 1972) leukemia. The differences in results could be due to recognized limitations inherent in either or both of the experimental designs. If both sets of results accurately reflect a real situation, alternative explanations could be proposed for the apparent differences. Different strains and subgroups of FeLV have different geographical distributions, and some readily infect human cells while others do not (Jarrett et al., 1972, 1973).

The Bross studies have been criticized for use of the rather vague description of "sick cats" as a reference rather than "leukemic" cats (Heath, 1971). Our current knowledge of FeLV seroepidemiology indicates, however, that cats with many severe illnesses (other than leukemia) harbor and excrete FeLV (Section VIII,G). An interpretation that would fit all the present epidemiologic evidence is that FeLV transmission could not account for many cases of human leukemia or other cancers, but the possibility of FeLV acting in an unusual case cannot be excluded.

A few studies using serologic procedures have also addressed the question of human infection with viruses of the FeLV–FeSV group. Using immunodiffusion, Hardy (1971) found no FeLV core antigen in tissues from more than 100 people. Most were leukemia, sarcoma, or carcinoma patients. More than 300 sera were also tested and found negative for antibody to the FeLV antigen. With passive hemagglutination, a more sensitive test, antibody to FeLV was detected in 3 sera of 200 from malignancy cases and in 6 of 189 from nonmalignant sources (Fink et al., 1971). In another study, all of 36 sera from veterinarians and all of 33 from laboratory personnel were negative for virus-neutralizing antibodies (Sarma et al., 1974b). About 600 samples from veterinarians were tested for antibody by indirect membrane immunofluorescence, and 1 was positive (Schneider and Riggs, 1973). Sutherland and Mardiney (1973) found FeLV antigen deposited in immune complexes in the kidney of a patient with acute myelocytic leukemia. Other studies have reported finding antibodies for oncornavirus determinants in human materials, but such reactivities are not specific for FeLV (Yohn, 1973; Schafer, 1973; Olsen et al., 1974c). Negative results in such studies seem reassuring regarding any possible transmission. Yet it must be recognized that postnatal monkeys and dogs with tumors induced by FeSV or FeLV are almost always "nonproducers" and negative by the same tests. The isolated and infrequent positive results must also be reviewed with suspicion until confirmed in other laboratories.

In final analysis, it appears that further studies in this area are important. We now know that many pet cats become either transiently or persistently infected with, and excretors of, FeLV. It has been estimated that about 30% of the households in a suburban–rural area of California contained 1 or more cats (Franti and Kraus, 1974). Considering the intimate contact that many people, especially children, have with pet cats, it seems safe to assume that exposure to FeLV is not infrequent. Generally accepted recommendations for laboratory workers exposed to the FeLV–FeSV group include such precautions as handling all virus preparations in biohazard-type hoods, wearing protective gloves, and disallowing pregnant women or children exposure to the laboratory environment (Hellman et al., 1973). In view of this it seems derelict, or at least hypocritical, if similar thought is not given to the detection and handling of analogous situations where people are exposed to viremic pet cats. Although the risk must be considered low in most pet-exposure situations, the degree of FeLV exposure in some leukemia cluster households is probably at least as high as in the laboratory.

As for the RD-114-endogenous feline oncornavirus, from our present knowledge there appears to be little need for concern about natural human exposure. The virus is not yet known to be oncogenic in any species (McAllister, personal communication) and producer-excretor cats have not been found. This agent deserves extensive investigation for many other reasons. Evidence that a closely related endogenous virus exists in primates (Sherr et al., 1974) suggests that information gained about RD-114 evolution and natural history may help clarify many unanswered questions concerning endogenous oncornaviruses of all species.

XI. Summary and Conclusions

Two distinct groups of oncornaviruses have been found in cats. One group, the RD-114-endogenous viruses, are vertically transmitted and found in a latent unexpressed form in all cats, both healthy and neoplastic. No evidence for oncogenic activity has been found for this group. They are xenotropic. They do not replicate under normal circumstances in feline cells, but replicate efficiently in cells from other species.

The FeLV–FeSV group of feline viruses differs from the RD-114 group in several ways. The FeLV–FeSV group has different virus core, virus envelope, and cell membrane antigens. They replicate efficiently in most cat cells, as well as cells from most other mammalian species. The FeLV's, unlike the RD-114 group, are efficiently transmitted horizontally. Current evidence does not support a role for vertical chromosomal transmission of the FeLV–FeSV group of viruses. Extrachromosomal vertical transmission of FeLV, as when a mother infects the unborn fetus or neonate, almost certainly occurs to some extent. This type of spread is probably not as important as horizontal transmission in the sense of virus distribution for the domestic cat population as a whole. Yet acquisition of virus at the fetal or neonatal stage probably results in a higher frequency of neoplastic disease for those infected in this manner.

Many more adult pet cats become infected with FeLV than the number that actually develop leukemia. One probable reason for this is that most adult cats are naturally exposed to suboncogenic doses of FeLV at an immunocompetent age. Many presumably only become transiently infected, rapidly eliminating the virus owing to an efficient immune response. Another probable reason why many exposed cats do not become leukemic is the immunosuppressive nature of FeLV. When cats are naturally exposed to large virus doses, as in leukemic cluster households, persistent viremia occurs. Persistently viremic cats have a greatly increased risk for the development of other unrelated bacterial and viral diseases, such as infectious peritonitis, septicemia, enteritis, and pneumonia. Unlike leukemia, the latter diseases have short incubation periods, since the agents exert their lethal effects before FeLV.

The humoral immune response to the feline oncornavirus-associated cell membrane antigen (FOCMA) is inversely correlated with the progression of tumors induced by FeLV and FeSV. The same relationship appears with field cases of feline leukemia.

The natural history and seroepidemiology of the FeLV–FeSV group parallels that of many other oncogenic or potentially oncogenic viruses that are found under natural conditions. These include the Marek's disease and group A oncornaviruses of chickens, the gibbon ape lymphoma virus, the Epstein–Barr virus associated with Burkitt's lymphoma, and polyoma virus of wild mice. The natural history of the RD-114 group is similar to that seen with nononcogenic group E avian oncornaviruses and the endogenous viruses of mice.

The public health significance of FeLV exposure is unknown. Many pet owners are exposed to the virus. The epidemiologic studies that have been done indicated either little or no increase in cancer risk for owners of leukemic or "sick" cats.

The FeLV–FeSV group of feline oncornaviruses provides an ideal system for the study of several questions central to cancer virology and immunology. One example is FeLV-induced leukemia of neonatal dogs. That model provides an ideal opportunity to study a nonproducer leukemia (rather than sarcoma), where reference reagents to detect unexpressed genomes are available or can be prepared. A second example is the opportunity to study different stages of the immune response to both the oncogenic virus and developing tumor following natural exposure to the agent.

Domestic cats are outbred, as is man. The lack of inbred strains creates significant problems when trying to circumvent or diminish that portion of an effect due to homograft rejection or individual variation. These disadvantages are offset, at least to some degree, by reassurance that knowledge gained with the feline system is more representative of the field situation. In this respect the domestic cat is an ideal "model."

Acknowledgments

Much of the work described by the author has been done in collaboration with several groups in other laboratories, particularly those of Drs. Cotter, Deinhardt, Hardy, Jakowski, O. Jarrett, W. Jarrett, Snyder, and Yohn. I am also grateful to my other colleagues, particularly Drs. Bauer, Gardner, Gilden, Maruyama, McAllister, Noronha, and Velicer, who generously provided me with prepublication information. The help of A. Sliski, E. Jagher, and L. Taylor in various aspects of the work is gratefully acknowledged. The author is a Scholar of the Leukemia Society of America and has received research grants from the Anna Fuller Fund, the Jane Coffin Childs Fund for Medical Research, The National and Massachusetts branches of the American Cancer Society and the U. S. National Cancer Institute.

References

Aaronson, S. A. (1973). *Nat. Cancer Inst., Monogr.* **35**, 83–87.
Aaronson, S. A., and Stephenson, J. R. (1973). *Proc. Nat. Acad. Sci. U. S.* **70**, 2055–2058.
Aaronson, S. A., and Todaro, G. J. (1970). *Nature (London)* **225**, 458–459.
Aaronson, S. A., Parks, W. P., Scolnick, E. M., and Todaro, G. J. (1971). *Proc. Nat. Acad. Sci. U. S.* **68**, 920–924.
Anderson, L. J., and Jarrett, W. F. H. (1971). *Res. Vet. Sci.* **12**, 179–180.
Anderson, L. J., and McKeating, F. J. (1970). *Immunology* **19**, 935–943.
Anderson, L. J., Jarrett, W. F. H., and Crighton, G. W. (1969). *Nat. Cancer Inst., Monogr.* **32**, 343–352.
Anderson, L. J., Jarrett, W. F. H., Jarrett, O., and Laird, H. M. (1971). *J. Nat. Cancer Inst.* **47**, 807–817.
August, J. T., Bolognesi, D. P., Fleissner, E., Gilden, R. V., and Nowinski, R. C. (1974). *Virology* **60**, 595–600.
Baltimore, D. (1970). *Nature (London)* **226**, 1209–1210.
Baluda, M. A., and Nayak, D. P. (1970). *Proc. Nat. Acad. Sci. U. S.* **66**, 329–336.
Baluda, M. A., and Roy-Burman, P. (1973). *Nature (London), New Biol.* **244**, 59–62.
Bardell, D., and Essex, M. (1974). *Infec. Immunity* **9**, 824–827.
Bauer, H. (1974). *Advan. Cancer Res.* **20**, 275–341.
Baxt, W., Hehlmann, R., and Spiegelman, S. (1972). *Nature (London), New Biol.* **240**, 72–75.
Baxt, W., Yates, J. W., Wallace, H. J., Jr., Holland, J. F., and Spiegelman, S. (1973). *Proc. Nat. Acad. Sci. U. S.* **70**, 2629–2632.
Benveniste, R. E., and Todaro, G. J. (1973). *Proc. Nat. Acad. Sci. U. S.* **70**, 3316–3320.

Benveniste, R. E., Lieber, M. M., and Todaro, G. J. (1974). *Proc. Nat. Acad. Sci. U. S.* **71,** 602–606.
Blumenschein, G. R., and Moloney, J. B. (1969). *J. Nat. Cancer Inst.* **42,** 123–133.
Boone, C. W., Church, E. C., and McAllister, R. (1973a). *Virology* **55,** 157–163.
Boone, C. W., Gordin, F., and Kawakami, T. G. (1973b). *J. Virol.* **11,** 515–519.
Brodey, R. S. (1971). *J. Amer. Vet. Med. Ass.* **158,** 1123–1125.
Brodey, R. S., McDonough, S. K., Susan, K., Frye, F. L., and Hardy, W. D. (1970). *In* "Comparative Leukemia Research 1969" (R. M. Dutcher, ed.), pp. 333–342. Karger, Basel.
Bross, I. D. J., and Gibson, R. (1970). *J. Med. Exp. Clin.* **1,** 180–187.
Bross, I. D. J., Bertell, R., and Gibson, R. (1972). *Amer. J. Pub. Health Nat. Health* **62,** 1520–1531.
Bryan, W. R. (1946). *J. Nat. Cancer Inst.* **6,** 225–237.
Burger, C. L., and Noronha, F. (1970). *J. Nat. Cancer Inst.* **45,** 499–506.
Burger, C. L., Harris, W. W., Anderson, N. G., Bartlett, T. W., and Kniseley, R. M. (1964). *Proc. Soc. Exp. Biol. Med.* **115,** 151–156.
Burmester, B. R., and Purchase, H. G. (1970). *In* "Comparative Leukemia Research 1969" (R. M. Dutcher, ed.), pp. 83–95. Karger, Basel.
Cerny, J., McAlack, W. S., Ceglowski, W. S., and Friedman, H. (1971). *Proc. Nat. Acad. Sci. U. S.* **68,** 862–869.
Chan, E. W., Schiop-Stansly, P. E., and O'Connor, T. E. (1974a). *J. Nat. Cancer Inst.* **52,** 473–482.
Chan, E. W., Schiop-Stansly, P. E., and O'Connor, T. E. (1974b). *J. Nat. Cancer Inst.* **52,** 469–472.
Chang, R. S. (1971). *Nature (London), New Biol.* **233,** 124.
Chang, R. S., Golden, H. D., and Harrold, B. (1970). *J. Virol.* **6,** 599–603.
Chang, R. S., Hsieh, M. W., and Blankenship, W. (1971). *J. Nat. Cancer Inst.* **47,** 469–477.
Chapman, A. L., Bopp, W. J., Brightwell, A. S., Cohen, H., Nielsen, A. H., Gravelle, C. R., and Werder, A. A. (1967). *Cancer Res.* **27,** 18–25.
Chapman, A. L., Fischinger, P. J., and O'Connor, T. E. (1970). *J. Nat. Cancer Inst.* **45,** 1047–1053.
Chapman, A. L., Weitlauf, H. M., and Bopp, W. (1974). *J. Nat. Cancer Inst.* **52,** 583–586.
Cotter, S. M., Gilmore, C. E., and Rollins, C. (1973). *J. Amer. Vet. Med. Ass.* **162,** 1054–1058.
Cotter, S. M., Essex, M., and Hardy, W. D., Jr. (1974). *Cancer Res.* **34,** 1061–1069.
Crighton, G. W. (1968a). *Vet. Rec.* **83,** 122–126.
Crighton, G. W. (1968b). *Vet. Rec.* **83,** 155–157.
Crighton, G. W. (1969a). *J. Small Anim. Pract.* **10,** 571–577.
Crighton, G. W. (1969b). *Vet. Rec.* **84,** 329–331.
Dalton, A. J. (1972). *Cancer Res.* **32,** 1351–1353.
Dalton, A. J., and Haguenau, F., eds. (1973). "Ultrastructure of Animal Viruses and Bacteriophages: An Atlas," Ultrastructure in Biological Systems Series, Vol. 5, 400 pp. Academic Press, New York.
de Harven, E. (1968). *In* "Experimental Leukemia" (M. A. Rich, ed.), pp. 97–130. Appleton, New York.
Deinhardt, F., Wolfe, L. G., Theilen, G. H., and Snyder, S. P. (1970). *Science* **167,** 881.
Deinhardt, F., Wolfe, L. G., Northrop, R., Marczynska, B., Ogden, J., McDonald, R.,

Falk, L., Shramek, J., Smith, R., and Deinhardt, J. (1972). *J. Med. Primatol.* **1**, 29–50.
Deinhardt, F., Wolfe, L., Massey, R., Hoekstra, J., and McDonald, R. (1973). *In* "Unifying Concepts of Leukemia" (R. M. Dutcher and L. Chieco-Bianchi, eds.), pp. 258–262. Karger, Basel.
Dent, P. B. (1972). *Progr. Med. Virol.* **14**, 1–35.
Dmochowski, L., Taylor, H. G., Grey, C. E., Dreyer, D. A., Sykes, J. A., Langford, P. L., Rogers, T., Shullenberger, C. C., and Howe, C. D. (1965). *Cancer (Philadelphia)* **18**, 1345–1368.
Dorn, C. R., and Schneider, R. (1972). *Amer. J. Pub. Health Nat. Health* **62**, 1460–1462.
Dorn, C. R., Taylor, D. O. N., and Hibbard, H. H. (1967). *Amer. J. Vet. Res.* **28**, 993–1001.
Dorn, C. R., Taylor, D. O. N., Schneider, R., Hibbard, H. H., and Klauber, M. R. (1968). *J. Nat. Cancer Inst.* **40**, 307–318.
Dougherty, E. (1971). *J. Amer. Vet. Med. Ass.* **158**, 1116–1118.
Dougherty, E., and Rickard, C. G. (1970). *J. Ultrastruct. Res.* **32**, 472–477.
Dougherty, E., Post, J. F., and Rickard, C. G. (1969). *Can. Vet. J.* **10**, 291–293.
East, J. L., Knesek, J. E., Allen, P. T., and Dmochowski, L. (1973). *J. Virol.* **12**, 1085–1091.
Ellerman, V., and Bang, O. (1908). *Centralbl. Bakteriol.* **46**, 595–609.
Essex, M. (1972). *Oncology* **26**, 345–354.
Essex, M. (1974). *In* "Viruses, Evolution and Cancer" (E. Kurstak and K. Maramorosch, eds.), pp. 513–548. Academic Press, New York.
Essex, M., and Snyder, S. P. (1973). *J. Nat. Cancer Inst.* **51**, 1007–1012.
Essex, M., Klein, G., Snyder, S. P., and Harrold, J. G. (1971a). *Int. J. Cancer* **8**, 384–390.
Essex, M., Klein, G., Snyder, S. P., and Harrold, J. G. (1971b). *Nature (London)* **233**, 195–196.
Essex, M., Kawakami, T. G., and Kurata, K. (1972a). *Proc. Soc. Exp. Biol. Med.* **139**, 295–299.
Essex, M., Klein, G., Deinhardt, F., Wolfe, L., Hardy, W., Jr., Theilen, G., and Pearson, L. (1972b). *Nature (London), New Biol.* **238**, 187–189.
Essex, M., Cotter, S. M., and Carpenter, J. L. (1973a). *Amer. J. Vet. Res.* **34**, 809–812.
Essex, M. Snyder, S. P., and Klein, G. (1973b). *In* "Unifying Concepts of Leukemia" (R. M. Dutcher and L. Chieco-Bianchi, eds.), pp. 771–777. Karger, Basel.
Essex, M., Hardy, W. D., Jr., Cotter, S. M., and Jakowski, R. M. (1974). *Proc. Int. Symp. Comp. Leuk. Res., 6th, Nagoya, Jap, 1973* pp. 431–436.
Essex, M., Cotter, S. M., Hardy, W. D., Jr., Hess, P., Jarrett, W., Jarrett, O., Mackey, L., Laird, H., Perryman, L., Olsen, R. G., and Yohn, S. D. (1975a). Submitted for publication.
Essex, M., Cotter, S. M., Carpenter, J. L., Hardy, W. D., Jr., Hess, P., Jarrett, W., and Yohn, D. S. (1975b). *J. Nat. Cancer Inst.* **54**, in press.
Essex, M., Hardy, W. D., Jr., Cotter, S. M., Jakowski, R. M., and Sliski, A. (1975c). *Infec. Immunity* **11**, in press.
Essex, M., Jakowski, R. M., Hardy, W. D., Jr., Cotter, S. M., Hess, P., and Sliski, A. (1975d). *J. Nat. Cancer Inst.* **54**, in press.
Feldman, D. G., and Gross, L. (1971). *Cancer Res.* **31**, 1261–1267.
Fenner, F. (1968). "The Biology of Animal Viruses," 844 pp. Academic Press, New York.

Filbert, J. E., McAllister, R. M., Nicolson, M. O., and Gilden, R. V. (1974). *Proc. Soc. Exp. Biol. Med.* **145**, 366–370.
Fink, M. A., Sibal, L. R., and Plata, E. J. (1971). *J. Amer. Vet. Med. Ass.* **158**, 1070–1075.
Fischinger, P. J., and Moore, C. O. (1971). *J. Gen. Virol.* **12**, 59–63.
Fischinger, P. J., and O'Connor, T. E. (1970). *J. Nat. Cancer Inst.* **44**, 429–438.
Fischinger, P. J., Peebles, P. T., Nomura, S., and Haapala, D. K. (1973). *J. Virol.* **11**, 978–985.
Franti, C. E., and Kraus, J. F. (1974). *J. Amer. Vet. Med. Ass.* **164**, 166–178.
Fujinaga, K., and Green, M. (1971). *J. Gen. Virol.* **12**, 85–93.
Fujinaga, K., Rankin, A., Yamazaki, H., Sekikawa, K., Bragdon, J., and Green, M. (1973). *Virology* **56**, 484–495.
Gardner, M. B. (1971). *J. Nat. Cancer Inst.* **46**, 281–290.
Gardner, M. B., Arnstein, P., Rongey, R. W., Estes, J. D., Sarma, P. S., Rickard, C. F., and Huebner, R. J. (1970). *Nature (London)* **226**, 807–809.
Gardner, M. B., Rongey, R. W., Johnson, E. Y., DeJournett, R., and Huebner, R. J. (1971). *J. Nat. Cancer Inst.* **47**, 561–568.
Gardner, M. B., Johnson, E. Y., Rasheed, S., and McAllister, R. M. (1973). *Int. J. Cancer* **12**, 563–567.
Gardner, M. B., Rasheed, S., Rongey, R. W., Charman, H. P., Alena, B., Gilden, R. V., and Huebner, R. J. (1974). *Int. J. Cancer* **14**: 97–105.
Geering, G., Hardy, W. D., Jr., Old, L. J., and deHarven, E. (1968). *Virology* **36**, 678–707.
Geering, G., Aoki, T., and Old, L. J. (1970). *Nature (London)* **226**, 265–266.
Gelderblom, H., Bauer, H., and Graf, T. (1972). *Virology* **47**, 416–425.
Gilden, R. V., and Oroszlan, S. (1971). *J. Amer. Vet. Med. Ass.* **158**, 1099–1103.
Gilden, R. V., and Oroszlan, S. (1972). *Proc. Nat. Acad. Sci.* **69**, 1021–1025.
Gilden, R. V., Oroszlan, S., and Huebner, R. J. (1971). *Nature (London), New Biol.* **231**, 107–108.
Gilden, R. V., Lee, Y. K., and Long, C. (1972). *Int. J. Cancer* **10**, 458–462.
Gilden, R. V., Oroszlan, S., and Hatanaka, R. (1974). *In* "Viruses, Evolution and Cancer" (E. Kurstak and K. Maramorosch, eds.), pp. 235–257. Academic Press, New York.
Gillespie, D., Gillespie, S., Gallo, R. F., East, J. L., and Dmochowski, L. (1973). *Nature (London), New Biol.* **224**, 51–54.
Gilmore, C. E., and Holzworth, J. (1971). *J. Amer. Vet. Med. Ass.* **158**, 1013–1025.
Graves, D. C., and Velicer, L. F. (1974). *J. Virol.* **14**: 349–365.
Green, R. W., Bolognesi, D. P., Schaffer, W., Pister, L., Hunsmann, G., and de Noronha, F. (1973). *Virology* **56**, 565–579.
Gross, L. (1951). *Proc. Soc. Exp. Biol. Med.* **76**, 27–32.
Hackett, A. J., and Manning, J. S. (1971). *J. Amer. Vet. Med. Ass.* **158**, 948–954.
Hackett, A. J., Priester, A., and Arnstein, P. (1970). *Proc. Soc. Exp. Biol. Med.* **135**, 899–904.
Hampar, B., Kelloff, G. J., Martos, L. M., Oroszlan, S., Gilden, R. V., and Walker, J. L. (1970). *Nature (London)* **228**, 857–859.
Hampar, B., Derge, J. G., Martos, L. M., and Walker, J. L. (1972). *Proc. Nat. Acad. Sci U. S.* **69**, 78–82.
Hampar, B., Rand, K. H., Lerner, R. A., del Villano, B. C., Jr., McAllister, R. M., Maftos, L. M., Derge, J. G., Long, C. W., and Gilden, R. V. (1973). *Virology* **55**, 453–464.

Hanes, B., Gardner, M. B., Loosli, C. G., Heidbreder, G., Kogan, B., Marylander, H., and Huebner, R. J. (1970). *J. Nat. Cancer Inst.* **45**, 1155–1162.
Hardy, W. D., Jr. (1971). *J. Amer. Vet. Med. Ass.* **158**, 1060–1069.
Hardy, W. D., Jr. (1974). *Vet. Clin. N. Amer.* **4**, 133–146.
Hardy, W. D., Jr., and Hurvitz, A. I. (1971). *J. Amer. Vet. Med. Ass.* **158**, 994–1002.
Hardy, W. D., Jr., Geering, G., Old, L. J., deHarven, E., Brodey, R. B., and McDonough, S. (1969). *Science* **166**, 1019–1021.
Hardy, W. D., Jr., Hirshaut, Y., and Hiss, P. (1973a). *In* "Unifying Concepts of Leukemia" (R. M. Dutcher and L. Chieco-Bianchi, eds.), pp. 778–799. Karger, Basel.
Hardy, W. D., Jr., Old, L. J., Hess, P. W., Essex, M., and Cotter, S. M. (1973b). *Nature (London)* **244**, 266–269.
Hardy, W. D., Jr., Hess, P. W., Essex, M., Cotter, S., McClelland, A. J., and MacEwen, G. (1974). *Int. Symp. Comp. Leuk. Res., 6th, Nagoya, Jap. 1973* (in press).
Harvey, J. J. (1964). *Nature (London)* **204**, 1104–1105.
Hatanaka, M., and Gilden, R. V. (1970). *J. Nat. Cancer Inst.* **45**, 87–89.
Hatanaka, M., and Hanafusa, H. (1970). *Virology* **41**, 647–652.
Hatanaka, M., Huebner, R. J., and Gilden, R. V. (1969). *J. Nat. Cancer Inst.* **43**, 1091–1096.
Heath, C. W. (1971). *J. Amer. Vet. Med. Ass.* **158**, 1119–1122.
Hehlmann, R., Kufe, D., and Spiegelman, S. (1972). *Proc. Nat. Acad. Sci.* **69**, 1727–1731.
Hehlmann, R., Baxt, W., Kufe, D., and Spiegelman, S. (1973). *Amer. J. Clin. Pathol.* **60**, 65–79.
Hellman, A., Oxman, M. N., and Pollack, R. (1973). "Biohazards in Biological Research," 369 pp. Cold Spring Harbor Lab., Cold Spring Harbor, New York.
Herz, A., Theilen, G. H., Schalm, O. W., and Munn, R. J. (1970). *J. Nat. Cancer Inst.* **44**, 339–348.
Hilgers, J., Nowinski, R. C., Geering, G., and Hardy, W. (1972). *Cancer Res.* **32**, 98–106.
Holzworth, J. (1960a) *J. Amer. Vet. Med. Ass.* **136**, 47–69.
Holzworth, J. (1960b). *J. Amer. Vet. Med. Ass.* **136**, 107–121.
Hoover, E. A., McCullough, C. B., and Griesemer, R. A. (1972). *J. Nat. Cancer Inst.* **48**, 973–983.
Hoover, E. A., Perryman, L. E., and Kociba, G. J. (1973). *Cancer Res.* **33**, 145–152.
Howard, E. B., Clark, W. J., and Hackett, P. L. (1968). *In* "Leukemia in Animals and Man. Proceedings 3rd International Symposium on Comparative Leukemia Research" (H. J. Bendixen, ed.), pp. 255–262. Karger, Basel.
Hsiung, G. D. (1972). *J. Nat. Cancer Inst.* **49**, 567–570.
Huebner, R. J., and Todaro, G. J. (1969). *Proc. Nat. Acad. Sci.* **64**, 1087–1094.
Huebner, R. J., Kelloff, G. J., Sarma, P. S., Lane, W. T., Turner, H. C., Gilden, R. V., Oroszlan, S., Meier, H., Myers, D. D., and Peters, W. L. (1970). *Proc. Nat. Acad. Sci.* **67**, 366–376.
Huebner, R. J., Sarma, P. S., Kelloff, G. J., Gilden, R. V., Meier, H., Myers, D. D., and Peters, R. L. (1971). *Ann. N. Y. Acad. Sci.* **181**, 246–271.
Ioachim, H. L. (1970). *Cancer Res.* **30**, 2661–2664.
Ishizaki, R., and Vogt, P. K. (1966). *Virology* **30**, 375–387.
Jarrett, O. (1970). *Advan. Cancer Res.* **13**, 39–62.
Jarrett, O. (1971). *J. Amer. Vet. Med. Ass.* **158**, 1032–1036.
Jarrett, O. (1973). *In* "Unifying Concepts of Leukemia" (R. M. Dutcher and L. Chieco-Bianchi, eds.), pp. 810–812. Karger, Basel.

Jarrett, O., Laird, H. M., Crighton, G. W., Jarrett, W. F. H., and Hay, D. (1968a). In "Leukemia in Animals and Man. Proceedings 3rd International Symposium on Comparative Leukemia Research" (H. J. Bendixen, eds.), pp. 244–254. Karger, Basel.
Jarrett, O., Laird, H. M., Hay, D., and Crighton, G. W. (1968b). Nature (London) **219**, 521–522.
Jarrett, O., Laird, H. M., and Hay, D. (1969a). Nature (London) **224**, 1208–1209.
Jarrett, O., Laird, H. M., Jarrett, W. F. H., and Hay, D. (1969b). J. Small Anim. Pract. **10**, 599–603.
Jarrett, O., Laird, H. M., and Hay, D. (1970). In "Comparative Leukemia Research 1969" (R. H. Dutcher, ed.), pp. 387–392. Karger, Basel.
Jarrett, O., Pitts, J. D., Whalley, J. M., Clason, A. E., and Hay, J. (1971). Virology **43**, 317–320.
Jarrett, O., Laird, H. M., and Hay, D. (1972). Nature (London) **238**, 220–221.
Jarrett, O., Laird, H. M., and Hay, D. (1973). J. Gen. Virol. **20**, 169–177.
Jarrett, W. F. H. (1971). Int. Rev. Exp. Pathol. **10**, 243–263.
Jarrett, W. F. H. (1972). J. Clin. Pathol. **25**, 43–45.
Jarrett, W. F. H. (1974). Brit. J. Cancer (in press).
Jarrett, W. F. H., Crawford, E., Martin, W. B., and Davie, F. (1964a). Nature (London) **202**, 567–569.
Jarrett, W. F. H., Martin, W. B., Crighton, G. W., Dalton, R. G., and Stewart, M. F. (1964b). Nature (London) **202**, 566–567.
Jarrett, W. F. H., Crighton, G. W., and Dalton, R. G. (1966). Vet. Rec. **79**, 693–699.
Jarrett, W. F. H., Anderson, L. J., Jarrett, O., Laird, H. M., and Stewart, M. F. (1971). Res. Vet. Sci. **12**, 385–387.
Jarrett, W. F. H., Essex, M., Mackey, L., Jarrett, O., and Laird, H. (1973a). J. Nat. Cancer Inst. **51**, 261–263.
Jarrett, W. F. H., Jarrett, O., Mackey, L., Laird, H., Hardy, W. D., Jr., and Essex, M. (1973b). J. Nat. Cancer Inst. **51**, 833–841.
Jarrett, W. F. H., Mackey, L. J., Jarrett, O., and Laird, H. M. (1973c). In "Unifying Concepts of Leukemia" (R. M. Dutcher and L. Chieco-Bianchi, eds.), pp. 93–101. Karger, Basel.
Jarrett, W. F. H., Mackey, L., Jarrett, O., Laird, H. M., and Hood, C. (1974). Nature (London) **248**, 230–232.
Kawakami, T. G., Theilen, G. H., Dungworth, D. L., Munn, R. J., and Beall, S. G. (1967). Science **158**, 1049–1050.
Kawakami, T. G., Moore, A. L., Theilen, G. H., and Munn, R. J. (1970). In "Comparative Leukemia Research 1969" (R. M. Dutcher, ed.), pp. 471–475. Karger, Basel.
Kawakami, T. G., Buckley, P. M., and McDowell, T. S. (1973). Nature (London), New Biol. **246**, 105–107.
Kelloff, G., Huebner, R. J., Oroszlan, S., Toni, R., and Gilden, R. V. (1970). J. Gen. Virol. **9**, 27–33.
Klein, G. (1973). Transplant. Proc. **5**, 31–41.
Klein, G., and Dombos, L. (1973). Int. J. Cancer **11**, 327–337.
Klement, V., and McAllister, R. M. (1972). Virology **50**, 305–308.
Klement, V., Rowe, W. P., Hartley, J. W., and Pugh, W. E. (1969). Proc. Nat. Acad. Sci. U. S. **63**, 753–758.
Klement, V., Nicholson, M. O., and Huebner, R. J. (1971). Nature (London), New Biol. **234**, 12–14.
Koprowski, H. (1972). In "The Nature of Leukaemia. Proceedings of the International Cancer Conference 1972" (P. C. Vincent, ed.), pp. 61–64. Blight, Sydney.

Kung, H. J., Bailey, J. M., Davidson, N., Nicolson, M. O., and McAllister, R. M. (1974). *J. Virol.* **14**, 170–173.
Kurth, R., and Bauer, H. (1972). *Virology* **47**, 426–433.
Laird, H. M., Jarrett, O., Crighton, G. W., and Jarrett, W. F. H. (1968a). *J. Nat. Cancer Inst.* **41**, 867–878.
Laird, H. M., Jarrett, O., Crighton, G. W., Jarrett, W. F. H., and Hay, D. (1968b). *J. Nat. Cancer Inst.* **41**, 879–893.
Laird, H. M., Jarrett, O., and Whalley, J. M. (1973). In "Unifying Concepts of Leukemia" (R. M. Dutcher and L. Chieco-Bianchi, eds.), pp. 133–138. Karger, Basel.
Lamon, E. (1974). *Biochim. Biophys. Acta* **355**, 149–176.
Lee, K. M. (1971). *J. Amer. Vet. Med. Ass.* **158**, 1037–1039.
Lee, K. M., Nomura, S., Bassin, R. H., and Fischinger, P. J. (1972). *J. Nat. Cancer Inst.* **49**, 55–60.
Levine, P. H., Horoszewicz, J. S., Grace, J. T., Jr., Chai, L. S., Ellison, R. R., and Holland, J. F. (1967). *Cancer (Philadelphia)* **20**, 1563–1577.
Levy, S. B. (1974). *New Engl. J. Med.* **290**, 513–514.
Livingston, D. M., and Todaro, G. J. (1973). *Virology* **53**, 142–151.
McAllister, R. M., Filbert, J. E., Nicolson, M. O., Rongey, R. W., Gardner, M. B., Gilden, R. M., and Huebner, R. J. (1971a). *Nature (London), New Biol.* **230**, 279–282.
McAllister, R. M., Nelson-Rees, W. A., Johnson, E. Y., Rongey, R. W., and Gardner, M. B. (1971b). *J. Nat. Cancer Inst.* **47**, 603–611.
McAllister, R. M., Nicolson, M., Gardner, M. B., Rongey, R. W., Rasheed, S., Sarma, P. S., Huebner, R. J., Hatanaka, M., Oroszlan, S., Gilden, R. V., Kabigting, A., and Vernon, L. (1972). *Nature (London), New Biol.* **235**, 3–6.
McAllister, R. M., Nicolson, M., Gardner, M. B., Rongey, R. W., Rasheed, S., Sarma, P. S., Huebner, R. J., Hatanaka, M., Oroszlan, S., Gilden, R. V., Kabigting, A., and Vernon, L. (1973). *Nature (London), New Biol.* **242**, 75–78.
McDonough, S., Larsen, S., Brodey, R. S., Stock, N. D., and Hardy, W. D., Jr. (1971). *Cancer Res.* **31**, 953–956.
Mackey, L. J., and Jarrett, W. F. H. (1972a). *J. Nat. Cancer Inst.* **49**, 853–865.
Mackey, L. J., Jarrett, W. F. H., Jarrett, O., and Laird, H. M. (1972). *J. Nat. Cancer Inst.* **48**, 1663–1670.
Malmquist, W. A., Van der Maaten, M. J., and Boothe, A. D. (1969). *Cancer Res.* **29**, 188–200.
Maruyama, K., and Dmochowski, L. (1969). *Tex. Rep. Biol. Med.* **27**, 437–456.
Maruyama, K., Wagner, S. H., and Dmochowski, L. (1974). *Proc. Int. Symp. Comp. Leuk. Res., 6th, Nagoya, Jap. 1973* (in press).
Melendez, L., Hunt, R., Daniel, M., Fraser, C., Barahona, H., Garcia, F., and King, N. (1972). "Oncogenesis and Herpesviruses," pp. 451–461. Int. Ag. Res. Cancer, Lyon.
Melnick, J. L., Altenburg, B., Arnstein, P., Mirkovic, R., and Tevethia, S. (1973). *Intervirology* **1**, 386–398.
Miller, J. M., Miller, L. D., Olson, C., and Gillette, K. G. (1969). *J. Nat. Cancer Inst.* **43**, 1297–1305.
Monti-Bragadin, C., and Ulrich, K. (1972). *Int. J. Cancer* **9**, 383–392.
Morgan, H. R., and Ganapathy, S. (1963). *Proc. Soc. Exp. Biol. Med.* **113**, 312–315.
Nadel, E., Banfield, W., Burstein, S., and Tousimis, A. J. (1967). *J. Nat. Cancer Inst.* **38**, 979–982.
Nazerian, K. (1973). *Advan. Cancer Res.* **17**, 279–316.
Neiman, P. E. (1973). *Nature (London)* **244**, 62–64.

Nielsen, S. W. (1969). *Nat. Cancer Inst., Monogr.* **32**, 73-94.
Nilsson, K., Klein, G., Henle, W., and Henle, G. (1971). *Int. J. Cancer* **8**, 443-450.
Nonoyama, M., and Pagano, J. S. (1971). *Nature (London), New Biol.* **233**, 103-106.
Noronha, F., Post, J. E., Norcross, N. L., and Rickard, C. G. (1972). *Nature (London), New Biol.* **235**, 14-15.
Noronha, F., Dougherty, E., Poco, A., Gries, C., Post, J., and Rickard, C. (1974). *Arch. Gesamte Virusforsch.* **45**, 235-248.
Notkins, A. L., Mergenhagen, S. E., and Howard, R. J. (1970). *Annu. Rev. Microbiol.* **24**, 525-538.
Nowinski, R. C., Old, L. J., Sarkar, N. H., and Moore, D. H. (1970). *Virology* **42**, 1152-1157.
Nowinski, R. C., Fleissner, E., Sarkar, N. H., and Aoki, T. (1972). *J. Virol.* **9**, 359-366.
O'Connor, T. E., Rauscher, F. J., and Ziegel, R. F. (1964). *Science* **144**, 1144-1147.
Okabe, H., Gilden, R. V., and Hatanaka, M. (1973a). *J. Virol.* **12**, 984-994.
Okabe, H., Gilden, R. V., and Hatanaka, M. (1973b). *Nature (London)* **244**, 54-56.
Oksanen, A., Strandstrom, H., and Hatakka, M. (1971). *Acta Vet. Scand.* **12**, 604-606.
Olsen, R. G., and Yohn, D. S. (1972). *J. Nat. Cancer Inst.* **49**, 395-403.
Olsen, R. G., Kahn, D. E., Hoover, E. A., Saxe, N. J., and Yohn, D. S. (1974a). *Infec. Immunity* **10**, 375-380.
Olsen, R. G., Krakowka, S., Mathes, L. E., and Yohn, D. S. (1974b). *Amer. J. Vet. Res.* **35**, 1389-1394.
Olsen, R. G., Mathes, L. E., and Yohn, D. S. (1974c). *Proc. Int. Symp. Comp. Leuk. Res. 6th Nagoya, Jap. 1973* (in press).
Oroszlan, S., Huebner, R. J., and Gilden, R. V. (1971). *Proc. Nat. Acad. Sci. U. S.* **68**, 901-904.
Oroszlan, S., Bova, D., White, M. H., Toni, R., Foreman, C., and Gilden, R. V. (1972). *Proc. Nat. Acad. Sci. U. S.* **69**, 1211-1215.
Oroszlan, S., Copeland, T., Summers, M. R., and Gilden, R. V. (1973). *Science* **181**, 454-455.
Oshiro, L. S., Riggs, J. L., Taylor, D. O. N., Lennette, E. H., and Huebner, R. J. (1971). *Cancer Res.* **31**, 1100-1110.
Oshiro, L. S., Taylor, D. O. N., Riggs, J. L., and Lennette, E. H. (1972). *J. Nat. Cancer Inst.* **48**, 1419-1424.
Oshiro, L., Riggs, J., Lennette, E., and McAllister, R. (1974). *J. Gen. Virol.* **22**, 277-280.
Pal, B., Gardner, M. B., and Roy-Burman, P. (1975). Submitted for publication.
Parks, W. P., and Scolnick, E. M. (1972). *Proc. Nat. Acad. Sci.* **69**, 1766-1770.
Pearson, L. D., Snyder, S. P., and Aldrich, C. D. (1973). *Amer. J. Vet. Res.* **34**, 405-409.
Perryman, L. E., Hoover, E. A., and Yohn, D. S. (1972). *J. Nat. Cancer Inst.* **49**, 1357-1365.
Pope, J. H., Horne, M. K., and Scott, W. (1969). *Int. J. Cancer* **4**, 255-260.
Porter, G. H., III, Dalton, J. S., Moloney, J. B., and Mitchell, E. Z. (1964). *J. Nat. Cancer Inst.* **33**, 547-566.
Post, J. E., Noronha, F., Hong, C., Poco, A., and Rickard, C. G. (1971). *J. Amer. Vet. Med. Ass.* **158**, 1088-1092.
Price, P. M., Hirschhorn, K., Gabelman, N., and Waxman, S. (1973). *Proc. Nat. Acad. Sci. U. S.* **70**, 11-14.
Priester, W. A., and Hayes, H. M. (1973). *J. Nat. Cancer Inst.* **51**, 289-293.
Priester, W. A., and Mantel, N. (1971). *J. Nat. Cancer Inst.* **47**, 1333-1344.

Quintrell, N., Varmus, H. E., Bishop, J. M., Nicolson, M. O., and McAllister, R. G. (1974). *Virology* **58**, 568–575.
Rabin, H. (1971). *Lab. Anim. Sci.* **21**, 1032–1049.
Rabin, H., Theilen, G. H., Sarma, P. S., Dungworth, D. L., Nelson-Rees, W. A., and Cooper, R. W. (1972). *J. Nat. Cancer Inst.* **49**, 441–450.
Rabin, H., Theilen, G. H., Dungworth, D. L., Sarma, P. S., Nelson-Rees, W. A., and Cooper, R. W. (1973). In "Unifying Concepts of Leukemia" (R. M. Dutcher and L. Chieco-Bianchi, eds.), pp. 244–250. Karger, Basel.
Rabotti, G. F., and Blackham, E. (1970). *J. Nat. Cancer Inst.* **44**, 985–991.
Rand, K. H., and Long, C. W. (1973). *J. Gen. Virol.* **21**, 523–532.
Rangan, S. R. S., Moyer, P. P., Cheong, M. P., and Jensen, E. M. (1972a). *Virology* **47**, 247–250.
Rangan, S. R. S., Wong, M. C., Moyer, P. P., and Jensen, E. M. (1972b). *Appl. Microbiol.* **23**, 628–636.
Rangan, S. R. S., Ueberhorst, P. J., and Wong, M. C. (1973). *Proc. Soc. Exp. Biol. Med.* **142**, 1077–1082.
Rickard, C. G. (1968). In "Experimental Leukemia" (M. Rich, ed.), pp. 173–188. Appleton, New York.
Rickard, C. G. (1969). *J. Small Anim. Pract.* **10**, 615–617.
Richard, C. G., Barr, L. M., deNoronha, F., Dougherty, E., and Post, J. E. (1967). *Cornell Vet.* **57**, 302–307.
Rickard, C. G., Gillespie, J. G., Lee, K. M., Noronha, F., Post, J. E., and Sarate, E. L. (1968). In "Leukemia in Animals and Man. Proceedings 3rd International Symposium on Comparative Leukemia Research" (H. J. Bendixen, ed.), pp. 282–284. Karger, Basel.
Rickard, C. G., Post, J. F., deNoronha, F., and Barr, L. M. (1969). *J. Nat. Cancer Inst.* **42**, 987–1014.
Rickard, C. G., Post, J. E., Noronha, F., and Barr, L. M. (1973a). In "Unifying Concepts of Leukemia" (R. M. Dutcher and L. Chieco-Bianchi, eds.), pp. 102–112. Karger, Basel.
Rickard, C. G., Post, J. E., Noronha, F., Dougherty, E., III, and Barr, L. M. (1973b). In "Biohazards in Biological Research" (A. Hellman, M. N. Oxman, and R. Pollack, eds.), pp. 166–178. Cold Spring Harbor Lab., Cold Spring Harbor, New York.
Riggs, J. L. (1971). *J. Amer. Vet. Med. Ass.* **158**, 1085–1087.
Riggs, J. L., Oshiro, L. S., Taylor, D. O. N., and Lennette, E. H. (1969). *Nature (London)* **222**, 1190–1191.
Riggs, J. L., Oshiro, L. S., Taylor, D. O. N., and Lennette, E. H. (1973). *J. Nat. Cancer Inst.* **51**, 449–455.
Riggs, J. L., McAllister, R. M., and Lennette, E. H. (1974). *J. Gen. Virol.* **25**, 21–30.
Robison, R. L., Holzworth, J., and Gilmore, C. E. (1971). *J. Amer. Vet. Med. Ass.* **158**, 981–986.
Rodgers, R., Merigan, T. C., Hardy, W. D., Jr., Old, L. J., and Kassel, R. (1972). *Nature (London), New Biol.* **237**, 270–271.
Rosenthal, P. N., Robinson, H. L., Robinson, W. C., Hanafusa, T., and Hanafusa, H. (1971). *Proc. Nat. Acad. Sci. U. S.* **68**, 2336–2340.
Roth, F. K., Meyers, P., and Dougherty, R. M. (1971). *Virology* **45**, 265–274.
Rous, P. (1910). *J. Exp. Med.* **12**, 695–705.
Rowe, W. P. (1973). *Cancer Res.* **33**, 3061–3068.
Rowe, W. P., Pugh, W. E., and Hartley, J. W. (1970). *Virology* **42**, 1136–1139.
Roy-Burman, P. (1971). *Int. J. Cancer* **7**, 409–415.

Roy-Burman, P., and Kaplan, M. B. (1972). *Biochem. Biophys. Res. Commun.* **48**, 1354–1360.
Rubin, H. T., Cornelius, A., and Fanshien, L. (1961). *Proc. Nat. Acad. Sci. U. S.* **47**, 1058–1069.
Ruprecht, R. M., Goodman, N. C., and Spiegelman, S. (1973). *Proc. Nat. Acad. Sci. U. S.* **70**, 1437–1441.
Sarma, P. S., and Log, T. (1971). *Virology* **44**, 352–358.
Sarma, P. S., and Log, T. (1973a). *In* "Unifying Concepts of Leukemia" (R. M. Dutcher and L. Chieco-Bianchi, eds.), pp. 113–124. Karger, Basel.
Sarma, P. S., and Log, T. (1973b). *Virology* **54**, 160–170.
Sarma, P. S., Log, T., and Huebner, R. J. (1970a). *Proc. Nat. Acad. Sci. U. S.* **65**, 81–87.
Sarma, P. S., Huebner, R. J., Baskar, J. F., Old, L. J., and Hardy, W. D., Jr. (1970b). *In* "Comparative Leukemia Research 1969" (R. H. Dutcher, ed.), pp. 368–378. Karger, Basel.
Sarma, P. S., Huebner, R. J., Baskar, J. R., Vernon, L., and Gilden, R. V. (1970c). *Science* **168**, 1098–1100.
Sarma, P. S., Huebner, R. J., Baskar, J. F., Vernon, L., Gilden, R. V., and Toni, R. (1970d). *Virology* **41**, 377–381.
Sarma, P. S., Baskar, J. F., Gilden, R. V., Gardner, M. B., and Huebner, R. J. (1971a). *Proc. Soc. Exp. Biol. Med.* **137**, 1333–1336.
Sarma, P. S., Gilden, R. V., and Huebner, R. J. (1971b). *J. Amer. Vet. Med. Ass.* **158**, 1055–1060.
Sarma, P. S., Gilden, R. V., and Huebner, R. J. (1971c). *Virology* **44**, 137–145.
Sarma, P. S., Log, T., and Theilen, G. H. (1971d). *Proc. Soc. Exp. Biol. Med.* **137**, 1444–1448.
Sarma, P. S., Sharar, A. L., and McDonough, S. (1972). *Proc. Soc. Exp. Biol. Med.* **140**, 1365–1368.
Sarma, P. S., Tseng, J., Lee, Y. K., and Gilden, R. V. (1973). *Nature (London), New Biol.* **244**, 56–59.
Sarma, P. S., Sharar, A., Tseng, J., Price, P. J., and Gardner, M. (1974a). *Proc. Soc. Exp. Biol. Med.* **145**, 757–762.
Sarma, P. S., Sharar, A., Walter, V., and Gardner, M. (1974b). *Proc. Soc. Exp. Biol. Med.* **145**, 560–564.
Schafer, W. (1973). *In* "Unifying Concepts of Leukemia" (R. M. Dutcher and L. Chieco-Bianchi, eds.), pp. 1182–1193. Karger, Basel.
Schafer, W., and Noronha, F. (1971). *J. Amer. Vet. Med. Ass.* **158**, 1092–1098.
Schafer, W., Lange, J., and Bolognesi, D. P. (1971). *Virology* **44**, 73–82.
Schafer, W., Pister, J., Hunsmann, G., and Maennig, V. (1973). *Nature (London)* **245**, 75–77.
Schaller, J. P., Olsen, R. G., Yohn, D. S., and Essex, M. (1974). *Annu. Meet. Amer. Soc. Microbiol.* (Abstr.)
Schalm, O. W., and Theilen, G. H. (1970). *J. Amer. Vet. Med. Ass.* **157**, 1686–1696.
Schneider, R. (1970). *J. Amer. Vet. Med. Ass.* **157**, 1753–1755.
Schneider, R. (1971). *J. Amer. Vet. Med. Ass.* **158**, 1125–1129.
Schneider, R. (1972a). *Int. J. Cancer* **10**, 338–344.
Schneider, R. (1972b). *Int. J. Cancer* **10**, 345–350.
Schneider, R. S., and Riggs, J. L. (1973). *J. Amer. Vet. Med. Ass.* **162**, 217–219.
Schneider, R., Frye, F. L., Taylor, D. O. N., and Dorn, C. R. (1967). *Cancer Res.* **27**, 1316–1322.

Scolnick, E. M., Parks, W. P., and Livingston, D. M. (1972). *J. Immunol.* **109**, 570–577.
Scott, F. W. (1971). *J. Amer. Vet. Med. Ass.* **158**, 944–945.
Scott, F. W., Csiza, C. K., and Gillespie, J. H. (1970). *J. Amer. Vet. Med. Ass.* **156**, 439–453.
Sherr, C. J., Lieber, M. M., Benveniste, R. E., and Todaro, G. J. (1974). *Virology* **58**, 492–503.
Sibal, L. S., Fink, M. A., Plata, E. J., Kohler, B. E., Noronha, F., and Lee, K. M. (1970). *J. Nat. Cancer Inst.* **45**, 607–611.
Slauson, D. O. (1973). *Fed. Proc., Fed. Amer. Soc. Exp. Biol.* **32**, 851a. (Abstr.)
Snyder, S. P. (1971). *J. Nat. Cancer Inst.* **47**, 1079–1085.
Snyder, S. P., and Dungworth, D. L. (1973). *J. Nat. Cancer Inst.* **51**, 781–792.
Snyder, S. P., and Theilen, G. H. (1969). *Nature (London)* **221**, 1074–1075.
Snyder, S. P., Theilen, G. H., and Richards, W. P. (1970). *Cancer Res.* **30**, 1658–1667.
Spiegelman, S., Burny, A., Das, M. R., Keydar, J., Schalm, J., Travnicek, M., and Watson, K. (1970a). *Nature (London)* **227**, 563–567.
Spiegelman, S., Burny, A., Das, M. R., Keydar, J., Schalm, J., Travnicek, M., and Watson, K. (1970b). *Nature (London)* **228**, 430–432.
Squire, R. A. (1966a). *Cancer (Philadelphia)* **19**, 447–453.
Squire, R. A. (1966b). *Cornell Vet.* **54**, 97–150.
Stenback, W. A., Van Hoosier, G. L., and Trentin, J. J. (1968). *J. Virol.* **2**, 1115–1121.
Stephens, R., Traul, K., Lowry, G., Zelljadt, I., and Mayyashi, S. (1972). *Nature (London)* **240**, 212–214.
Strand, M., and August, J. T. (1974). *J. Virol.* **13**, 171–180.
Sutherland, J. C., and Mardiney, M. R., Jr. (1973). *J. Nat. Cancer Inst.* **50**, 633–644.
Temin, H. M. (1968). *Int. J. Cancer* **3**, 273–282.
Temin, H. M. (1971). *Annu. Rev. Microbiol.* **25**, 639–648.
Temin, H. M., and Baltimore, D. (1972). *Advan. Virus Res.* **17**, 129–186.
Temin, H. M., and Mizutani, S. (1970). *Nature (London)* **226**, 1211–1213.
Theilen, G. H. (1971). *J. Amer. Vet. Med. Ass.* **158**, 1040–1045.
Theilen, G. H., Kawakami, T. G., Dungworth, D. L., Switzer, J. W., Munn, R. J., and Harrold, J. B. (1968). *J. Amer. Vet. Med. Ass.* **153**, 1864–1872.
Theilen, G. H., Kawakami, T. G., Rush, J. D., and Munn, R. J. (1969). *Nature (London)* **222**, 589–590.
Theilen, G. H., Dungworth, D. L., Kawakami, T. G., Munn, R. J., Ward, J. M., and Harrold, J. B. (1970). *Cancer Res.* **30**, 401–408.
Theilen, G. H., Gould, D., Fowler, M., and Dungworth, D. L. (1971). *J. Nat. Cancer Inst.* **47**, 881–890.
Theilen, G. H., Hall, J. G., Pendry, A., Glover, D. J., and Reeves, B. R. (1974). *Transplantation* **17**, 152–155.
Todaro, G. J., and Huebner, R. J. (1972). *Proc. Nat. Acad. Sci. U. S.* **69**, 1009–1019.
Todaro, G. J., Benveniste, R. E., Lieber, M. M., and Livingston, D. M. (1973a). *Virology* **55**, 506–515.
Todaro, G. J., Tevethia, S. S., and Melnick, J. L. (1973b). *Intervirology* **1**, 399–404.
Tooze, J., ed. (1973). "The Molecular Biology of Tumor Viruses," 743 pp. Cold Spring Harbor Lab., Cold Spring Harbor, New York.
Ubertini, T., Noronha, F., Post, J. E., and Rickard, C. G. (1971). *Virology* **44**, 219–222.
Vogt, P. K. (1970). *In* "Comparative Leukemia Research 1969" (R. M. Dutcher, ed.), pp. 153–167. Karger, Basel.
Ward, J. M. (1970). *Virology* **41**, 191–194.

Weijer, K., Calafat, J., Daams, J. H., Hagerman, P. C., and Misdorp, W. (1974). *J. Nat. Cancer Inst.* **52**, 673–679.
Weinstein, R. S., and Moloney, W. C. (1965). *Proc. Soc. Exp. Biol. Med.* **118**, 459–461.
Weiss, R. A., and Biggs, P. M. (1972). *J. Nat. Cancer Inst.* **49**, 1713–1725.
Weiss, R. A., Friis, R. R., Katz, E., and Vogt, P. K. (1971). *Virology* **46**, 920–938.
Whalley, J. M. (1973). *In* "Unifying Concepts of Leukemia" (R. M. Dutcher and L. Chieco-Bianchi, eds.), pp. 125–132. Karger, Basel.
Wolfe, L. G., and Griesemer, R. A. (1966). *Pathol. Vet.* **3**, 255–270.
Wolfe, L. G., and Griesemer, R. A. (1971). *J. Amer. Vet. Med. Ass.* **158**, 987–993.
Wolfe, L. G., Marczynska, B., Rabin, H., Smith, R., Tischendorf, P., Gavitt, F., and Deinhardt, F. (1971). *In* "Medical Primatology. Proceedings 2nd International Conference Experimental Medicine and Surgery in Primates 1971" (H. I. Goldsmith and J. Moor-Jankowski, eds.), pp. 671–682. Karger, Basel.
Wolfe, L. G., Smith, R. D., Hoekstra, J., Marczynska, B., Smith, R. K., McDonald, R., Northrop, R. L., and Deinhardt, F. (1972). *J. Nat. Cancer Inst.* **49**, 519–539.
Wright, B. S., and Korol, W. (1969). *Cancer Res.* **29**, 1886–1887.
Yohn, D. S. (1973). *Ohio J. Sci.* **73**, 3–10.
Yohn, D. S., and Olsen, R. G. (1973). *In* "Unifying Concepts of Leukemia" (R. M. Dutcher and L. Chieco-Bianchi, eds.), pp. 744–754. Karger, Basel.
Yoshiki, T., Mellors, R. C., and Hardy, W. D., Jr. (1973). *Proc. Nat. Acad. Sci. U. S.* **70**, 1878–1882.
Yoshiki, T., Mellors, R. C., Hardy, W. D., Jr., and Fleissner, E. (1974). *J. Exp. Med.* **139**, 925–942.
Zeigel, R. F., and Clark, H. F. (1969). *J. Nat. Cancer Inst.* **43**, 1097–1099.
Zook, B. C., King, N. W., Robison, R. L., and McCombs, H. L. (1968). *Pathol. Vet.* **5**, 91–95.
Zur Hausen, H., and Schulte-Holthausen, H. (1970). *Nature (London)* **227**, 245–248.

EPITHELIAL CELLS: GROWTH IN CULTURE OF NORMAL AND NEOPLASTIC FORMS[1]

Keen A. Rafferty, Jr.

Department of Anatomy, The University of Illinois at the Medical Center, Chicago, Illinois

I. Introduction	249
A. Cell Contamination in Culture	249
B. Normal and Neoplastic Human Cell Lines	250
II. Aging Revisited	251
A. Species-Related Phenomena	251
B. The Theory of Cellular Senescence	252
III. Senescence and Cell Type	253
A. Stromal Cells or "Fibroblasts" in Culture	254
B. Lymphoid Cells in Culture	255
C. Normal Epithelial Cells in Culture	256
D. Human Carcinoma Cells in Culture	259
E. General Principles	260
IV. Epithelial Cells *in Vivo* and Limits on Division Potential	261
A. Logarithmic (Expanding) Cell Populations	261
B. Linear (Renewing) Cell Populations	262
V. Summary and Conclusions	268
References	270

I. Introduction

A. CELL CONTAMINATION IN CULTURE

It is widely accepted that few examples of human carcinoma cell lines are in existence, despite numerous attempts to establish them. Among widely disseminated lines there may in fact be only one, the HeLA cell. This surmise is the result of Gartler's (1967, 1968) well-known finding that all the human epithelial cell lines listed in the catalog of the Cell Culture Collection Committee have the characteristic isozyme of glucose-6-phosphate dehydrogenase, which is confined to blacks. The HeLa line on the other hand was derived from cervical adenocarcinoma of a black patient, Henrietta Lacks

---

[1] Supported by NIH Research Grant No. CA06008 from the Division of Research Grants, by Institutional General Research Support Grant 485, and by American Cancer Society Institutional Grant 9M-1.

(Jones et al., 1971). The easiest explanation for this finding is that all the commonly used permanent human epithelial lines have been contaminated at some time during their history with HeLA cells, with the result that the cultures were dominated and replaced by them. Initially a startling conception, it has become easier to accept with the passage of time. This is partly because alternative explanations seem even less likely, and partly because most tissue culturists have in fact encountered accidental cell contamination at one time or another in their own laboratories. In retrospect, it is not difficult to imagine such an accident occurring as a result of forgetting to change a pipette when aspirating medium from a group of cultures — a procedure usually carried out three times a week for prolonged periods. Replacement of a culture by contaminating cells is further fostered by the investigator's quite understandable tendency to select for subculture those flasks or dishes that contain the most rapidly proliferating cells.

B. Normal and Neoplastic Human Cell Lines

If this is indeed the situation, an interesting corollary presents itself: either that HeLA cells grow more rapidly than any other epithelial cell type and/or that establishment of human carcinoma in culture is quite an unusual event. In many reports of the establishment of such cell lines, primary cultures undergo an initial burst of mitosis and then remain static for more-or-less protracted periods. A typical report then chronicles the sudden appearance of a single focus of rapidly proliferating cells, which subsequently dominate the culture. The original (and understandable) interpretation generally was that a rare transformation event occurred in a single cell. In the light of present information it may well be that spontaneous transformation events are even more seldom seen than even these observations would indicate.

This corollary — that spontaneous transformation of human cells is extremely unusual — also creates a paradox in that carcinoma cells are the least controlled *in vivo* and on the face of it ought to be the ones most able to develop into permanent cell lines. The paradox is compounded by numerous authenticated reports of the establishment of permanent epithelial cell lines from carcinoma and from normal organ parenchymal tissues of some nonprimate vertebrates. Moreover, the ease with which human diploid fibroblast lines are established, self-limited in division potential as they are, is well known. To complete the confusion there is good evidence from *in vivo* studies that some normal epithelial cells may be in continuous division throughout the life of the organism: in at least one *in vitro* system, relatively prolonged growth of normal human epithelial cells has been reported (Lagerholm, 1966; Flaxman *et al.*, 1967).

This review deals with division potential of different cell types *in vivo*, and with the factors that may be responsible for some of the unexplained differences that we find in culturing cells of different origins.

II. Aging Revisited

A. Species-Related Phenomena

The generally poor success in propagation of normal and abnormal epithelial cells prompts a brief consideration of the nonepithelial culture systems in which initiation of cell strains is routine. In some of these the vigorous growth that begins after a short lag period in primary culture is followed by degeneration of the culture after a predictable number of cell divisions. The most thoroughly studied of such systems is that of the human diploid fibroblast, which appears to be limited to about 50–70 cell divisions when cultured from lung of first trimester abortuses (for review, see Hayflick, 1974; also see Swim and Parker, 1957; Puck *et al.*, 1959). Spontaneous transformation of such cell strains to yield permanent cell lines is an exceedingly rare event (Moorhead, 1965).

Other laboratories have found that primates in general tend to be limited in division potential, although with a number of exceptions. Aderca and Iftimovici (1971) obtained at least two permanent cell lines from 11 strains initiated from kidney of African green monkeys (*Cercopithecus aethiops*). This form, however, is associated with a number of viruses which frequently appeared in the cultures, leading to their degeneration in early passages.

Wallace *et al.* (1973) initiated 27 permanent or long-term lines from African green monkeys and rhesus monkeys (*Macaca mulatta*), and followed their culture history until senescence or development into long-term or permanent lines occurred. Seven of the lines were epithelial, of which three spontaneously deteriorated after 5–12 doublings, and the remaining four became permanent lines which were also shown to be heteroploid. Of the 20 fibroblastic lines developed, all except two (one from each species) degenerated. The latter, however, persisted for 141 doublings before being lost, a figure considerably higher than that expected on the basis of the lifetime of the animals. These two lines were also shown to be heteroploid.

Rafferty (1973) made a similar study of several species of *Macaca* (*mulatta, speciosa,* and *iris*); of the spider monkey (*Ateles geoffroi*);

and of the baboon (*Papio* sp.). Of seven strains initiated from lung and other tissues of these forms, all were fibroblastic and all spontaneously degenerated after 22–62 doublings.

The results of Aderca and Iftimovici and of Wallace *et al.* clearly establish that cultures of normal primate cells occasionally give rise to permanent lines, accompanied by heteroploid transformation. On the other hand, these forms are well known to be hosts of a number of viruses, including such highly oncogenic agents as SV_{40}. The animals used in the study by Wallace's group were serologically screened, and an effort was made to select virus-free individuals. The possibility cannot be ruled out, however, that endemic and latent agents were responsible for the apparently spontaneous transformation sometimes observed.

The other well-studied system in which spontaneous degeneration is routinely seen comprises cultures derived from the chick embryo. This observation, now well confirmed, is in contradistinction to the numerous and much publicized reports from Carrel's laboratory during the 1930s which resulted in the claim of continous propagation of a line of chick heart cells for 34 years [related by Parker (1961)]. Other workers have been unable to duplicate these results, and it is now generally conceded that chick embryo cells are quite limited in their ability to grow in culture. Haff and Swim (1956) and Harris (1957) described spontaneous degeneration of cultured rabbit and chick cells. Hay and Strehler (1967) were perhaps the first to make a quantitative study of this behavior, with the result that chick embryo cells were found to decline after some 25 generations in culture. A similar report by Hayflick (1972) found decline after 15–35 doublings. These cells are fibroblastic in morphology.

B. The Theory of Cellular Senescence

There is much other evidence to suggest that limited potential for *in vitro* growth of some cells may be an expresssion of events that result in senescence in intact animals. These have been extensively reviewed elsewhere (Hayflick, 1970, 1972, 1974) and will not be treated in detail here. Evidence that is at least consistent with the senescence theory is as follows:

1. Decline in growth of cell strains seems to be an inherent cell property. Cultures resurrected from frozen storage decline repeatedly after the predicted number of cell generations. Activation of latent viruses seems to be ruled out by Hayflick's (1965) experiments in which identifiable aged cells of one sex were cocultivated with younger cells of the other sex. On further propagation, cells of the older group disappeared first from the cultures.

2. Long-lived animals should produce relatively long-lived cell strains. In addition to the *in vitro* life-spans of primate and chick cells, Goldstein (1975) is reported to have found that cultures of the Galapagos tortoise, which has a confirmed maximum life-span in excess of 100 years (Comfort, 1964), survived for 72–114 doublings in different attempts. Todaro and Green (1963) showed that crisis of growth occurs in mouse cell cultures after 14–28 generations.

3. Cells from aged individuals, in which division potential is presumably diminished, also have a shortened *in vitro* growth potential (Hayflick, 1965; Goldstein, 1969; Martin *et al.*, 1970).

4. Cells from human patients with premature aging diseases (progeria, Goldstein, 1969; Werner's syndrome, Martin *et al.*, 1970) are severely limited in their growth potential.

5. Individual tissues seem to have a finite life-span of their own. Skin (Krohn, 1962) and mammary gland (Daniel *et al.*, 1968) survive as isologous transplants for predictable times, based upon the life expectancy of the donor.

It is important to remember, however, that these observations apply only to fibroblastic cell lines.

III. Senescence and Cell Type

One of the observations that must be reconciled with the theory of aging as proposed by Hayflick is the widely known fact that cells from many animals are by no means limited in their *in vitro* division potential. Rather they are perhaps more the rule than is limitation, which has been shown to be systematically effective only in some primates and in birds. Thus mouse cell cultures essentially always give rise to permanent cell lines, following a crisis in growth, when propagated by usual culture techniques. Lines have also been established repeatedly from cells of rats, rabbits, fish, amphibians, and various other vertebrates. In some instances transformation through the action of latent oncogenic viruses is a sensible explanation for this effect. This is particularly true in the case of the mouse, which in the laboratory form is highly inbred and known to be contaminated with numerous potentially oncogenic agents. The same should be true to a lesser extent, however, in the case of domestic fowl, which never produces permanent cell lines. Moreover, cultures initiated from a house mouse trapped wild in Downers Grove, Illinois, also gave rise to permanent cell lines [W. A. Clark, Jr. and K. A. Rafferty, Jr, unpublished experiments].

It is generally understood that permanent cell lines are karyotypically heteroploid and often if not always potentially capable of forming tumors when the cells are reintroduced into the donor species. Of greater interest, however, is the observation that a number of well-documented cases have been reported in which euploid cell lines were produced and propagated for considerably more cell generations than can be explained on the basis of the life expectancy of the donor. This point deserves discussion in some detail.

A. STROMAL CELLS OR "FIBROBLASTS" IN CULTURE

Appreciation of the fact that fibroblasts from some organisms are limited in *in vitro* growth potential, while remaining diploid, developed slowly and was first clearly enunciated and systematically pursued by Hayflick and Moorhead (1961). This realization, however, brought forth several publications from various laboratories in which long-term cell lines of predominantly normal karyotype had been developed, as well as some others in which only chromosome counts (but not karyotype analyses) were done, or reports in which a sizable proportion of heteroploid cells were present in predominantly euploid lines. On balance, however, there emerged from the reports the finding that karyotypically normal cells can be propagated for long periods in selected instances, usually when derived from hamster or rat tissues.

In an early report of this kind, Yerganian and Leonard (1961) noted some success in selecting long-term diploid lines of Chinese hamster cells by cloning, although the proportion of diploid cells (55–80%) was somewhat low. MacPherson (1963), in studies of polyoma virus transformation, reported development of a permanent control cell line from the hamster in which 90% of the cells were diploid. Homologous transfer of these in large inoculum (10^6 cells) resulted in tumors. Since karyotype analysis was not done, it is possible that the cells were cryptic heteroploids, in having duplication of chromosome segments through translocation, or that the tumors arose from the relatively small number of heteroploid cells present. Using rat tissues, Peturssen *et al.* (1964) reported an apparently permanent cell line in which 60% of the cells were euploid by karyotype analysis. Tumorigenicity was not tested. In another report involving rat cells, in this case derived from rhabdomyosarcomas, Basrur and Gilman (1963) observed the reverse of most experiences, that is, the transformation of a heteroploid into a diploid cell line. In these observations the heteroploid line, which was also permanent and tumorigenic, also lost the ability to produce tumors. Another report involving rat tissues is that of Krooth *et al.* (1964) in which cells of a permanent line were diploid in more than 80% proportion.

Karyotype analysis was completed in this case, and the cells were shown to be euploid. In a case of human origin Moore and Sandberg (1964) established an interesting monolayer cell strain from a pleural effusion derived from a patient with squamous cell carcinoma. At the time of their writing this strain had undergone 35 subcultures and was still viable but had a normal karyotype. It also produced tumors in cancer patients and in conditioned animals.

Rabbit cells were added to the list of those that can produce long-term and apparently normal cell lines, through the report of Valenti and Friedman (1968). Earlier, Swim and Parker (1957) had developed some permanent (but heteroploid) rabbit cell lines, noting, however, that in most instances spontaneous degeneration occurred after about 12 subcultures. Shiratori et al. (1968) developed a cell line from papillomas of rabbit skin induced by Shope virus. The line had undergone 55 subcultures at the time of the report and was still vigorous. Most cells were euploid at the twentieth subculture although 28% were heteroploid.

Prunieras et al. (1969) developed several cell lines from guinea pig skin. Initially epithelial in morphology, these became spindled in appearance. Some lines were predominantly heteroploid, but some were shown to be 80% diploid on long-term culture. A potentially interesting point is that the cells of the long-term lines may be epidermal and not fibroblasts, since like epidermal cells they were naphthylamidase negative whereas fibroblasts are positive (Jacquemont and Prunieras, 1969), and lacked large ergastoplasmic cisternae, unlike fibroblasts (Gazzolo and Prunieras, 1969). The hazard of using morphological criteria as the sole indicator of cell origin is discussed in a later section.

B. Lymphoid Cells in Culture

In the foregoing instances of predominantly diploid permanent or long-term lines, the cells are of spindled morphology. A second group of established diploid lines is represented by lymphoid cells that grow in suspension. Development of the first permanent lymphoblastoid lines was reported by Paul (1958). Subsequently other groups, notably that headed by Moore (for reviews, see Moore and McLimans, 1968; Moore et al., 1967) repeatedly established permanent lymphoblastoid lines from diseased and normal human sources. This group and others (i.e., Steele and Edwards, 1971) described procedures by which a permanent line can be established from peripheral blood of virtually any individual. In a karyological study, Macek et al. (1971) found that most such lines are diploid or nearly diploid and that some are euploid. To the author's knowledge all human lymphoblastoid lines that have been appropriately examined have been shown to contain DNA of the Epstein–Barr virus and hence are probably neoplastic.

C. NORMAL EPITHELIAL CELLS IN CULTURE

As noted, there is general agreement that development of culture lines by routine methods results in lines of fibroblasts, or at least of spindled cells, in virtually every instance. Hence examples of the development of lines of epithelial morphology are of particular interest.

1. *Permanent Euploid Epithelial Cell Lines*

Rafferty (1969) reported development of an epithelial line from teased fragments of tadpoles of the frog, *Rana sylvatica*. In early establishment of the line, fragments attached to the surface of the culture vessel and epithelial cells continuous with the skin of the fragments migrated over the surface. Spindled cells were also present but did not divide rapidly. Subcultures were made over a period of months, with the result that spindled cells rapidly disappeared. In subsequent subcultures all cells were epithelial in appearance and the morphology did not change greatly during the time the cell line was under observation. Because of the circumstances of the initial outgrowth, the line was assumed to be derived from epidermis. It underwent 90 subcultures and was still vigorous when lost to bacterial contamination. A detailed karyotype analysis was carried out on cells of the 79th subculture, comparing the chromosome measurements with those of chromosomes prepared from marrow. On the basis of general morphology, arm ratio, and relative length, no appreciable differences were found. About 80% of the cells were diploid after 79 cell generations, with most of the remainder being subtetraploid. In the development of this line, the trend was seen to be toward slowly increasing heteroploidy with relatively high (subtetraploid) chromosome numbers, while cells varying from the major mode by only one or a few chromosomes became less frequent. The result was that the proportion of diploid cells actually increased slightly during the culture history. The presumption was, however, that prolonged culture would eventually have resulted in a line dominated by heteroploid cells. This is probably also true of most long-term diploid lines, since it will be seen that the majority of these have sizable proportions of heteroploid cells. In the case of human diploid fibroblasts, on the other hand, usually fewer than 10% of the cells deviate from the normal karyotype.

As already noted, Prunieras *et al.* (1969) developed long-term, evidently permanent, cell lines from guinea pig skin, and of these 80% of the cells of some strains were diploid and karyotypically normal.

Rafferty (1973) initiated several permanent cell lines from fetal lung tissue of the rat and ferret. Of two lines from the rat, one remained karyotypically normal for more than 100 cell generations, when subcultivation was terminated. In the case of the ferret, three lines were initiated from different individuals and two of these remained euploid at the time subcultivation was stopped, again at more than 100 divisions. All three lines were distinctly epithelial in morphology.

As has been noted previously, prolonged growth of epithelial cells does not readily succeed, even when attempts are made to initiate cultures from carcinoma. Some animals, however (rat, ferret, guinea pig and frog), do tend to yield epithelial cell cultures, and occasionally—as in the case of fibroblasts from related forms—long-term, predominantly euploid cultures may result. In all probability these slowly accumulate heteroploid cells, but it seems clear that karyotypically normal cells do not invariably die after a fixed number of cell divisions. The question is thus raised whether some rapidly dividing cell populations *in vivo* exceed the Hayflick limit on division potential, and whether such limits may vary with cell type or with species. This possibility is consonant (see below) with the rather compelling indications that epithelial cells of some rapidly renewing systems may not have reserve stem cell compartments *in vivo* but may instead be in rapid, more-or-less continuous, division throughout the life of the organism.

2. *Normal Epithelial Cells in Short-Term Culture*

Before considering division potential of epithelial cells *in vivo*, it should be noted that considerable success has in recent years attended efforts to cultivate epithelial cells on at least a short-term basis. This success may well be due to the use of efforts to prevent fibroblast overgrowth and to the development of more suitable media. Many such epithelial cell lines seem to show the Hayflick limit on division, but these to date have been derived from epithelia in which renewal is not rapid. These are discussed below.

Retinal pigment cells were cultured from chick embryos (Cahn and Cahn, 1966) with the result that senescence occurred at about the time expected for chick cells. A somewhat remarkable, and more recent, observation was made with human retinal cells (Mannagh et al., 1973). In about 100 cultures, deterioration occurred in all except seven, which were found to be heteroploid. Hence, it appears to be possible for normal human cells to transform spontaneously, and possibly the frequency is a function of cell type. HeLa cell contamination seems to be eliminated as a possible explanation for these results, since some of the late passage cells contained pigment.

Another interesting example of human epithelial cell culture derives from the work of Pontén and Macintyre (1968), who cultured human brain tissue acquired from surgery for wound debridement, hematoma, or aneurism. Ten epithelial lines were developed from normal tissue and had the appearance of glia. All deteriorated spontaneously, in an average of about 16 cell generations, a figure compatible with their derivation from adults. Of further interest is the observation that 25 of 29 lines from gliomas also had finite life-spans, of the same general range, while four became permanent. In other work involving brain tissue, Lim and Mitsunobu (1974) have developed a number of epithelioid lines from embryonic rat brain tissue, and report a prevailing view that these are also glial in origin. A feature of these particular lines is that they may be "transformed" morphologically into populations of cells that resemble astrocytes. In this case, the transforming agent is a protein extracted from adult brains. These lines were not propagated serially for prolonged periods.

Liver has been cultured with surprising success, beginning with the attempts of Coon (1968) and of Coon and Weiss (1969) using adult rat material. These lines, which are strikingly epithelial, were shown by immunoelectrophoretic analysis to produce several rat serum albumins after protracted culture. In cases where karyology was investigated, some were shown to be diploid or near-diploid, but it is believed that most or all gradually become heteroploid as culture progresses.

Kaighn and Prince (1971) developed a line of human liver cells which produced a number of serum albumins during serial subculture and hence must be derived from hepatocytes in spite of the fact that their morphology is spindled. These cells cannot be propagated indefinitely, and are lost at about the time expected for adult human fibroblasts [M. E. Kaighn, personal communications].

Castor and Naylor (1969) developed epithelial cell lines seemingly from normal human mesothelium obtained through aspirating pericardial effusions. These were predominantly diploid in early passage, but were not followed for a prolonged period.

Chick embryo thyroid cells were also propagated in monolayer culture (Spooner, 1970), but, like chick cells from other tissues, could not be propagated indefinitely.

Lewis *et al.* (1973) have initiated several lines of endothelial cells, derived from human umbilical vein: these have ABO blood group antigens and are immunofluorescence positive for thrombosthenin. They seem to deteriorate at various periods and an effort has not been made to maintain them permanently in culture. However, they have undergone at least 13 doublings in culture, in addition to the number of doublings required to establish the original monolayer. In other work, Douglas and Kaighn (1974) have cultured differentiated rat lung cells which are epithelial and seem to produce pulmonary surfactant. These often seem to deteriorate, however, after a few subcultures. At the sixth subculture the karyotype was normal [M. E. Kaighn, personal communication]. Van Venrooij *et al.* (1974) have repeatedly established epithelial monolayer cultures from dissociated calf lens epithelium. These deteriorate after about 50 subcultures at a split ratio of 1:3, or about 65 doublings [W. J. van Venrooij, personal communication]. Finally, Lycette and Whyte (1973) have initiated monolayer lines of epithelial cells from bovine colon, and showed that they produce PAS-positive mucin. Once again, however, these were not followed to determine whether spontaneous deterioration occurs.

These results appear to indicate that deterioration of at least some epithelial cells occurs, and at about the expected time in culture. As noted, it is problematical whether such deterioration takes place in rapidly renewing epithelial cells.

D. HUMAN CARCINOMA CELLS IN CULTURE

The curious fact has already been noted that most of the available cell lines purported to have been established from human carcinoma are probably HeLa cells. This situation points up the difficulty in initiating such lines, a problem confirmed in the author's laboratory, where attempts to begin lines from some 30 surgical specimens have all failed. A typical result, observed also in other laboratories, is that epithelial cell colonies form in the primary cultures, and vigorous cell division is often seen within them. After a rather low number of doublings, however, division ceases and the cells become vacuolated and eventually detach and die. Within recent years there has been renewed interest in initiating new human carcinoma lines, in part the result of appreciating that so few lines exist. As a result, a few successes are being reported. Since workers are now generally alerted to the danger of HeLa cell contamination there is every reason for confidence that the lines in question are bona fide: many laboratories avoid having other established human cell lines in culture at all. Some examples of recent success in carcinoma cell culture are discussed.

Sykes *et al.* (1970) developed an apparently permanent epithelioid cell line from cervical carcinoma.

Bassin and co-workers (1972) isolated an established epithelioid cell line from human breast carcinoma. Giard *et al.* (1973) and Kersey *et al.* (1973) cultured some 200 tumors, including some sarcomas. Of these, eleven epithelial lines were established, comprising seven carcinomas (two renal, two bronchogenic, and three epidermoid), two brain tumors, and two melanomas. Leibovitz (1973) has reported development of a cell line from small cell carcinoma of the adrenal cortex, and a few other such reports are in the current literature.

The remarkable feature of these reports is their paucity, leading to the speculation that epithelial malignancy may be difficult to establish in culture for the same reasons that normal epithelial cell lines present problems: a transformation process may be involved, while there is no reason why carcinoma cells *in vivo* might not be limited in their growth potential, just as fibroblasts and some normal epithelial cells seem to be. Problems in culture of human carcinoma may also stem from the fact that most specimens are necessarily derived from aged individuals and so might have even more foreshortened division potential. A further possible source of difficulty has to do with the quality of material available for initiation of human carcinoma cell culture. Anyone who has examined sections of surgical specimens of carcinoma is struck by the fact that many of them consist predominantly of connective tissue and of regions of normal epithelia. In the absence of criteria for positive identification of cell type, one cannot be certain that the cells in question are indeed carcinomatous in origin unless histological examination of the tissue shows it to be essentially free of other elements.

E. GENERAL PRINCIPLES

In summarizing a large number of observations, a few rather general statements can be defended, in application to cell culture by "standard" methods in current use.

1. In the culture of avian and some primate (including human)

tissues, the resulting cell lines are routinely fibroblastic, limited in growth potential, and karyotypically normal.

2. In the culture of cells from many rodent, lagomorph, carnivore, and amphibian sources, permanent cell lines may be karyotypically normal in terms of the prevailing cell type and may also be tumorigenic or of neoplastic origin. These slowly develop into heteroploid lines.

3. Through the use of special procedures lymphoblastoid and epithelial lines may be established which are permanent or relatively long-term, and karyotypically normal in terms of the prevailing cell type. In some instances (human) these are derived from a source that normally yields cell lines of limited division potential.

4. Cells of many carcinomas behave as though they are limited in their division potential and require intervention of a transformation process for their establishment as permanent cell culture lines.

IV. Epithelial Cells *in Vivo* and Limits on Division Potential

A. LOGARITHMIC (EXPANDING) CELL POPULATIONS

In a logarithmically expanding cell population, the 50–70 limit on the number of possible doublings of human cells (taken at the end of the first trimester of fetal life) presents no obstacle to the imagination since simple calculation reveals that such a process would produce many tons of cells. Perhaps a more meaningful way of perceiving a limit on division potential is in terms of stem cell populations, which presumably exist for each cell type of the adult. Thus if the clonal selection theory of Burnet (1960) is correct, each lymphocyte can be programmed for a specific response to only one or two antigens, and therefore each antigen to which the organism can respond must initially be represented by a rather small stem cell population within the organism. Even in this case, however, calculation indicates no theoretical difficulties resulting from a human cell doubling limit. Hence, even if only 0.01% of the cells of the body were capable of division the entire body could be renewed from such a population every 3 weeks for 100 years and still require only 33 divisions from the end of the first trimester. In the case of lymphoid stem cell populations, even if the stem population for any one antigen producer cell line amounted to only 1000 cells, 40 logarithmic divisions would produce more than 10^{15} cells, which would weigh about 260 tons.

There is evidence, moreover, that clonal senescence does occur in mouse lymphoid elements. Siminovitch *et al.* (1964) transplanted lymphoid cells into irradiated mouse hosts and demonstrated that formation of dividing colonies in the spleens resulted. On serial transfer, the ability to form colonies disappeared, apparently as the result of the loss of cell viability. No attempt was made to estimate the number of cell generations undergone by the transplanted cells. Williamson and Askonas (1972) serially transplanted isologous clones of specific antibody-producing cells and noted that antibody-producing capacity was eventually lost in the later transfers. Taking into account the fact that transfers were made from a small proportion of the stem cell population the authors calculated that some 90 cell divisions were involved. This value seems quite high for the mouse, with its small body size and short life-span, but the nature of the experiment required that a number of assumptions had to be made in order to arrive at an estimated value for doubling capacity. In this respect, however, it is of interest to note that Martin *et al.* (1970) estimated that the actual doubling limit for cultured human diploid fibroblasts is nearer 90 than 50. This figure was arrived at by taking into account such factors as cell loss on transfer, the presence of inviable cells in the culture, and so forth. In a similar study, Good (1972) concluded that the human limit is even higher, at a value of 140–180. Thus, the apparently high limit obtained for mouse cells *in vivo* may reflect lowered viability *in vitro*. Whatever the case, Kay (1965) noted that about 5% of marrow cells may be stem cells. He also noted that all the red and white cells required in 60 years could be supplied by logarithmic division beginning from a single cell, if 54 cell generations are possible. Burnet (1970) theorizes that senescence of dividing lymphoid elements may be the principle cause of aging *in vivo*.

B. Linear (Renewing) Cell Populations

In dividing cell populations in which the progeny differentiate and so cease division, difficulties are rapidly introduced when a limit on division potential is postulated. The extent of these depends in turn upon the degree to which progenitor cells can divide serially before the onset of differentiation. The ultimate limitation is that of the strict "renewal" population (Leblond, 1964) or "tangential" division (Kay, 1965) in which each stem cell division results in one daughter cell that differentiates and one that remains a stem cell. In this case, an effective low limit on division potential, as applied to cell populations that are frequently renewed, is difficult to visualize since a stem cell division would be required for each differentiated cell produced. There is very suggestive evidence, however, that this is precisely what does occur in stratified squamous epithelia and perhaps in the cuboidal epithelia of intestinal crypts.

1. *Stratified Squamous Epithelia*

Skin and esophagus are organs in which mitoses are frequently observed in or near the basal layer of the epithelium. Moreover, the progeny are continually lost through keratinization and sloughing, placing unusual demands upon the division potential of the progenitor cells. Leblond's group (Leblond, 1964; Marques-Pereira and Leblond, 1965) studied cell renewal in them, with particular emphasis on the esophagus of the rat. The choice of esophagus was felicitous because the basal layer of cells is a monolayer, unlike skin, in which "basal" cells are often several layers thick. The simple nature of esophageal epithelium, coupled with the fact that all mitosis occurs within the basal layer (references above), make it almost ideal for investigation of the question of limit on division potential *in vivo*. The basic approach was to inject tritiated thymidine at frequent intervals (i.e., shorter than the S phase of the cell cycle) and determine the cell cycle by autoradiographic analysis. Three hours after a single injection, virtually all the metaphases seen were labeled, indicating that analysis is not complicated in this case by production of differentiating cells from cells arrested in G_2. When essentially continuous exposure to the labeled compound was provided by injections at 3-hour intervals for prolonged periods it was seen that all cells of the basal layer were radioactive within 6 days (Leblond *et al.*, 1964). As noted, it was shown also that no mitoses occurred in any other layer. Cell cycle analysis gave a T_c value (generation time) of 82 hours in the rat, as a mean. It was also shown, however, that a subpopulation of the basal layer replicated in 54 hours, indicating a heterogeneous population. In study of the cells of more superficial layers, following a single pulse of the labeled compound, it was observed that labeled cells occurred either singly or in pairs. From a determination of the frequency distribution of these, it was shown that cells were randomly transferred from the basal layer (Marques-Pereira and Leblond, 1965; Nadler, 1965) Thus, division of a basal layer cell was followed by all three possible occurrences, determined by chance: ejection of one daughter cell and retention of the other, ejection of both, or retention of both daughter cells. The conclusion, therefore, was that all cells of the basal layer divide at least once every 6 days (Leblond *et al.*, 1964). If literally correct, this finding strongly suggests that these cells undergo at least 60 divisions a year and that a Hayflick-like limit could not be possible. Because of the importance of the implications this topic deserves further discussion.

A finite low-level limit on the division potential of basal cells would require periodic repopulation of the layer, presumably either by (1) logarithmic division of a quiescent subpopulation, however small; or, (2) migration of stem cells into the basal layer, either from the dermis or from strata overlying the basal layer. Both of these possibilities will be examined.

a. Quiescent Subpopulation. Occurrence of a population of reserve cells would seem to be eliminated quite simply by the observations, already noted, that all cells of the basal layer become labeled (and presumably divide) at least once every 6 days. On the other hand, it was also seen that very large numbers of cells could be produced by a few cells dividing logarithmically if the progeny were to repopulate the basal layer from time to time. Thus epithelia might be renewed at this rate in the human, even for 100 years, if only 1 cell in 1000 acted as a reserve cell with a division potential of about 70 cell generations. It is also evident that a proportion of unlabeled cells this small might reasonably be overlooked unless specifically sought after. A further point is that unlabeled cells do seem to occur in mouse skin under these circumstances. Hegazy and Fowler (1973) reported that 96 hours after beginning thymidine injections at 3-hour intervals, the proportion of cells labeled is not significantly different from unity. Inspection of the plotted data indicates, however, that about 3% of the cells were unlabeled after the 4-day period. Moreover, at the end of 150 hours about 2% remained unlabeled, and the curve appeared to be approaching unity asymptotically at this time, when the experiment was terminated. In a similar experiment, Potten (1974) and Potten *et al.* (1974) found that some 11% remained unlabeled after 150 hours of continuous exposure. In addition, these workers determined, through cell cycle studies, that a slowly cycling cell is present in skin. Because of ambiguous results in some experiments, the possibility was investigated that experimental manipulation stimulates division: many experiments of this type utilize dorsal skin, and the possibility was evidenced that picking up the animals at 3-hour intervals in order to give injections could affect the division rate. Potten *et al.* (1974) did in fact show that the rate of entry into S rises during the experimental period and concluded that little significance should be attached to results under these circumstances. There is no question, however, that division is very extensive under normal circumstances *in vivo:* such labeling is evident in rats given thymidine in the drinking water (Leblond *et al.*, 1964) and in epithelia which should not be affected by handling, i.e., plantar and ear skin, and esophagus.

To return momentarily to consideration of a reserve cell population in these epithelia, Chopra and Flaxman (1974) cultured human skin for 7 days, to allow time for a monolayer outgrowth of epidermal cells to occur around the explant, and then exposed the cultures continuously to radioactive thymidine for an additional 5 days. At this time, 34% of the cells remained unlabeled. The authors did not attribute the labeling failure of this relatively large fraction to a lengthy cell cycle, since the cycle for the population as a whole was 59 hours. On the other hand, it is clear for the purposes of the present topic that the finding is of limited significance, since it might simply indicate the existence of poorly viable cells in culture, or inadequacy of the medium.

The studies of Potten (1974), combining morphological study with cell cycle analysis in mouse skin, do appear to have significant implications for this subject. Potten defined an organization unit of about 20 cells, hexagonal in shape, of which a mean of 10.6 were found in the basal layer, which may be two or three cells thick. In addition, the cell cycle studies showed that the central nucleus cycles more slowly and responds slightly earlier to stimulation, as is accomplished by plucking the fur. Moreover, of the 11% of cells remaining unlabeled after 150 hours, half are in the central position of the organizational unit, which Potten designated the epidermal proliferative unit. Further morphological studies indicated that the central cell differs also from the rest in that it has no desmosomes and is not attached to the basement membrane. Thus it need not be carried into the upper layers as differentiation progresses, but could remain behind to repopulate the basal layer.

In experiments on human skin, Penneys et al. (1970) injected ^{3}H-TdR intradermally and removed the area by biopsy procedures 45 minutes later. Autoradiographic analysis of this material indicated that 32% of the labeled cells were located above the basal cell layer, and the authors concluded that cell division is not confined to the layer. The analysis was three-dimensional in that it took into account the fact that cells may appear to be superficial to the basal layer in some sections, as a result of the undulations in the dermal-epidermal line which accommodate the dermal papillae.

As suggestive as these findings are, they do not in themselves indicate that the basal cells are of low division potential. Further, in application to esophageal epithelia there are mechanical and other problems in periodic repopulation of the one-cell-thick basal layer. Since all or virtually all basal cells seemingly divide at brief intervals, any reserve cell population, as noted, would need to be present as quite a small minority. This in turn would imply that repopulation through logarithmic division of reserve cells would give rise to clones of considerable extent. A consequence of this process would be that mitoses would occur in regional clusters. The analyses performed by Leblond *et al.* (1964) showed, however, that labeled cells are randomly distributed in the basal layer of the rat esophagus after administration of a single dose of thymidine. Thus, while it is possible that a reserve cell arrangement occurs in skin of the mouse, the evidence is very good, although not conclusive, that all basal cells of most forms divide frequently. In the case of esophageal epithelium, however, there is no evidence for existence of a reserve cell group, and the evidence seems to indicate that the stem cells are in continuous rapid division.

  b. External Augmentation. The possibility must also be considered that stem cells are added from time to time to stratified squamous epithelia by migration from the dermis or from sequestered groups of cells within the basal layers, which would not be detected in the usual labeling experiments. Although this may happen in mouse skin, random labeling seems to indicate that addition of reserve cells that form clones of basal cells does not occur. Although random labeling could occur if every large numbers of reserve cells entered the basal layer from the dermis without giving rise to clones, this seems unlikely. Tissue culture experiments with adult human skin are instructive in this regard and deserve additional attention. Flaxman and Chopra (1972) have extensively cultured split thickness skin explants, which can be introduced into culture in such a manner that outgrowth of fibroblasts is prevented. The result is that a pure epithelial layer migrates out and populates the culture dish. Initially this cell population (presumably derived from the basal layer) is one cell thick. When the dish becomes confluent, however, or when the migrating edge of the cell sheet expands to a point sufficiently remote from the initiating explant, differentiation begins to occur in the central region. Since these cultures lack a dermal component, migration of reserve cells from the dermis *in vivo* seems unlikely. In addition, many cell divisions obviously occur in the cultures without the increase afforded by such cells. Unfortunately, although cell division is vigorous and extensive in this system, it has not been possible so far to accomplish subculture reliably, and thus the division capacity of the cells is undetermined, although clearly considerable.

  On balance it would appear that the division potential of stem cells in stratified squamous epithelia is probably considerably in excess of the division potential of fibroblasts, although it is at present not possible to conclusively affirm this. As suggested by others, an interesting experiment for this point, and one which in all probability is feasible, would be to culture human epidermal cells on cover slips, transferring the slip and its attached cells to a new dish each time the culture surface is completely populated. If subculture could be accomplished in this manner the question of division potential could readily be settled.

2. *Intestinal Epithelium*

The other situation in which rapid continuous proliferation takes place in a relatively defined population occurs within the crypts of Lieberkühn, particularly those of the small intestine (Messier, 1960; Messier and Leblond, 1960). In this site, the intestinal epithelium of the mouse is completely replaced every 3 days through cell division which is confined to the small crypts, each containing some 250 cells (Kovacs and Potten, 1973). Pulse-labeling experiments showed that the transit time from the crypts is only 16.5 hours (Potten *et al.*, 1974), an indication of the intense level of generative activity in this location. Of the cell population of the crypt, an upper region of about 72 cells constitutes the zone of maturation, in which labeled cells occur later on in pulse experiments but in which division does not occur (Kovacs and Potten, 1973). A central region of some 135 cells is that in which all division takes place, while in a lower Paneth zone of 47 cells division seldom occurs. Potten *et al.* (1974) note that cells of this zone could comprise a stem cell population for the replacement of Paneth cells (and, in the colon, of goblet cells) which have a longer life than do absorptive cells of the small intestine. On the other hand, these authors also recognize that the Paneth zone might contain reserve cells by which the proliferative zone could be repopulated from time to time. In continuous labeling experiments (injection of tritiated thymidine every 3 hours for 7 days) the Paneth zone shrinks by about 10 cells, indicating that the cells located at the upper margin of the Paneth zone, where it is continuous with the proliferative zone, enter mitosis in a more leisurely fashion and therefore constitute a subpopulation of more slowly cycling cells, which clearly could constitute a compartment of fundamental stem cells. On the basis of earlier calculations, Kay (1965), however, felt it unlikely that the small number of cells in the mouse crypts could include an effective stem cell population, and postulated that if epithelial cells of the mouse are limited in their capacity to divide (presumably to about 15 cell divisions) then replacement of the intestinal epithelium would require immigration of stem cells, a process that seems unlikely but is possible. Based upon earlier data which indicated that the cycle of human crypt cells is 100 hours, Kay assumed that epithelial replacement was relatively slow in this instance and that the cells could be limited in division capacity and still not require augmentation from external sources. More recent data, in which modern and more dependable techniques have been used, indicate, however, that human cell turnover times are quite comparable to those of experimental animals. Thus, Bertalanffy and Nagy (1961) estimated that the turnover time of human duodenal epithelium is 2 days. Cell turnover in colonic epithelium was determined to be 6–8 days (Cole and McKalen, 1961) and 4–6 days in the rectum (Cole and McKalen, 1963). Richart (1963) estimated the turnover rate of stratified squamous epithelial cells of the cervix to be 5.7 days. These values, as noted, are quite comparable with those obtained in rodents and suggest that epithelial replacement poses the same problems for man, in terms of constraints imposed by limited division potential, as they do for experimental animals.

These results, taken together, clearly suggest that the limits of the division potential of fibroblasts may not apply in the case of all cell types.

V. Summary and Conclusions

Tissue cultures begun from dissociated tissues of human and avian origin are usually dominated by fibroblasts, even though epithelial cells may be present at first. The fibroblastic cultures are limited in their growth potential to about 50 divisions when a human fetal tissue source is employed. This limit appears to depend at least partly, however, upon the longevity and life-expectancy of the donor, so that individual and species-specific factors are important in the evolution and history of a cell line.

Fibroblast dominance of mixed cell cultures could result from more rapid proliferation of fibroblasts than of epithelial cells, leading to their completely populating the culture after a few subcultivations. More seems to be involved than a simple competitive advantage, however, because in human and avian cultures epithelial cells usually undergo only a few divisions and then become quiescent. As a result, epithelial cell lines have not been developed from these sources (with one or two exceptions), even through the expediency of low density plating followed by clonal isolation of epithelial colonies. The lack of growth by these cells might be due either to specific medium inadequacy or to intrinsic low-level limitation on division potential, perhaps reflecting low division potential *in vivo*—as in the case of kidney epithelial cells, for example, The latter explanation would seem more probable in view of success in propagating human liver and epidermal cells for relatively prolonged periods: both of these cell types are known to have substantial division potential *in vivo*. On the other hand, various epithelial cell types from some forms (notably hamster, rat, rabbit, ferret, and frog) can often be propagated successfully and even give rise to permanent cell lines.

It seems unlikely *a priori* that fundamental or deep-seated species differences occur, and it is concluded that prolonged cultivation of human and avian epithelial cells might attend revision of techniques or of medium composition. The second possibility becomes more attractive in view of the fact that virtually all readily available media have been developed using growth of rodent fibroblasts as the criterion for selection and concentration of medium components.

The relation between karyology and growth potential is also of interest, especially since lines which are limited in division potential are also of normal karyotype, and transformation of human cell lines to heteroploid form with retention of viability is exceedingly rare in the absence of oncogenic agents. The obverse—that cells which retain normal karyotype are also limited in division potential—is not necessarily true, however: the special forms mentioned (rodent, etc.) can produce rapidly growing long-term cell lines in which the prevailing cell type is euploid. With the passage of time these eventually become heteroploid, but there seems no doubt that euploid cells of selected species can divide for substantially longer than expected on the basis of the diploid limit for human cells.

The behavior of cultured normal epithelial cells is of particular importance for the *in vitro* study of carcinoma, since it is only occasionally that permanent human carcinoma cell lines can be established, using present day methodology. Moreover, all such lines are heteroploid and therefore should be considered "transformed," since carcinoma *in vivo* is basically euploid. The question, therefore, arises whether carcinoma cells *in vivo* have unlimited growth potential, as is usually assumed to be the case. Biologically and kinetically there is no need for such an assumption, since a limited number of cell divisions in an expanding population of logarithmically dividing cells is quite sufficient for very large amounts of tumor tissue. The difficulty in establishment of human carcinoma cell lines could therefore be the result of a requirement for a secondary transformation occurring as a random spontaneous event at very low frequency.

Finally, division potential in renewing epithelia (in which differentiating cells are a product of cell division) is potentially instructive in understanding the biology of the carcinoma cell. There is evidence that some stem cell populations (notably intestinal and stratified squamous epithelia) may be in continuous rapid division throughout the lifetime of the organism, requiring a very high limit on division potential, and perhaps no limit at all. This possibility is subject to study in human material, and might yield very instructive results.

A justifiable conclusion is that care should be taken to avoid ascribing to neoplastic cells as a whole properties that are not clearly biological necessities. In particular it may be improper and highly misleading to assume that they are "transformed" in the usually understood *in vitro* sense: neoplastic cells may be karyotypically normal and sharply limited in division potential, as well as being normal in many other key biological parameters. It is possible that technical refinements in culture approaches will permit examination of these factors in epithelial and in carcinoma cells.

References

Aderca, I., and Iftimovici, M. (1971). *Rev. Roum. Inframicrobiol.* 8, 123–128.
Basrur, P. K., and Gilman, J. P. (1963). *J. Nat. Cancer Inst.* 30, 163–201.
Bassin, R. H., Plata, E. J., Gerwin, B. I., Mattern, C. F., Haapala, D. K., and Chu, E. W. (1972). *Proc. Soc. Exp. Biol. Med.* 141, 673–680.
Bertalanffy, F. D., and Nagy, K. P. (1961). *Acta Anat.* 45, 362–370.
Burnet, F. M. (1960). *Perspect. Biol. Med.* 3, 447–458.
Burnet, F. M. (1970). *Lancet* ii, 358–360.
Cahn, R. D., and Cahn, M. B. (1966). *Proc. Nat. Acad. Sci. U. S.* 55, 106–114.
Castor, C. W., and Naylor, B. (1969). *Lab. Invest.* 20, 437–443.
Chopra, D. P., and Flaxman, B. A. (1974). *Cell Tissue Kinet.* 7, 69–76.
Cole, J. W., and McKalen, A. (1961). *Gastroenterology* 41, 122–125.
Cole, J. W., and McKalen, A. (1963). *Cancer* 16, 998–1002.
Comfort, A. (1964). "Ageing: The Biology of Senescence." Routledge & Kegan Paul, London.
Coon, H. G. (1968). *J. Cell Biol.* 39, 29a.
Coon, H. G., and Weiss, M. C. (1969). *Wistar Inst. Symp. Monogr.* 9, 83–96.
Daniel, C. W., deOme, K. B., Young, J. T., Blair, P. B., and Faulkin, L. J., Jr. (1968). *Proc. Nat. Acad. Sci. U. S.* 61, 53–60.
Douglas, W. H. J., and Kaighn, M. E. (1975). *In Vitro* (in press).
Flaxman, B. A., and Chopra, D. P. (1972). *J. Invest. Dermatol.* 59, 102–105.
Flaxman, B. A., Lutzner, M. A., and Van Scott, E. J. (1967). *J. Invest. Dermatol.* 49, 322–332.
Gartler, S. M. (1967). *Nat. Cancer Inst., Monogr.* 26, 167–181.
Gartler, S. M. (1968). *Nature (London)* 217, 750–751.
Gazzolo, L., and Prunieras, M. (1969). *Pathol. Biol.* 17, 251–259.
Giard, D. J., Aaronson, S. A., Todaro, G. J., Arnstein, P., Kersey, J. H., Dosik, H., and Parks, W. P. (1973). *J. Nat. Cancer Inst.* 51, 1417–1424.
Goldstein, S. (1969). *Lancet* i, 424.

Goldstein, S. (1975). *Exp. Cell Res.* (in press).
Good, P. I. (1972). *Cell Tissue Kinet.* **5**, 319–323.
Haff, R. F., and Swim, H. E. (1956). *Proc. Soc. Exp. Biol. Med.* **93**, 200–204.
Harris, M. (1957). *Growth* **21**, 149–166.
Hay, R. J., and Strehler, B. (1967). *Exp. Gerontol.* **2**, 123–135.
Hayflick, L. (1965). *Exp. Cell Res.* **37**, 614–636.
Hayflick, L. (1970). *Exp. Gerontol.* **5**, 291–303.
Hayflick, L. (1972). *In* "Aging and Development" (H. Bredt and J. W. Rohen, eds.), Vol. 4, pp. 1–15. Schattauer, Stuttgart.
Hayflick, L. (1974). *J. Amer. Geriat. Soc.* **22**, 1–12.
Hayflick, L., and Moorhead, P. S. (1961). *Exp. Cell Res.* **25**, 585–621.
Hegazy, M. A. H., and Fowler, J. F. (1973). *Cell Tissue Kinet.* **6**, 17–33.
Jacquemont, C., and Prunieras, M. (1969). *Pathol. Biol.* **17**, 243–249.
Jones, H. W., McKusick, V. A., Harper, P. S., and Wuu, K.-D. (1971). *Obstet. Gynecol.* **38**, 945–949.
Kaighn, M. E., and Prince, A. M. (1971). *Proc. Nat. Acad. Sci. U. S.* **68**, 2396–2400.
Kay, H. E. M. (1965). *Lancet* ii, 418–419.
Kersey, J. H., Yunis, E. J., Todaro, G. J., and Aaronson, S. A. (1973). *Proc. Soc. Exp. Biol. Med.* **143**, 453–456.
Kovacs, L., and Potten, C. S. (1973). *Cell Tissue Kinet.* **6**, 125–134.
Krohn, P. L. (1962). *Proc. Roy. Soc., Ser. B* **157**, 128–147.
Krooth, R. M., Shaw, M., and Campbell, B. (1964). *J. Nat. Cancer Inst.* **32**, 1031–1044.
Lagerholm, B. (1966). *Acta Dermato-Venereol.* **46**, 231–236.
Leblond, C. P. (1964). *Nat. Cancer Inst. Monogr.* **14**, 119–150.
Leblond, C. P., Greulich, R., and Marques-Pereira, J. P. (1964). *Advan. Biol. Skin* **5**, 39–67.
Leibovitz, A. (1973). *J. Nat. Cancer Inst.* **51**, 691–697.
Lewis, L. J., Hoak, J. C., Maca, R. D., and Fry, G. L. (173). *Science* **181**, 453–454.
Lim, R., and Mitsunobu, K. (1974). *Science* **185**, 63–66.
Lycette, R. R., and Whyte, S. (1973). *Res. Vet. Sci.* **14**, 121–122.
Macek, M., Seidel, E. H., Lewis, R. T., Brunschwig, J. P., Wimberly, I., and Benyesh-Melnick, M. (1971). *Cancer Res.* **31**, 308–321.
MacPherson, I. (1963). *J. Nat. Cancer Inst.* **30**. 795–816.
Mannagh, J., Arya, D. V., and Irvine, A. R., Jr. (1973). *Invest. Ophthalmol.* **12**, 52–64.
Marques-Pereira, J. P., and Leblond, C. P. (1965). *Amer. J. Anat.* **117**, 73–74.
Martin, G. M., Sprague, C. A., and Epstein, E. J. (1970). *Lab. Invest.* **23**, 86–92.
Messier, B. (1960). *Amer. J. Dig. Dis.* **5**, 833–835.
Messier, B., and Leblond, C. P. (1960). *Amer. J. Anat.* **106**, 247–285.
Moore, G. E., and McLimans, W. F. (1968). *J. Theor. Biol.* **20**, 217–226.
Moore, G. E., and Sandberg, A. (1964). *Cancer (Philadelphia)* **17**, 170–175.
Moore, G. E., Gerner, R. E., and Franklin, H. A. (1967). *J. Amer. Med. Ass.* **199**, 510–524.
Moorhead, P. S. (1965). *Exp. Cell Res.* **39**, 190–196.
Nadler, N. J. (1965). *Amer. J. Anat.* **117**, 87–88.
Parker, R. C. (1961). "Methods of Tissue Culture." Hoeber, New York.
Paul, J. (1958). *Nature (London)* **182**, 808.
Penneys, N. S., Fulton, J. E., Weinstein, G. D., and Frost, P. (1970). *Arch. Dermatol.* **101**, 323–327.
Peturssen, G., Coughlin, J. I., and Meylon, C. (1964). *Exp. Cell Res.* **33**, 60–67.
Ponten, J., and Macintyre, E. H. (1968). *Acta Pathol. Microbiol. Scand.* **74**, 465–486.

Potten, C. S. (1974). *Cell Tissue Kinet*, **7**, 77–88.
Potten, C. S., Kovacs, L., and Hamilton, E. (1974). *Cell Tissue Kinet.* **7**, 271–284.
Prunieras, M., Delescluse, C., and Regnier, M. (1969). *Pathol. Biol.* **17**, 235–241.
Puck, T. T., Cieciura, S. J., and A. Robinson. (1959). *J. Exp. Med.* **108**, 945–955.
Rafferty, K. A., Jr. (1969). *In* "Biology of Amphibian Tumors" (M. Mizell, ed.), pp. 52–81. Springer-Verlag, Berlin and New York.
Rafferty, K. A., Jr. (1973). *Differentiation* **1**, 363–372.
Richart, R. M. (1963). *Amer. J. Obstet. Gynecol.* **86**, 925–930.
Shiratori, O., Osato, T., Utsumi, K. R., and Ito, Y. (1968). *Proc. Soc. Exp. Biol. Med.* **128**, 12–18.
Siminovitch, L., Till, J. E., and McCulloch, E. A. (1964). *J. Cell. Comp. Physiol.* **64**, 23–32.
Spooner, B. S. (1970). *J. Cell Physiol.* **75**, 33–47.
Steel, C. M., and Edwards, E. (1971). *J. Nat. Cancer Inst.* **47**, 1193–1201.
Swim, H. E., and Parker, R. F. (1957). *Amer. J. Hyg.* **66**, 235–243.
Sykes, J. A., Whitescarver, J., Jernstrom, P., Nolan, J. F., and Byatt, P. (1970). *J. Nat. Cancer Inst.* **45**, 107–122.
Todaro, G. J., and Green, H. (1963). *J. Cell Biol.* **17**, 299–314.
Valenti, C., and Friedman, E. A. (1968). *Texas Rep. Biol. Med.* **26**, 363–380.
van Venroij, W. A., Groeneved, A. A., and Bloemendal, H. (1974). *Int. Soc. Eye Res.* (*Abstr.*) (in press).
Wallace, R. E., Vasington, P. J., Petricciani, J. C., Hopps, H. E., Lorenz, D. E., and Kadanka, Z. (1973). *In Vitro* **8**, 333–341.
Williamson, A. R., and Askonas, B. A. (1972). *Nature* (*London*) **238**, 337–339.
Yerganian, G., and Leonard, N. J. (1961). *Science* **133**, 1600–1601.

SELECTION OF BIOCHEMICALLY VARIANT, IN SOME CASES MUTANT, MAMMALIAN CELLS IN CULTURE*

G. B. Clements†

Department of Tumor Biology, Karolinska Institute, Stockholm, Sweden

I. Introduction	274
II. Selection and Characterization of Variant Cells	282
A. Selection	282
B. Characterization	286
III. Drug-Resistant Variants	289
A. Purine Base Analogs	289
B. Purine Nucleoside Analogs	314
C. Thymidine and Its Analogs	318
D. Deoxycytidine Analogs	331
E. Uracil and Uridine Analogs	334
F. Folic Acid Analogs	335
G. Puromycin	343
H. Actinomycin D	346
I. Carbohydrate Analogs	348
J. Steroids	349
K. Miscellaneous Compounds	350
IV. Variants with Altered Expression of Antigenic Surface Components or Immunoglobulin Production	358
V. Variants with Altered Nutritional Requirements	364
A. Auxotrophs	364
B. Variants That Can Utilize a Wider Range of Metabolites Than Can Wild-Type Cells	368
C. Variants with Reduced Requirements	369
VI. Temperature-Sensitive Conditionally Lethal Cells	370
VII. Variants Resistant to Physical Agents	376
VIII. Spontaneous Variants	379
IX. Conclusions	379
References	380

* This review was written during the tenure of a British Medical Research Council Travelling Fellowship and subsequently a Fellowship in Cancer Immunology, Cancer Research Institute, Inc. and incorporates work published up to the end of 1973.

† Present address: Pathology Department, Western Infirmary, Glasgow G11 6NT, Scotland.

I. Introduction

Brockman (1963) and Hutchinson (1963) incorporated information on biochemical variants of mammalian cells in culture as part of more general reviews for this publication. Since then the field has developed very rapidly and is having a major impact on diverse areas of biology and medicine. The multiplicity of applications has resulted in a scattered, and at times incomplete, literature relating to the actual production and characterization of the variants. This review will pay particular attention to the conditions of selection, and document as far as possible the resulting phenotypic modifications permitting the survival and growth of the variant cells. It cannot encompass the production of cell variants during passage in animals, selection of chromosomal segregants from hybrid somatic cells, the establishment of cells in culture from individuals known to have biochemical genetic defects or the modification of cell behavior by viruses. Although highly relevant, it is not possible to discuss in detail the biochemical properties of drugs used to select drug-resistant variant cells. Biochemical variation in cultured cells has been reviewed previously, notably by Klein (1963), Davidson (1964), Harris (1964), Gartler and Pious (1966), Chu (1970, 1971), Ruddle (1972), and Thompson and Baker (1973). These sources have been of invaluable assistance in gathering the information for this review.

Puck and Fischer (1965) showed by cloning that within a population of HeLa cells there were spontaneous variants with different growth requirements. Hsu (1961), Klein (1963), and Harris (1964) emphasized the importance of considering cultured cells as populations of individuals capable of exhibiting subtle differences, and considered evolution in the cell populations relevant to the problems of cell differentiation and carcinogenesis. Populations of bacteria growing in a fully defined medium may exhibit continual alterations leading to the replacement of the original strain by ones having successively superior abilities to survive. Termed orthoselection or periodic selection, it has been suggested that the phenomenon must also apply to mammalian cells in culture (Ryan, 1962; Harris, 1964). Mammalian cells are not routinely grown in fully defined media, but require the addition of serum or fractions of serum, which imposes a degree of uncontrollable variation during the passage of established cell lines. Although orthoselection has not been detected by a systematic examination of a cultured mammalian cell line over many generations of continuous passage, it is well established that spontaneous alterations in cell behavior and karyotype may take place under standard growth conditions. Deliberate selective pressure may be applied to cultured cells only against the background of this variation.

The control of expression of their genetic information by mammalian cells is at present an area for speculation. Both novel mechanisms (for example, Littlefield, 1970) and those similar to those of prokaryotic organisms (for example, Ohno, 1972) have been proposed. It may be impossible to distinguish mutations, which are changes in the base sequence of DNA and therefore in the informational content, from stable alterations to epigenetic systems. Epigenetic systems may be considered as selecting the information to be expressed from that potentially available to the cell.

Mutation of a structural gene might be expected to exhibit the following traits: (1) occurrence at a low frequency, with the mutant phenotype usually remaining stable in the absence of selection; (2) increase in the rate of appearance of the variant phenotype, and also in some cases the rate of reversion, after exposure to mutagens; (3) association of the phenotypic change with the production of an altered gene product (the changes that may take place are discussed in more detail later); (4) lastly, the altered phenotype should behave in a Mendelian fashion, being capable of assignment to a specific region in the genome by linkage studies with other known genetic loci.

Mutation in a regulatory gene might be expected to exhibit similar characteristics, except that the structure of the product of the associated structural gene(s) would be unmodified; the gene product being either absent or produced in abnormal quantities. Epigenetic events, if stable, might be indistinguishable on these criteria from mutation in a control process. To leave the distinction between the above possibilities open, the term "variant" will be used to describe cells surviving a selective procedure. In a few cases there is very strong evidence on the above criteria that the phenotypic change is the result of a mutation in a structural gene.

The details of the conditions used for selection are important in determining the properties of the variant cell produced. Some variants have been isolated using a single-step procedure by one exposure to a rigorous set of selective conditions. In other cases cells have been exposed to increasingly stringent conditions during multiple selective procedures, each raising the level of resistance. A single-step selective procedure is most likely to isolate variants whose resistance is caused by one change. A multi-step selective procedure on the other hand, will favor the production of variants by successive changes for resistance, each enhancing resistance.

The following general approaches have been used to derive variant cells in culture: (1) selection for drug-resistant variants; (2) selection for an altered expression of surface antigens; (3) selection for altered nutritional requirements; (4) selection for temperature-sensitive conditionally lethal cells; (5) selection for resistance to physical agents; (6) isolation of spontaneous variants without selection; either by cloning or by a chance overgrowth of the wild-type population.

1. *Selection of Drug-Resistant Variants*

One or more of the following adaptations may lead to the production of drug-resistant variants (adapted from Hutchinson, 1963): (a) decreased conversion of the inhibitor to an active form. (b) increased degradation of the inhibitor to an inactive compound; (c) increased synthesis (or decreased degradation) of an inhibited enzyme; (d) modification of an inhibited enzyme; (e) decreased permeability to the inhibitor; (f) the activation of alternative pathways to bypass the metabolic block; (g) increased synthesis of a normal metabolite to compete out the inhibitor; (h) decreased requirement for the product of an inhibited enzyme.

The particular mode of adaptation taken will be influenced both by the drug and the cells.* For example 6-thioguanine (TG), an analog of the purine base hypoxanthine, is itself nontoxic, but is metabolized to compounds capable of exerting inhibitory effects; a phenomenon which has been termed lethal synthesis (Peters, 1951). TG is converted to its active metabolite 6-thioguanylic acid (TGMP) by the enzyme hypoxanthine/guanine phosphoribosyltransferase (HGPRT, EC 2.4.2.8). TGMP has been quoted as inhibiting three en-

---

* Abbreviations: AA, 8-azaadenine; AAR, 8-azaadenosine; AG, 8-azaguanine; AGR, 8-azaguanosine; AK, adenine kinase; APRT, adenine phosphoribosyltransferase; APRT⁻, APRT-deficient cells; AZH, 8-azahypoxanthine; 6-aza-UR, 6-azauridine; BUdR, 5-bromo-2′-deoxyuridine; But2cAMP, $N^6,O^{2'}$-dibutyryl adenosine 3′:5′-cyclic monophosphate; C′, complement; CAR, cytosine arabinoside; CDP, cytidine 5′-diphosphate; dCDP, deoxycytidine 5′-diphosphate; dCK, deoxycytidine kinase; CMP, cytidine 5′-monophosphate; dCMP, deoxycytidine 5′-monophosphate; Con A, concanavalin A; DAP, 2:6-diaminopurine; DDUG, 4:4′-diacetyl-diphenyl-urea-bisguanylhydrazone; 2DG, 2-deoxyglucose; 2DG6P, 2-deoxyglucose 6-phosphate; DNA, deoxyribonucleic acid; EMS, ethyl methane sulfonate; FA, 2-fluoroadenine; FAR, 2-fluoroadenosine; FU, 5-fluorouracil; FUR, 5-fluorouridine; FUdR, 5-fluoro-2′-deoxyuridine; HAT, Selective medium containing hypoxanthine, thymidine, and aminopterin; HGPRT, hypoxanthine/guanine phosphoribosyltransferase; HGPRT⁻, HGPRT-deficient cell; IUdR, 5-iodo-2′-deoxyuridine; K_m, Michaelis constant; MeMPR, 6-methylthiopurine ribonucleoside; MNNG, N-methyl-N′-nitro-N-nitrosoguanidine; MP, 6-mercaptopurine; RNA, ribonucleic acid; TdR, thymidine; TG, 6-thioguanine; TGR, 6-thioguanosine; TGMP, 6-thioguanylic acid; TK, thymidine kinase; TK⁻, TK-deficient cell; ts, temperature sensitive, TTP, thymidine triphosphate; Tub, tubercidin; UMP, uridine monophosphate; dUMP, deoxyuridine monophosphate.

zymes (Roy-Burman, 1970), phosphoribosylpyrophosphate amidotransferase which catalyzes the first step in the *de novo* pathway of purine synthesis, inosine monophosphate dehydrogenase, and a nucleotide monophosphokinase specific for the phosphorylation of guanosine 5'-monophosphate of guanosine 5'-diphosphate. TGMP may be phosphorylated and utilized for RNA and for DNA synthesis since small quantities of TG residues have been detected in the nucleic acid of cells grown in the presence of TG (LePage, 1963). The TG residues may increase the chance of mismatching and therefore lead to misreading of the nucleic acid. Lethal synthesis of TGMP may be prevented by a single modification at either of two steps in the metabolism of TG. The passage of TG through the cell membrane may be blocked, or alternatively synthesis of TGMP may be decreased by reducing the activity of HGPRT. Adaptation to avoid the effects of TGMP entails overcoming its several separate effects simultaneously. Since it is more probable that single rather than multiple modifications would occur, variants resistant to TG would be expected to prevent synthesis of TGMP. This is the case, HGPRT activity being absent in variant cells resistant to TG.

Aminopterin and amethopterin, both folic acid analogs, inhibit folic acid reductase (dihydrofolate reductase, 5,6,7,8-tetrahydrofolate:$NADP^+$ oxidoreductase, EC 1.5.1.3) preventing synthesis of reduced folic acid. No lethal synthesis is required in this case, the folic acid analog itself being the inhibitor. Hakala *et al.* (1961) reported that the folic acid reductase activity of two amethopterin-resistant variants was increased in proportion to their degree of resistance. The properties of the enzymes in the variant cells were unchanged with respect to kinetic characteristics, molecular weight, electrophoretic mobility, and rate of reaction. The authors suggested that the increase in folic acid reductase could bind the intracellular amethopterin owing to the high affinity of this enzyme for the drug. Since amethopterin can only enter cells slowly, they considered that there was always enough newly synthesized free folic acid reductase remaining to maintain adequate levels of reduced folic acid.

In the two examples quoted, opposite adaptations are found in the variant cells leading to drug resistance. Loss of HGPRT activity leading to TG resistance and increased activity of folic acid reductase leading to amethopterin resistance. Other alterations may also lead to the development of resistance to these or similar analogs and will be described in detail later. At the present time it is important to consider variants as unique, even those derived from the same population selected for the same traits, since similar phenotypic modifications may result from different causations.

In the presence of inhibitory concentrations of a folic acid analog, cells are rendered auxotrophic for both thymidine (TdR), a purine source (usually hypoxanthine is supplied) and also glycine. If the medium is supplemented with these compounds, and the cells can utilize them, the lethal effects of the folic acid analog are overcome (Hakala, 1957; Hakala and Taylor, 1959). Cell variants lacking HGPRT activity fail to grow in the presence of supplemented medium since they are unable to utilize hypoxanthine (Lieberman and Ove, 1960). Szybalski et al. (1962) used this selective system, which they termed HAT medium, both to estimate the rate at which revertants having HGPRT activity (and consequently the ability to grow in HAT) appeared from an HGPRT$^-$ variant and also to eliminate preexisting HGPRT$^-$ cells from the wild-type population before measuring the rate of appearance of 8-azahypoxanthine (AZH)-resistant variants. HAT will be used as a general term to describe selective media in which the inhibitory action of aminopterin (amethopterin) is reversed by hypoxanthine and TdR. The optimal concentrations of the components of HAT vary for different lines of cells.

Littlefield (1964a) utilized HAT for the selection of hybrid cells from parental cells, one of which was deficient in HGPRT and the other in thymidine kinase (TK, EC 2.7.1.75). For different reasons neither parent grew in HAT, those being HGPRT$^-$ not incorporating hypoxanthine and those being TK-deficient (TK$^-$) not incorporating TdR. Some of the cell hybrids formed after fusion between the different types of parental variants grew out in HAT to form lines of hybrid cells. The separate biochemical defects of the parental cells complemented each other in these hybrids.

2. Selection of Variants with Altered Expression of Antigenic Surface Components or Immunoglobins

Oda and Puck (1961) demonstrated specific killing of established cell lines of human and Chinese hamster cells by exposure in the presence of complement (C′) to an antiserum raised against intact washed cells. Isoantigenic expression can be detected in established cell lines (Cann and Herzenberg, 1963a), and selection may be directed against particular isoantigens. Cann and Herzenberg (1963b) showed that cells carrying an isoantigen may be killed when exposed in the presence of C′ to antibody made against the antigen. Death of susceptible cells, which bind the antigen, occurs by C′-mediated lysis. Coffino et al. (1970) using immunoglobulin-producing cells established a methodology for detecting and isolating variants which had lost the ability to produce some or all immunoglobulin moieties.

3. *Selection of Variants with Altered Nutritional Requirements*

This group of variants may be subdivided into the following classes with either: (a) additional requirements; (b) substitution of a different metabolite for the one normally used; (c) reduced requirements.

a. Additional Requirements. Variants having additional requirements to those of the parental cells are termed auxotrophs. Several systems have been developed for the isolation of auxotrophic mammalian cells. The general approach is to place wild-type cells in a medium lacking the metabolite for which auxotrophy is desired; auxotrophic cells are unable to grow under these conditions while wild-type cells continue to divide. The culture is then exposed to conditions that kill cells which are passing around the cell cycle (cycling cells). Auxotrophs survive and can be isolated by first removing the lethal agent and then adding back the metabolite for which auxotrophy is desired. DeMars and Hooper (1960) isolated HeLa cells auxotrophic for glutamine by killing cycling cells by prolonged exposure to aminopterin. Other systems that select against cycling cells are growth in tritiated thymidine or treatment with 5-bromo-2'-deoxyuridine (BUdR) followed by exposure to light; these are subsequently discussed in detail.

b. Substitution. In a few cases variants have been selected for the capacity to utilize a metabolite not normally used by substituting it for the normal metabolite. Much of the early work involved carbohydrate metabolism and it has been criticized by Bradley (1962). More recently, for clinical reasons, interest has centered on obtaining variants not requiring asparagine.

c. Reduced Requirements. The elimination of a nutritional requirement, though formally different from class b, is difficult to distinguish from it in biochemical terms. The nutritional requirements for the culture of mammalian cells have been extensively investigated, notably by Eagle. Although some lines of cells may require enriched media, a minimum of 28 defined factors are required for the sustained growth of cells *in vitro* (Eagle, 1959). The growth rate of the cells is critically dependent on the concentration of these factors (Cohen and Eagle, 1961). The cell density influences the nutritional requirements, since at low densities essential metabolites and metabolic intermediates may be lost to the medium at rates beyond the synthetic capacity of the cell and the intracellular concentration fall below the level needed to maintain growth. After conditioning of the medium and at high cell densities, these metabolites are present at concentrations sufficient to maintain effective levels within the cells; such growth requirements are population-density dependent and have been reviewed by Eagle (1965). It is not generally feasible to establish a selective system to obtain cell variants with reduced nutritional requirements against this background of variation. Population density-dependent cell behavior has other important implications for the isolation of biochemically variant cells and will be discussed in detail in Section II.

4. *The Isolation of Temperature-Sensitive Conditionally Lethal Cells*

The configuration or stability of a polypeptide chain may be critically temperature dependent. The structural alterations consequent upon a missense mutation may modify the polypeptide chain in such a way that it functions normally at one temperature (the permissive temperature) but abnormally at a second temperature (the nonpermissive temperature). If the behavior of a polypeptide chain is severely altered at the nonpermissive temperature and the normal function is essential for viability, the temperature-sensitive (*ts*) phenotype will be conditionally lethal and the variant cells will survive and grow only at the permissive temperature. Alterations in the structure of nucleic acids have also been reported to lead to a *ts* phenotype (Smith *et al.*, 1970).

Temperature sensitivity is the only general conditional lethal phenotype available at present in mammalian cells. Its use provides flexibility not available to other selective systems. Since stocks of cells can be produced under permissive conditions and studied under nonpermissive conditions, proteins carrying out essential functions can be investigated. Initial selection of *ts* cells does not require prior knowledge of the nature of the function selected for. Cells growing under permissive conditions supply a good control for experiments carried out on the same cells under nonpermissive conditions.

5. *Selection for Resistance to Physical Agents*

Variant cells have been selected with increased resistance to transient exposure to elevated temperature (Harris, 1969). The nature of the modifications leading to this change are unknown.

Much work has been carried out in the course of investigating the acute response of cells to irradiation and cannot be covered in this review. Cell variants have been selected for increased resistance to ultraviolet (Uv), beta (β), gamma (γ), and X-irradiation. One possible mode of adaptation used by such variants is to increase the efficiency of DNA repair. Initially described by Elkind and Sutton (1960), the split-dose effect is one manifestation of these repair mechanisms; cells survive a total dose of X-irradiation much better if it is fractionated than if given as a single exposure. The gap between doses allows time for the repair to be effected. The sensitivity of cells to irradiation varies with the phase of the cell cycle they are passing through, being lowest during S phase (Terasima and Tolmach, 1963; Sinclair and Morton, 1963, 1965). The variation is perhaps a reflection of differences in the efficiency of repair through the cycle, although other factors seem to be involved also (Sinclair, 1973).

Another aspect of the response of cells to ionizing radiation is a great increase in the proportion of cells forming abnormally small colonies (Puck, 1960; Elkind and Sutton, 1960; Sinclair, 1964; Todd, 1968). Such cells are slow growing, have a low oxygen consumption, and are radiosensitive; the alterations in behavior are heritable although the cells gradually revert to normal on prolonged growth.

6. *The Isolation of Variants without Selection*

A great number of well-documented examples exist of spontaneous changes occurring in populations of cells during passage in culture. In these cases, perhaps for reasons other than the observed change, the variant was at a selective advantage and overgrew the original wild-type cells. As already noted, even while growing under constant and favorable circumstances there will be spontaneous variation and continual shifts in the constitution of any culture when regarded as a population. In addition there are inevitably many factors that exert continuous, cyclic, or short-term influences both on the behavior of individual cells and the distribution of subpopulations of cells within the culture. For example, if cells are passaged as monolayers the cells in suspension being discarded at each passage, only those cells that attach to the glass remain in the population. It is often possible to convert a cell line from growing as a monolayer to a suspension culture simply by retaining and passaging only those cells free in the medium. Many parameters cannot be continuously rigorously controlled during the growth of cells in culture. In particular there is variation between batches of serum, and each batch will exert a unique selective effect on a cell population. Instances where variation due to the serum used has been observed during the use of selective systems will be noted.

No attempt will be made to review all the examples of spontaneous changes taking place during culture of cells, but several will be referred to during the course of the review since the spontaneous variants have been used as parental cells in selective procedures. Isolation of numerous clones may by chance yield a variant that was present in the wild-type population at a low frequency. Thompson *et al.* (1971) obtained variants *ts* for growth by this procedure. Replica-plating techniques have been developed (Goldsby and Zipster, 1969; Suzuki *et al.*, 1971) that allow large number of clones to be handled. This approach will prove most valuable, for it allows variants to be isolated without prior exposure to selective conditions. Therefore variants may be isolated in cases where (a) there is no selective system available for the phenotype desired; (b) the selective system itself influences the behavior of the cell in general ways or is mutagenic: for example, selection for resistance to BUdR.

II. Selection and Characterization of Variant Cells

There follows a comprehensive review of the systems that have been used for the selection of variant mammalian cells. For reasons of space, comment in particular cases will be reduced to a minimum. Each variant should be examined in the light of the possibilities listed in Section I, and information may be complemented by data available using other lines of cells selected in a similar manner. In several cases the yield of variants has been shown to be increased by mutagenesis, and from other sources there is additional evidence that many of the variants are the result of mutations. Epigenetic mechanisms will be found to be the underlying cause of other variants, indeed since many of the variants are the product of multistep selection procedures, some may be the result of both mutation and epigenetic changes.

The conditions of selection have in some cases been systematically examined and shown to influence both the yield and also the phenotypes of the variants obtained. A detailed description of the practical details of selection is to be found in a recent review (Thompson and Baker, 1973).

A. SELECTION

The definition of the selective system is crucial both when the yield of variants is being quantitated and also when a detailed study of the phenotypic changes permitting the survival of the variants under the selective conditions is being examined. The following parameters are of importance.

1. The Number of Steps Used

Some comments have already been made on this point in Section I. To obtain firm quantitation of the frequency with which variants are obtained, a single-step procedure is mandatory. The number of steps involved in any particular selection is in general pointed out in the text or a table, wherever applicable. Some systems permit single-step selections whereas other do not, either because selection pressure is relatively weak or because several independent changes are required for the development of resistance.

2. The Cell Density during Selection

The cell density during selection is one of the parameters that has not always been well controlled. As noted previously, Eagle has shown that during normal growth the behavior of cells may be density dependent for general reasons. These effects will be enhanced during the crisis imposed on a culture during a selective procedure in which only about 1×10^{-6} of the originally wild-type cells survive.

Some mammalian cells in culture are capable of interacting in a way that has been shown to be particularly relevant to the selection of variant cells. This is termed metabolic cooperation and was originally demonstrated using polyoma-transformed baby hamster kidney 21/C13 (BHK21/C13) cell variants (Subak-Sharpe *et al.*, 1966, 1969; Subak-Sharpe, 1969). Two different variant cell lines were used, PyY AA/AAR (resistant to both 8-azaadenine and 8-azaadenosine and unable to incorporate exogenously supplied adenine) and PyY TG/TGR (resistant to both 6-thioguanine and 6-thioguanosine and as a result HGPRT$^-$). In mixed culture, when in contact with a cell capable of incorporating the purine supplied in the medium, variant cells normally unable to incorporate that purine were shown by autoradiography to have had their biochemical defects corrected. Intimate contact is required, since variant cells in the same preparation not in contact with cells capable of incorporating the purine supplied retained their variant phenotype. On application of selective pressure for HGPRT$^-$ to a dense culture (for example, by exposure to TG), potentially variant cells would probably arise while in contact with a wild-type cell. By virtue of metabolic cooperation the phenotype of the potential variant would continue to be wild type and the cell would remain susceptible to the effects of the analog and be killed. The variants of PyY cells were originally selected from sparsely seeded cultures, and consequently metabolic cooperation did not affect the outcome. Fujimoto *et al.* (1971) and Clements (1972) showed by reconstruction experiments that metabolic cooperation prevents the recovery of variants from mixtures of cells grown at high densities under selective conditions. Not all cells are capable of participating in metabolic cooperation; for example, an HGPRT⁻ variant of mouse L cells, A9 (Littlefield, 1963), is unable to cooperate either with wild-type L cells or wild-type BHK cells (Pitts, 1971), and it is possible to select variants of L cells resistant to purine and pyrimidine analogs even if plated at high density.

Khalizev *et al.* (1966, 1969) noted that the yield of Chinese hamster cells resistant to purine analogs ceased to be proportional to the number of cells inoculated at high cell densities. Shapiro *et al.* (1972) investigated this "concentration effect" more closely. During selection for resistance to 6-mercaptopurine (MP), adherent Chinese hamster cells yielded a constant proportion of variants at densities up to 1.8×10^3 cells cm^{-2}. The yield was reduced rapidly on further increase in density during selection. A similar effect was observed during the selection of a glucose-independent variant, but at lower cell concentration. In addition to the effects of metabolic cooperation, Shapiro and co-workers proposed that two other factors, exhaustion of the medium and the accumulation of unidentified toxic substances originating from death of sensitive cells, contributed to the depressed yield of variants when selected at high cell densities. Shapiro *et al.* (1972) reported that diploid human fibroblasts behaved differently from Chinese hamster cells when selected for resistance to MP, yielding relatively few variants at low cell densities, owing probably to a reduction in the plating efficiency. At high density there was no toxic effect of MP on the culture. Survival of confluent human fibroblasts in MP may be related to the decrease in metabolism accompanying contact inhibition of growth with little incorporation of MP.

3. *The Concentration of the Analogs*

The concentration of the analog, or, in more general terms, the severity of the selective conditions, may influence both the yield and the phenotypes of the variants obtained. The degree of inhibition in any particular case will be expressed as the concentration of inhibitor producing a 50% reduction in growth of cells (ID_{50}) first applied to this particular problem by Harris (1961). The shape of the dose-response curves obtained varies, some being very flat with a large tail of highly resistant cells while others drop very steeply. The shape of a dose-response curve gives some indication of the heterogeneity within the population with respect to the response to the selective conditions and has been discussed in some detail by

Thompson and Baker (1973). In the face of this variability the ID_{50} is a good parameter to use for comparison between different curves. In many cases the ID_{50} has been extracted from published data and at times may be an approximation. As an internal reference to the degree of resistance of a particular variant the ID_{50} of the wild-type population is given when available. Various criteria have been used to determine the ID_{50} by different workers (for example, cloning efficiency, increase in cell number, increase in protein), and so, strictly speaking, they may not be comparable. It is of interest to compare ID_{50}s of identical systems obtained independently and gratifying to find good agreement in many cases. Even in closely matched cases there are factors, such as variability in purity of different batches of the inhibitor used, that cannot be controlled. To enable the inhibitory effects of different analogs to be compared all data have been converted to a molar basis.

4. *The Duration of Exposure of the Cells to Selective Conditions*

The duration of exposure to selective conditions may influence both the yield and phenotype of surviving variants. Cells may be retained within the selected population if they were in a refractory state during exposure to selective conditions. For example, BUdR can exert no selective pressure against a cell that fails to pass through S phase during the time of exposure to the drug. Survival of refractory cells will be encouraged under weakly selective conditions. The proportion of refractory cells in a culture will be influenced by the treatment the culture has received prior to selection. A culture in the logarithmic phase of growth will have a lower probability of containing cells refractory to BUdR than a stationary one. As already noted, confluent human fibroblasts were refractory when exposed to MP (Shapiro *et al.*, 1972). It is of importance to note that selection for auxotrophs and *ts* variants is designed to enrich also for refractory cells. Chu *et al.* (1972) thoroughly investigated a selective system for the production of auxotrophs with reference to the timing and duration of exposure to selective conditions.

Another factor that may be of importance in some situations is loss of variant cells due to the elimination of a conditioning effect by frequent changes of the medium during selection. Changing the medium would also eliminate any toxic products of dead cells, which would tend to operate in the opposite direction. Frequent changes of medium may also cause other changes; the inhibitor may be unstable, degraded, or competed out by metabolites released from the dead cells, effects that would be reduced or eliminated if the medium was changed during selection.

5. Mutagenesis

Early work on mutagenesis of mammalian cells in culture provided no evidence to indicate that exposure to known mutagens increased the frequency of drug-resistant variants (Szybalski et al., 1964). Later, however, simultaneous and independent studies showed that after brief exposure to alkylating agents the incidence of biochemically variant cells was increased (Chu and Malling, 1968a,b) and Kao and Puck (1968). There is now a voluminous literature concerned with the effects of known mutagens on cultured mammalian cells, and systems have been developed for testing potentially mutagenic compounds as a routine procedure. Discussion of this aspect of the field is beyond the scope of this review. However, data on nonmutagenized control cultures obtained during the course of these studies will be incorporated into the tables.

Some of the selective systems used to obtain variants are known to be mutagenic (Chu et al., 1972), but for many no data are yet available. Any selective system may be tested for mutagenicity using one of the now standard systems referred to above. Huberman and Heidelberger (1972) have shown that, while hydroxyurea and 5-fluoro-2'-deoxyuridine (FUdR) are not mutagenic to cultured Chinese hamster cells, cytosine arabinoside (CAR) and BUdR are mutagenic. This line of study may give important insights into the relative frequencies of mutations and epigenetic changes.

B. CHARACTERIZATION

It is only relatively recently that the study of the range of phenotypes expressed by variants obtained independently under a particular set of defined conditions has been pursued, the initial investigations in this direction having been carried out by Littlefield (1963, 1964b).

1. *The Rate of Appearance of Variants*

The rate of appearance of variants may be estimated using the fluctuation test (Luria and Delbrück, 1943), which also indicates whether they appear independently of, or as a result of, exposure to the selective conditions. A fluctuation test compares the variance (a measure of the variability between samples) of the number of cells resistant to the selective conditions present in two different groups of samples. Those of the first group are taken from a single culture. The second group comprises several populations each originating as clones (or small samples) of one culture, which also gave rise to the population from which the first group of samples was taken. The data obtained from a fluctuation test may be analyzed in several different ways (e.g., Shapiro et al., 1972) some of which involve making assumptions about the behavior of the variants. In several selective systems more than one type of phenotypic change has been shown to lead to the development of resistance. Consequently the observed rates of appearance of the variants will in these cases be the sum of the frequencies of several separate events. The frequency of a particular variant phenotype within a given culture at any particular time is only partially dependent on the rate of appearance of the variants. Also of influence are the time at which the variant appeared relative to the time of sampling, the sampling of the population during splitting, and the relative growth rates of variant and parental cells. Single estimates of the frequency of variants within a culture give no indication of the rate of appearance of the variants, being analogous to single samples in a fluctuation test. It is most important to distinguish between the rate of appearance and the frequency of variants within a population.

2. Biochemical Changes

The biochemical changes accompanying variant selection have been much studied. In many cases the alterations that have occurred in the behavior of cells surviving selective conditions are those that would have been expected. Two examples of alterations in enzyme activity associated with drug resistance have been quoted in Section I, and extensive tabulation follows in subsequent sections. In some cases, unexpected alterations have been noted and in many instances have yet to be explained. Their further investigation may shed light on unknown areas of cellular behavior in a few cases, but in many the explanation may be more mundane, though nonetheless of interest. Where loss of an enzyme activity in cell-free extracts is unaccompanied by loss of the activity in intact cells, the possibility of there being an unstable, but active, enzyme present must be considered. The conditions of the assay, though optimal for the wild-type activity, may require modification to allow demonstration of the variant activity. In particular, *ts* variants could be screened for by reducing the temperature of the assay system. The conditions of extraction may destroy activity of a very labile enzyme. Addition of substrate to the extraction buffer may allow recovery of activity since it is well established that in some cases enzymes are stabilized in the presence of substrate (e.g., Littlefield, 1965). The demonstration of altered specificity or a change in the kinetics of an enzyme activity in variant cells may not be the result of a mutation affecting the structural gene but may be due to the expression of an enzyme activity that is either not expressed or present only in small amounts in parental cells. For example, residual TK activity in a line of BUdR-resistant cells has a different electrophoretic mobility to that of parental cells (Kit and Minekawa, 1972). The residual activity is due to a mitochondrial TK that is present in wild-type cells but masked by a vast excess of cytoplasmic TK activity which is not present in the variant cells.

3. *Chromosomal Changes*

The investigation of chromosomal changes during selection of biochemically variant cells has yielded little consistent information until recently owing both to the use of aneuploid cell lines and the insensitivity of methods for karyotypic analysis. Now that karyotypic analysis has improved so much in sensitivity and variants can be derived from diploid material (Albertini and DeMars, 1970), this approach may bear fruit. Rappaport and DeMars (1973) noted consistent changes in the karyotypes of several human fibroblast variants selected for resistance to 2:6-diaminopurine (DAP). Karyotypic analysis may prove useful in the discrimination between different classes of variants although it must be emphasized that the finest detectable changes probably involve hundreds of loci. One serious disadvantage of using diploid human fibroblasts as parental cells for selection is that they have a very low cloning efficiency and a limited life-span.

4. *Cross-Resistance and Collateral Sensitivity*

Investigation of cross resistance and collateral sensitivity of variant cells are complementary to biochemical characterization. Such studies are extensive and have not been covered systematically in this review, being mentioned only in cases where the information obtained affords insights into the mechanism of resistance not obtained by other means. Studies on cross-resistance and collateral sensitivity in cultured cells link with those using both clinical material and experimental tumors passaged in animals.

5. *Fusion Studies on Variants*

The production of somatic cell hybrids almost at will has permitted the investigation of many aspects of cell behavior, one or both of the parental cells used for hybridization usually being biochemically marked. The rationale of the selective system most commonly used, HAT, has been described in the preceding section. A drawback to the use of hybrid cells is the abnormal dosage effects which may be introduced in near-tetraploid cells hindering interpretation of the results. Although it should strictly be reserved for diploid situations, the term complementation has been used to describe the correction of biochemical defects of variant cells after hybridization. Complementation has in some cases been observed between independently isolated variant cells of the same phenotype indicating genetic nonidentity of the lesions causing the biochemical defect. It has been shown in many cases that fusion of an HGPRT$^-$ variant with a TK$^-$ variant yields hybrids capable of growth in HAT, both defects being complemented. To rigorously prove the existence of noncomplementing combinations, it is necessary to isolate hybrids without the use of HAT and show them to be TK$^-$ and/or HGPRT$^-$, requiring the use of an independent selection system and thus, in most parental combinations, multiply marked cells. The inability of a particular combination of parental cells to complement may be due to trivial reasons or reasons other than the noncomplementation of the TK and HGPRT markers. The same is true for every marker and selective system analyzed using somatic cell hybrids, the markers being investigated should ideally not themselves be used to select the hybrids. Chasin (1973) has used multiply marked cells in the analysis of HGPRT$^-$ variants by cell fusion.

6. Reversion of Variants

The investigation of the reversion characteristics of variants is an area that will provide much information about their etiology, particularly the reversion rate, the effect of mutagens and biochemical characterization of the revertants. This information is covered in detail in subsequent sections. Some variant phenotypes, for example TK$^-$, HGPRT$^-$, and auxotrophs, can be selected against and permit easy quantitation of reversion rates and selection of revertants. The ability to select revertants is an important factor in the choice of a system to use for the investigation of biochemically variant cells.

III. Drug-Resistant Variants

A. Purine Base Analogs

1. 8-Azaguanine (AG)

The biochemistry of purine analogs has recently been reviewed by Brockman (1969) and Roy-Burman (1970). Several analogs of hypoxanthine have been used to select biochemically variant cells and all are considered to behave in an essentially similar manner, requiring a lethal synthetic step to be rendered toxic as described for TG in Section I. To date the choice of analog has been largely empirical. It will be noted that there are many reports of 8-azaguanine(AG)-resistant cells that retain HGPRT activity while no report exists of a TG-resistant cell retaining HGPRT activity. However, few comparisons have been carried out using both AG and TG in the same system. Subak-Sharpe (1965) found AG to be relatively innocuous for polyoma-transformed BHK cells whereas TG was toxic and could be used to select variants. Recently Gillin et al. (1972) using Chinese hamster cells, and Sharp et al. (1973) using L cells have investigated this matter in some detail.

a. Mouse (Table I). Lieberman and Ove (1959a) selected AG-resistant variants from a cloned line of L cells (Sanford et al., 1948). Variants were derived by exposure of logarithmic phase cells seeded as a monolayer in 6.6×10^{-6} M AG. After the death of about 95% of the cells, the selective medium was replaced by fresh normal medium and the culture was allowed to grow to confluence. Cycles of selection and growth were repeated until a culture of cells was obtained whose growth was no longer affected by 6.6×10^{-6} M AG (Table I). There was no detectable loss of resistance after growth of the variant for more than 50 generations in the absence of AG. Lieberman and Ove (1960) found the variant cross-resistant to MP, and cell extracts lacked HGPRT activity. The variant was unable to grow in HAT but could grow in the presence of aminopterin if the purine source was adenine instead of hypoxanthine.

Littlefield (1963, 1964a,b) selected variants of L cells resistant to 2.0×10^{-6} M, 6.6×10^{-6} M, and 1.3×10^{-5} M AG. In the case of cultures containing more than 10^4 cells, it was found necessary to refeed with AG-containing medium on the second day and subsequently at 2–3 day intervals. Without feeding, extensive growth took place, perhaps because of incorporation or catabolism of AG or release of competing purines by dead cells. At 10–20 days after the initiation of selection, colonies could be picked and propagated independently. Whenever tested, resistance persisted after removal of AG, one clone, AG3, having been grown for over two years in the absence of AG without losing resistance. AG3 was one of a group of variants, also including A9, that were selected for resistance to 1.3×10^{-5} M AG, cell extracts of which lacked detectable HGPRT activity. Mass selection was also carried out in suspension culture using three levels of AG, 6.6×10^{-8} M, 6.6×10^{-7} M, and 6.6×10^{-6} M. Assays of HGPRT activity in cell free extracts of the variants showed three distinct groups having levels of activity correlating with the degree of AG resistance, having, respectively, 67%, 35%, and 1% or less of wild-type activity (Littlefield, 1964b). Two of the partially resistant lines were recloned and retained their partial enzyme deficiency, eliminating the possibility that they might be composed of mixtures of cells with high and low activity. There was no evidence for the presence of an activator or an inhibitor of HGPRT in cell extracts. In two variants of intermediate HGPRT activity the heat inactivation curve and in one case the Michaelis constant (K_m) of the HGPRT were not significantly different from the wild-type enzyme, indicating that a reduction of the quantity of wild-type enzyme present might be the basis of the reduction in HGPRT activity. Reversion of the variant phenotype was studied by growing the cells in HAT medium (Littlefield, 1964a). Variants of intermediate levels of resistance grew as well as wild-type cells under these conditions. Of three variants containing virtually no HGPRT activity, one variant, AG3, had a reversion rate of less than 5×10^{-6}, but two others were found to have reversion rates of 10^{-2} and 3×10^{-3}, respectively. These revertants contained intermediate levels of HGPRT both prior to and after cloning. One variant, A9 has been widely used and has a very low spontaneous reversion rate. Scaletta et al. (1967) reported one revertant, and Klein et al. (1971) selected what was almost certainly a revertant of A9 having 60% HGPRT activity of wild-type cells and a marker chromosome characteristic of A9.

Watson et al. (1972) detected an HGPRT activity electrophoretically identical to that of L cells in four out of five hybrids between A9 cells with either human lymphocytes or human fibroblast or lymphoblast cell lines. McBride and Ozer (1973) obtained two revertants with HGPRT activity having the same electrophoretic mobility as that derived from wild-type L cells after plating 1.4×10^9 cells in HAT. After treating A9 cells with DNA obtained either from A9, L (wild type) or HeLa cells, Shin et al. (1973) obtained clones that grew in HAT and contained HGPRT activity having the same heat stability and electrophoretic mobility as that from wild-type L cells. The frequency with which such clones appeared was variable, but in one series of experiments an overall frequency of 1.8×10^{-8} was obtained. Analogous results have been obtained after fusion of other HGPRT$^-$ cell lines that have low or undetectable reversion rates. Bakay et al. (1973) showed that after fusion of IR cells (HGPRT$^-$ L cells, qv) with chick embryo fibroblasts, HGPRT activity with the same mobility as the mouse enzyme was present in the hybrid cells. Croce et al. (1973a) fused FU5AH cells (HGPRT$^-$ rat cells, qv) with

TABLE I
Mouse Cells Selected for Resistance to 8-Azaguanine (AG)

Cell type and reference	Selection level (M)	Frequency of variants	ID_{50} (M)	Reversion rate
L cells				
Lieberman and Ove (1959a)	Wild type	—	6.6×10^{-7}–2.2×10^{-6}	—
	6.6×10^{-6}	—	6.6×10^{-5}–2.2×10^{-4}	—
Littlefield (1963, 1964a,b)	Wild type	—	$<2.0 \times 10^{-7}$–6.6×10^{-7}	—
	2.0×10^{-6}	—	—	Grow in HAT
	6.6×10^{-6}	—	—	$3 \times 10^{-3}, 10^{-3}$
	1.3×10^{-5}	5×10^{-7}	2.6×10^{-5}–6.6×10^{-5}	$5 \times 10^{-6}, >10^{-9}$
Morrow (1964, 1970)	Wild type	—	1.2×10^{-7}	—
	1.3×10^{-6}	—	2×10^{-6}	—
	2.0×10^{-5}	1.5–$5.7 \times 10^{-6\,a}$	3×10^{-5}	$>10^{-7}$
Ignatova et al. (1968a)	2.0×10^{-4}	—	—	—
Adomaitiene et al. (1970)	6.0×10^{-4}	2.6×10^{-4}	—	—
Adomaitiene (1971)	6×10^{-4}	$6.9 \times 10^{-6\,b}$	—	—
Miggiano et al. (1969)	1×10^{-4}	—	—	$>5 \times 10^{-7}$
Shows (1970, 1971, 1972)	1st step 3.3×10^{-5}	—	—	—
	2nd step 1.3×10^{-4}	—	—	—
LMTK$^-$				
Murayama-Okabayashi et al. (1971)	6.6×10^{-5}	—	—	—
Spurna and Nebola (1971)	Wild type	—	3.3×10^{-5}	—
	1.2×10^{-4}	—	—	4.6×10^{-5} (uncloned)
	3.3×10^{-4}	—	4.5×10^{-5}	8.7×10^{-7} (uncloned)
Sharp et al. (1973)	2.0×10^{-5}	10^{-6}	—	Variable

P388 (Dawe and Potter, 1957)				
Roosa et al. (1961)	Wild type	—	2×10^{-7}–5×10^{-7}	
	1×10^{-6}	—	2×10^{-6}	
Roosa et al. (1962)	2×10^{-5}	—	5×10^{-6}–1×10^{-5}	
	1×10^{-4}	—	2×10^{-3}–5×10^{-3}	
L120				
Bach (1969)	Wild type	—	2.1×10^{-7}	
	1.3×10^{-6}	—	1.5×10^{-5}	
NCTC-2472-6				
Scaletta et al. (1967)	2.0×10^{-6}	—	—	0.5–1.0×10^{-5}
RPC-5				
Mohit and Fan (1971)	1×10^{-4}	—	—	—
BALB/cd renal adenocarcinoma				
Klebe et al. (1970)	1st step 3.3×10^{-5}	—	—	Not detected, rare
	2nd step 1.3×10^{-4}	—	—	—
FM3A mammary carcinoma C3H (Nakano, 1966)				
Koyama et al. (1970)	2×10^{-4}	—	—	Not detected, rare
Diploid fibroblasts				
Van Zeeland et al. (1972)	Wild type	—	$<3.3 \times 10^{-6}$	—
	1.1×10^{-6}	—	Up to 2×10^{-4}	—

[a] Rate of appearance of variants determined by a fluctuation test, expressed per cell per generation.
[b] Pretreated by growth in selective medium containing hypoxanthine, thymidine, and aminopterin (HAT) in an attempt to remove preexisting variants.

human fibroblasts. Of 15 clones whose HGPRT activity was examined by electrophoresis eight expressed human enzyme only, one expressed both human and rat, and the remaining six expressed only the rat enzyme. Various explanations have been proffered for these results, the most simple being that the variant cells fail to express HGPRT by virtue of either alteration to or deletion of regulatory genes, retaining the structural gene for HGPRT intact. On fusion the defect is made good, regulatory genes of the second genome reactivating the expression of HGPRT by structural genes originating from the variant cell.

Morrow (1964, 1970) selected AG-resistant variants of a line M-MC which was of L-cell origin. Two levels of resistance were obtained, an intermediate level by selection in up to 1.3×10^{-6} M. AG, and a higher level after selection in AG at concentrations above this. Variants of intermediate resistance had HGPRT activities 30–50% that of wild-type cells while highly resistant variants had only about 1% of wild-type HGPRT activity. The latter could be grown in the absence of inhibitor for a year without losing resistance. Variants of intermediate resistance regained sensitivity to AG after growth for about 1 month in drug-free medium, the HGPRT activity returning in some cases to or near to wild-type levels. Revertants of the highly resistant clones were selected by plating cells in HAT, the reversion rate being less than 10^{-7} per cell per generation. Revertants regained wild-type HGPRT levels.

Spurna and Nebola (1971) selected variants of L cells resistant to several concentrations of AG up to 3.3×10^{-4} M. At 1 day after plating, fresh medium containing the desired level of inhibitor was added. Three times a week fresh medium containing AG was added. After 3–5 weeks, surviving colonies were trypsinized and passaged in medium containing AG at the same or in some cases a higher concentration. Eventually several clones were isolated from either 1.3×10^{-4} or 3.3×10^{-4} M AG. Selection in HAT yielded revertants at low frequency from the variants prior to cloning, but no revertants were obtained from cloned stocks.

In a recent investigation, Sharp et al. (1973) after mutagenesis with N-methyl-N'-nitro-N-nitrosoguanidine (MNNG) selected variants of L cells resistant to AG and also to a combination of AG and TG. Variants selected for resistance to AG were heterogeneous with respect to the ability to incorporate exogenously supplied hypoxanthine into intact cells. Some variants had no reduction in incorporation when compared to the wild type but about half, all independently isolated, had their incorporation of hypoxanthine reduced to less than 10% of wild-type cells. The majority of these variants, despite the presence of HGPRT, were unable to grow in HAT. Some variants that contained high levels of HGPRT were capable of growth both in HAT and AG. A series of variants isolated by selection simultaneously in 2.0×10^{-5} M AG and 3.0×10^{-5} M. TG were all unable to incorporate exogenously supplied hypoxanthine into intact cells and also lacked HGPRT activity in crude extracts. The variants were reexposed to MNNG and selected for reversion by growth in HAT. Many of the first set of variants, selected for resistance only to AG, had high spontaneous reversion frequencies, in one case as high as 10^{-2}. The MNNG-induced reversion frequencies ranged from 3×10^{-5} to 10^{-3}; the reversion rate of many of the frequently reverting variants was not increased after MNNG treatment. Those variants capable of growth in HAT were excluded from this part of the study. The frequency of MNNG-induced reversion in the second group, selected for resistance to both AG and TG ranged from 10^{-8} to 10^{-5} with a mode at 10^{-7}. Revertants of the second group had from 15 to 60% wild-type HGPRT activity. The thermal inactivation of the HGPRT derived from six independently selected revertants of a common parent was compared. Two were similar to the wild type, one was slightly more heat sensitive, and three were very sensitive. Heterogeneity in the behavior of different revertants from a single parental variant is most simply explained by their being due to different amino acid substitutions in a defective HGPRT leading to complete or partial restoration of function. The HGPRT activity in crude extracts of variants selected for resistance to AG and capable of growing both in AG or HAT was examined. One variant produced HGPRT that was markedly less inhibited by AG (but not by TG) than that of wild-type cells. The K_m of HGPRT derived from the variant was reduced by a factor of three compared to wild-type enzyme. The altered characteristics suggest that the HGPRT of this variant has an amino acid sequence different to the wild-type enzyme resulting from a mutation in the HGPRT structural gene.

Roosa et al. (1961, 1962) selected AG-resistant variants from a cloned line of P 388 murine lymphatic leukemia cells. For selection of variants a confluent sheet of cells was exposed to an inhibitory concentration of AG, the resistant survivors growing up to form colonies in the presence of the inhibitor. Independent selections were carried out using 10^{-6} M and 2×10^{-5} M AG. The latter variant was subsequently selected for resistance to 10^{-4} M AG. The variants resistant to 2×10^{-5} M and 10^{-4} M AG showed no loss of resistance after prolonged growth in the absence of the analog. After an extended period of growth in the absence of AG, the cloning efficiency of the second-step variant at 10^{-3} M AG was reduced, but not at 10^{-4} M. Roosa et al. (1961), Davidson et al. (1962), and Brockman et al. (1962) showed that at all three levels of resistance to AG there was essentially complete loss of HGPRT activity.

b. *Chinese Hamster* (Table II). Chu and Malling (1968a,b) and Chu et al. (1969b) selected variants from clone V79-4 of a line V79-122D1, derived from Chinese hamster lung, with a stable near-diploid karyotype (Ford and Yerganian, 1958). A resistant variant (225-1) was initially obtained by culturing wild-type cells in increasing concentrations of AG over 25 days. Cells selected for resistance to 6.6×10^{-5} M AG were found to be resistant to levels up to 6.6×10^{-3} M. The line 225-1 was found to have 23 chromosomes, the same as the parental line, but there was less variation in the karyotype, which indicated the probable origin from a single cell. No HGPRT activity was detectable in extracts of this variant. In later experiments a single-step procedure was used, selecting in 6.6×10^{-5} M AG and picking surviving clones after 2 weeks' growth. The frequency of appearance of AG-resistant variants was variable, and increased with time after the removal of pre-existing variants by passage in HAT. There was little difference in the rate of appearance of definitive colonies from wild-type cells over concentrations of AG ranging from 3.3×10^{-5} M to 2×10^{-4} M (Chu and Malling, 1968b). The rate of appearance of AG resistant variants was determined to be 1.5×10^{-8} per cell per generation both for parental cells and for reselection from a drug-sensitive revertant. By growth of the 225-1 variant in HAT, the rate of reversion was determined to be 2 to 5×10^{-7} per cell per generation. Of eight revertants isolated, only one (256-8) regained wild-type sensitivity to AG and was capable of utilizing exogenously supplied hypoxanthine when grown in normal medium. Two variants were capable of incorporating hypoxanthine into intact cells only if the *de novo* synthetic pathway was blocked with aminopterin. HGPRT assays were carried out on cell-free extracts of the revertants. One lacked detectable activity, six had reduced but significant activities due perhaps to a low level of normal HGPRT or alternatively to the production of a defective enzyme. The eighth, 256-8, had an approximately 8-fold increase in HGPRT activity over the wild-type though incorporation of exogenously supplied hypoxanthine by intact cells took place at the same rate in both revertant and wild type. The reversion rate was increased after exposure to mutagens (Chu et al., 1969a; Chu, 1970); however, some spontaneously occurring variants never gave rise to revertants. A hybrid was isolated between an AG-resistant variant and a glutamine auxotroph of V79 (qv). The hybrid was sensitive to AG and prototrophic for glutamine, both characters behaving in a recessive manner.

Gillin et al. (1972) isolated and characterized 35 independent AG-resistant variants also selected from a subclone of V79 cells. Near-confluent monolayers were mutagenized with either MNNG or ethyl methane sulfonate (EMS) and selected for resistance to 2×10^{-4} M AG. Resistant colonies were recloned after picking, one clone only being picked from each plate to ensure independence. The variants were investigated with respect to their abilities to grow in HAT, TG, or AG. Seventeen grew in both TG and AG, but not in HAT, and failed to incorporate exogenously supplied hypoxanthine into intact cells. Cell-free extracts of these clones contained no detectable HGPRT activity. Twelve clones grew under all three selective conditions, but only nine of these both had significant HGPRT activity when assayed in crude extracts and also incorporated exogenously supplied hypoxanthine into intact cells. Of the three clones lacking HGPRT activity in extracts, two incorporated hypoxanthine into intact cells, but the third had neither activity *in vitro* nor in intact cells. The six remaining clones grew in HAT and AG but not in TG, and all incorporated hypoxanthine in varying amounts into intact cells. Two of these clones had very low levels of HGPRT activity in crude extracts.

A group of clones, among which were some having less than 1% wild-type HGPRT activity and others with near wild-type activity, were capable of incorporating hypoxanthine into intact cells only in the presence of aminopterin. The HGPRT activity of cell-free extracts remained unchanged after growth in aminopterin.

AG-resistant clones not capable of growing in HAT were studied for spontaneous reversion and reversion induced by NMMG; frequencies of reversion ranged from 10^{-7} to 10^{-4}. The HGPRT activities of cell-free extracts of the revertants ranged from supra-wild type to very low levels. Some clones failed to give rise to revertants, indicating the possibility that their lesion might be due to a deletion. Immunologically detectable HGPRT was present (CRM+) in extracts of three clones having no HGPRT activity in crude extracts (Beaudet et al., 1973). These findings are most simply explained by there being a mutation in the structural gene for HGPRT at a site that destroys enzyme activity, but does not affect the recognition of the now defective enzyme by the antibody. Although the antibody was not monospecific for HGPRT, the assay was carried out in such a way

TABLE II
CHINESE HAMSTER CELLS SELECTED FOR RESISTANCE TO 8-AZAGUANINE

Cell type and reference	Selection level (M)	Frequency of variants	ID_{50} (M)	Reversion rate
V79-122D1				
Chu and Malling (1968a,b)	Wild type	—	$\simeq 6.6 \times 10^{-6}$	—
	3.3×10^{-5}	4×10^{-4}	—	—
	6.6×10^{-5}	4.5×10^{-4}	—	—
	2×10^{-4}	5.2×10^{-4}	—	—
Chu et al. (1969b)	6.6×10^{-5}	1.5×10^{-8a}	6.6×10^{-3}	$2.5 \times 10^{-7}, 5.5 \times 10^{-7}$, not detected
Gillin et al. (1972)	2×10^{-4}	—	—	10^{-4}–10^{-7}
Harris (1971a,b)	6×10^{-5}	—	—	—
	Diploid, 2×10^{-4}	2.2×10^{-5a}	—	—
	Tetraploid, 2×10^{-4}	4.7×10^{-5a}	—	—
	Octaploid, 2×10^{-4}	1.3×10^{-5a}	—	—
V79-4				
Bridges and Huckle (1970)	5×10^{-5}	1.9–3.8×10^{-4}	—	—
Bridges et al. (1970)	1×10^{-4}	2.4×10^{-5}	—	—
	2×10^{-4}	1.4×10^{-5}–1.1×10^{-6}	—	—
Huberman et al. (1971)	Wild type	—	8×10^{-6}	—
	1.3×10^{-4}	1×10^{-5}	$\simeq 5.3 \times 10^{-4}$	$<10^{-6}, 3 \times 10^{-6}$
Kelly-Garvert and Legator (1973)	2×10^{-4}	1×10^{-5}	—	—

Cell line / Reference				
Don, Chinese hamster fibroblast				
Westerveld et al. (1971)	Multistep, 2×10^{-4}	—	$>2.6 \times 10^{-3}$	Not detected
DC-3F/ADX (qv ACD)				
Berebbi and Barski (1971)	2.6×10^{-4}	—	—	Not detected
CHO/pro⁻ (qv auxotrophs)				
Morrow et al. (1973)	Wild type	—	2.0×10^{-5}	—
	2×10^{-4}	7.7×10^{-6}	4.2×10^{-5} to 3.6×10^{-4}	—
BIId(ii)-FAF28				
Shapiro et al. (1968, 1972)	2.0×10^{-4}	$4 \times 10^{-6\,a}$	—	—
	4.0×10^{-4}	—	—	—
Lung fibroblasts				
Sekiguchi and Sekiguchi (1973)	Multistep, 1.3×10^{-4}	—	—	—
CHW				
(Lin et al., 1971)	2×10^{-4}	—	—	—
Hamerton et al. (1973)				

[a] Rate of appearance of variants estimated by a fluctuation test, expressed per cell per generation.

that the other specificities present did not affect it. The anti-HGPRT antiserum inhibited Chinese hamster HGPRT specifically, and the assay was carried out by estimating the degree of blocking of this inhibitory activity after mixing with extract of the variant cell. Two of the CRM+ variants failed to incorporate hypoxanthine into whole cells and yielded revertants with detectable HGPRT activity. The third clone incorporated hypoxanthine into intact cells but had no HGPRT activity in crude extracts. The structure of HGPRT produced by this variant may have undergone a change due to a structural gene mutation rendering it highly unstable so that it was inactivated during extraction or assay.

Harris (1971b) found the frequency of appearance of AG-resistant variants of V79-122D1 cells, as determined by a fluctuation test, to be similar (about 2×10^{-5} per cell per generation) in diploid, tetraploid, and octaploid cells. Polyploidy was introduced by treatment with Colcemid (Harris, 1971a) and was confirmed by chromosome counts but not by detailed karyotypic analysis. The HGPRT activity, growth characteristics in selective media, and reversion of the variants were not examined.

Morrow *et al.* (1973) using a proline-requiring line of Chinese hamster ovary cells, CHO/pro$^-$ (Kao and Puck, 1967) selected clones resistant to AG in a single-step procedure. Without being picked, they were subjected to a second selective step by pouring off the AG-containing medium and substituting HAT medium. Of 217 AG-resistant clones, 36 were also HAT resistant, the phenotype of the latter clones was stable during subsequent growth either in nonselective medium or AG. Variants resistant to both HAT and AG arose at a frequency of 1.28×10^{-6}. The HGPRT activities of extracts of six doubly resistant variants ranged from 50% to nearly 300% of the wild-type level while the resistance to AG ranged from a 2-fold to a 20-fold increase above that of the wild-type cells. One variant examined that was AG resistant but not HAT resistant had no detectable HGPRT activity.

c. Human (Table III). Szybalski (1959), Szybalski and Smith (1959), Szybalski *et al.* (1962), and Szybalski and Szybalska (1962) selected AG-resistant variants from a clone of D98 cells (Table III), a line now considered to be derived from HeLa (Gey *et al.*, 1952) on the basis of isozyme pattern (Gartler, 1967) and karyotype (Matsuya and Green, 1969; Miller *et al.*, 1971). Less than 1% of wild-type cells grew to form clones at concentrations of AG above 6.6×10^{-6} M. The exact frequency varied between sublines. One variant, D98/AG, was stably resistant to AG, subculturing for over

150 generations either in the presence of 4×10^{-5} M AG or without the analog failed to alter the level of resistance. The HGPRT activity of extracts of D98/AG was unchanged when compared to that of extracts from wild-type cells (Szybalski et al., 1961), and the variant grew normally in HAT. After growth of D98 in HAT for 2 weeks before exposure to AG, the frequency of isolation of variants resistant to 4×10^{-5} M AG was reduced from 4.9×10^{-4} to 2×10^{-4}, possibly because of the elimination of some preexisting AG-resistant variants. A mutation rate of 3×10^{-4} per cell per generation was calculated from this figure, a value in agreement with that obtained by a fluctuation test. No increase in frequency of variants resistant to 4×10^{-5} M AG was found after exposure of D98 cells to a wide range of mutagens (Szybalski et al., 1964).

Albertini and DeMars (1970) isolated diploid AG-resistant variants from male human fibroblasts seeded at low densities after exposure to 220 r of X-rays (the 40% survival dose). Two lines were isolated; one, 199 AG^{r-1}, having a low HGPRT activity and being highly resistant to AG, while the second, 52 AG^{r-1}, was much less resistant with 50% of the HGPRT activity of wild-type cells and the ability to grow in HAT. Resistance persisted after many generations of growth in normal medium. DeMars and Held (1972) extended these studies and found two classes of variants; a minority (1 of 10) had a low HGPRT activity and an inability to utilize exogenously supplied hypoxanthine and grew in high levels of AG. The remaining nine variants investigated had HGPRT activities ranging from normal to undetectable and lower levels of resistance to AG, but all could grow in HAT. Albertini and DeMars (1973) investigated the effectiveness of the selective system in recovering AG-resistant variants. Reconstruction experiments indicated that at cell densities above 3.5×10^3 cells cm^{-2} the recovery of variants was dramatically reduced, perhaps due to metabolic cooperation. It is of interest to note that the figure for the critical cell density at which recovery of variants became poor is in close agreement with that obtained by Shapiro et al. (1972) (qv Section II). Variants isolated after X-irradiation were investigated with respect to the following parameters: growth in AG, the ability to utilize exogenously supplied hypoxanthine, and HGPRT activity. The HGPRT activity of independently isolated variants—some spontaneous, others after X-irradiation—ranged from negligible to supra-wild type.

Van Zeeland et al. (1972) selected AG-resistant variants of an aneuploid strain of fibroblasts derived from embryonic skin and muscle. A sparse culture of wild-type cells was exposed to 6.6×10^{-5} M

TABLE III
HUMAN, PIG, SYRIAN HAMSTER, AND RAT CELLS SELECTED FOR RESISTANCE TO 8-AZAGUANINE

Cell type and reference	Selection level (M)	Frequency of variants	ID_{50} (M)	Reversion rate
Human				
D98 (*HeLa*)				
Szybalski (1959)	Wild type	—	1.8×10^{-6}	—
Szybalski and Smith (1959)	6.6×10^{-6}–6.6×10^{-5}	1×10^{-2}–1×10^{-4}	—	—
	4.0×10^{-5} D98AG	—	$> 6.6 \times 10^{-5}$	Grow in HAT
	1.2×10^{-5}	1.0×10^{-4a}	—	—
	2.6×10^{-5}	$\leq 5.0 \times 10^{-4}$	—	—
	4.0×10^{-5}	$\leq 4.9 \times 10^{-4}$	—	—
	5.2×10^{-5}	$\leq 5.0 \times 10^{-4}$	—	—
Pekhov et al. (1970)	Wild type	—	3×10^{-7}	—
	2.6×10^{-5}	—	—	—
Diploid fibroblasts				
Albertini and DeMars (1970)	Wild type	—	$\leq 3 \times 10^{-7}$	—
	2×10^{-5} 199AG^r-1	—	$> 1 \times 10^{-4}$	None detected
	2×10^{-5} 52AG^r-1	—	2×10^{-6}	Grow in HAT
DeMars and Held (1972)	8×10^{-6}	4×10^{-7}–1×10^{-5}	2×10^{-5} to 1×10^{-4}	None detected
Shapiro et al. (1972)	4×10^{-4}	4.5×10^{-7a}	—	—
Aneuploid fibroblasts from WI38		6.6×10^{-5}–1.5×10^{-4a}		
Shapiro et al. (1972)	4×10^{-4}	6.6–9.1×10^{-5a}	—	—
Van Zeeland et al. (1972)	Wild type	—	6.6×10^{-6}	—
	6.6×10^{-5}	Up to 1.6×10^{-3}	—	—
WI18-VA2 cl.VA2-B				
(Pontén et al., 1963)				
Weiss et al. (1968);				
Attardi and Attardi (1972a)	2.0×10^{-6}	—	—	—

Cell line / Reference			Months after isolation ID$_{50}$ (M)		
			1	2	3
Raji (Pulvertaft, 1964; Nyormoi et al. (1973))	Multistep, 3.3 × 10^{-4}	—			1.3 × 10^{-6}
Pig					
PK15 (Harris and Ruddle (1960))	Wild type 6.6 × 10^{-4}	1.3 × 10^{-5}	—	3.3 × 10^{-5}	—
				>6.6 × 10^{-4}	—
Clone					
1			—	>6.6 × 10^{-4}	>6.6 × 10^{-4}
2			—	>6.6 × 10^{-4}	>6.6 × 10^{-4}
3			—	>6.6 × 10^{-4}	>6.6 × 10^{-4}
4			6.6 × 10^{-4}	—	>6.6 × 10^{-4}
6			>6.6 × 10^{-4}	2.3 × 10^{-4}	1.2 × 10^{-4}
7			—	>6.6 × 10^{-4}	>6.6 × 10^{-4}
9			6.6 × 10^{-4}	2.7 × 10^{-4}	1.6 × 10^{-4}
Syrian hamster					
RPM1-3460 Davidson et al. (1966, 1968)	2.6 × 10^{-5}	—			1 × 10^{-4} (1 clone)
Fu5 (Pitot et al. 1964); Croce et al. (1973a,b); Obtained from M. Siniscalco	1 × 10^{-5}	—			None detected

^{a} Rate of appearance of variants estimated by a fluctuation test, expressed per cell per generation.

AG in the presence of a feeder layer of AG-resistant mouse cells. No variants were obtained in the absence of a feeder layer.

d. Pig (Table III). Harris and Ruddle (1960) selected variants from a clone of pig kidney cells, PK15, either by exposing a population of cells to 6.6×10^{-4} M AG in a single-step procedure, or by cyclic treatment with the drug, surviving cells being allowed to grow up in normal medium between the selective steps. Sublines of the variant were then derived by cloning from single cells in the presence of 6.6×10^{-4} M AG. The clones varied in their behavior and may represent the progeny of two variants that arose independently. Two (6 and 9) (Table III) were of uniform morphology and grew rapidly. The remainder grew more slowly and were morphologically heterogeneous. The two rapidly growing clones retained a high level of resistance during growth for 1 month in nonselective medium after isolation, however the ID_{50} declined progressively over the next 2 months. The other clones all retained a high level of resistance to AG during growth in normal medium for 3 months.

e. Syrian Hamster (Table III). Davidson et al. (1966, 1968) selected an AG-resistant variant of the Syrian hamster melanoma RPMI-3460 (Moore, 1964). Davidson (1972) reported a variant of RPMI-3460 also resistant to AG, but with about double the number of chromosomes of the parental cell line, having 91 chromosomes.

2. *6-Thioguanine (TG)* (Table IV)

a. Mouse. Long et al. (1973) selected variants of 3T6 (Todaro and Green, 1963) resistant to TG. One clone was isolated which had no detectable HGPRT activity, and did not grow in HAT. The modal chromosome number soon after isolation was 49, but it doubled during passage. This variant was shown to excrete more hypoxanthine and xanthine into the medium than did wild-type cells (Chan et al., 1973).

b. Chinese Hamster. Chasin (1973) compared the frequency with which TG-resistant variants appeared from a CHO-K1 gly A^- auxotroph (qv) obtained after mutagenesis (Kao et al., 1969a) and a "tetraploid" clone obtained after exposure to Colcemid. After mutagenesis with EMS, TG-resistant variants appeared from the tetraploid cells 25 times less frequently than from the subdiploid CHO-K1 gly A^- cells. Some TG-resistant variants derived from the "tetraploid" clone had a reduction of up to five in their modal chromosome number. All the TG-resistant variants derived from both parents lacked detectable HGPRT activity in cell-free extracts. No difference was found in the reversion rate to prototrophy for glycine between the subdiploid and "tetraploid" lines.

Sekiguchi and Sekiguchi (1973) selected variants resistant to TG from Chinese hamster cells previously selected for resistance to 1.3×10^{-4} M AG (qv). Four clones which did not grow in HAT were chosen and fused in pairs in all combinations. Of the six possible combinations, only three yielded colonies capable of growth in HAT; such colonies appeared at very high frequencies in these cases. One variant was a common partner in all three of these HAT-resistant hybrids. The HGPRT activities in cell-free extracts of the three unique partners, relative to the HGPRT activity of similar extracts from wild-type cells, were 2.3%, 1.6%, and 1.2% while that of the common partner was 0.19%. The HGPRT activity of the hybrids ranged from 24% to 34% relative to that of wild-type cells. It is possible that the four variants fell into two complementation groups, three variants belonging to a single group while the fourth fell into a separate group.

c. *Human.* Sato et al. (1972) selected TG-resistant variants from a diploid clone of the established lymphoblast line PGLC-33H derived from a female patient with infectious mononucleosis. The line had been cloned in agarose in the presence of a feeder layer of human fibroblasts twice. For the selection of variants, cells were plated in agarose-containing medium in the presence of 3 to 5×10^{-5} M TG. The feeder layer used for selection consisted of fibroblasts derived from a patient with the Lesch-Nyhan syndrome, and therefore was resistant to the effects of TG. Resistant clones grew up and could be picked 3–4 weeks after plating. Reconstruction experiments indicated that there was a depressed recovery of variants when selection was applied to cultures at densities greater than 1×10^5 cells per milliliter. All variants were found to have 1% or less of the HGPRT activity present in wild-type cells. TG-resistant variants were also obtained from another human lymphoblastoid cell line, MG-57, at low frequency.

d. *Syrian Hamster.* Subak-Sharpe (1965, 1969) selected TG-resistant variants of polyoma-transformed BHK21/C13 cells (Stoker and Macpherson, 1964), PyY, and a variant of PyY previously selected for resistance to both AA and AAR (qv). Variants were selected by exposure to TG at low cell densities. Intact variant cells were neither unable to incorporate significant quantities of hypoxanthine, nor were they capable of growth in HAT. TG resistance was accompanied by the loss of HGPRT activity in cell-free extracts (Subak-Sharpe et al., 1969).

Marin and Littlefield (1968) selected variants of BHK21/C13 cells by exposing wild-type cells seeded at low densities to 6.6×10^{-7} M. TG. After 2 weeks colonies appeared and a pooled cell-free extract of

TABLE IV
CELLS SELECTED FOR 6-THIOGUANINE (TG) RESISTANCE

Cell type and reference	Selection level (M)	Frequency of variants	ID_{50} (M)	Reversion rate
Mouse				
Neuroblastoma C-1300				
Minna et al. (1971)	1st step, 1×10^{-6}	2×10^{-5}	—	—
	2nd step, 5×10^{-5}	4×10^{-6}	—	—
	3rd step, 1×10^{-4}	—	—	$1-5 \times 10^{-7}$
L cells				
Morrow (1972)	4.9×10^{-6}	—	—	—
Sharp et al. (1973)	3.0×10^{-5} (AG 2×10^{-5})	10^{-8}	—	—
T1M1C57BL/6 radiation leukemia virus-induced tumor				
Hyman (1973)	1×10^{-5}	—	—	—
3T6				
Long et al. (1973)	Wild type	—	$<5 \times 10^{-8}$	—
	Multistep selection	—	$>3.5 \times 10^{-5}$	$<10^{-7}$
Chinese hamster				
Fibroblasts				
Pontecorvo (1971) (from Westerfield)	2×10^{-5}	—	—	—
Sekiguchi and Sekiguchi (1973)	Multistep 2×10^{-4}	—	—	$<2 \times 10^{-7}$

Cell line / Reference	Type				
CHO-K1 Gly A⁻					
Chasin (1972, 1973)	Wild type	—	2×10^{-7}	—	
	5×10^{-5}	9×10^{-7}	5×10^{-5}	$<2 \times 10^{-7}$	
	(DAP resistant) 5×10^{-5}	—	2×10^{-6}	—	
Human					
PGLC-33H					
Sato et al. (1972)	Wild type	—	$<2.5 \times 10^{-6}$	—	
	2.5×10^{-6}	4×10^{-2}	—	—	
	5×10^{-6}	2×10^{-4}	—	$<5 \times 10^{-7}$	
Syrian hamster					
PyY BHK21/C13					
Subak-Sharpe (1965, 1969)	Single step	5×10^{-7}	—	—	
BHK21/13					
Marin and Littlefield (1968)	Wild type	—	2×10^{-7}	—	
	1st step, 6.6×10^{-7}	2.5×10^{-4}	—	—	
	2nd step, 4.2×10^{-5}	5×10^{-5}	$>1 \times 10^{-4}$	6×10^{-6}	
Rat					
c6 Wistar glioma					
Gilman and Minna (1973)	1st step, 6.6×10^{-6}	—	—	—	
	2nd step, 6.6×10^{-4}	—	—	—	

these first-step resistant variants had a reduced HGPRT activity compared to that of wild-type cells. In a second selective step, these partially resistant variants were exposed to 4.2×10^{-5} M TG. Colonies were isolated after 2 weeks, and cell-free extracts of cultures derived from them had no detectable HGPRT activity. One subline, which contained the lowest proportion of revertants (6×10^{-6}), was one hundredfold more resistant to TG after cloning than wild-type cells.

3. 6-Mercaptopurine (MP) (Table V)

a. Mouse. Tomizawa and Aronow (1960) obtained variants of L cells resistant to MP. Selection was accomplished by continuous exposure of wild-type cells to 10^{-6} M MP for 8 weeks. Then additional

TABLE V
CELLS SELECTED FOR 6-MERCAPTOPURINE (MP) RESISTANCE

Cell type and reference	Selection level (M)	Frequency of variants	ID_{50} (M)	Reversion rate
Mouse				
L cells				
Tomizawa and Aronow	Wild-type	—	1×10^{-6}	—
(1960)	Multistep 10^{-3}	—	1×10^{-3}	—
Chinese hamster				
BIId(ii)-FafJ28				
Shapiro et al. (1972)	1×10^{-4}	$1.0-2.4 \times 10^{-5}$ [a]	—	—
Human				
H.Ep. No. 2				
Kelley et al. (1961)	Wild type	—	1×10^{-6}	—
Brockman et al. (1961)	3.3×10^{-6}	—	2.1×10^{-3}	—
	6.6×10^{-6}	—	—	—
	6.6×10^{-5}	—	2.1×10^{-3}	—
KB				
Higgins et al. (1969)	Wild type	—	6.6×10^{-7}	—
	Variant	—	6.6×10^{-6}	—
Rat				
HTC				
(Thompson et al., 1966)				
Levisohn and Thompson	1×10^{-4}	—	—	—
(1973)				

[a] Rate of appearance of variants determined by a fluctuation test, expressed per cell per generation.

selective steps in 10^{-5} M, 10^{-4} M, and 10^{-3} M MP were used sequentially, resistance to each level taking 20 or more weeks to achieve. The variant selected at 10^{-5} M MP retained resistance after growth for one hundred generations in the absence of the drug. Variants resistant to 10^{-4} M MP were unable to synthesize mercaptopurine ribotide from MP and unable to grow in HAT, suggesting a lack of HGPRT activity.

b. *Human.* Kelley et al. (1961) selected MP-resistant H.Ep. No. 2 cells (Moore et al., 1955). Clonal lines of wild-type cells were established and found to be completely inhibited at 3.3×10^{-6} M MP. Variant clones were isolated after growth in the presence of various concentrations of MP either in suspension or attached to a glass surface. Unlike wild-type cells after incubation of the variants resistant to 6.6×10^{-6} M and 6.6×10^{-5} M MP with either radioactive guanine, MP, or hypoxanthine there was no incorporation of labeled material into nucleic acid. Assay of HGPRT activity in extracts confirmed these observations; the clone isolated in 3.3×10^{-6} M MP had a very much reduced activity while the more highly resistant variants had no detectable activity (Brockman et al., 1961). The variant resistant to 6.6×10^{-5} M MP retained this lack of HGPRT activity after growth for 50 generations in the absence of the drug. Purine metabolism and cross-resistance of two of these variants were further studied (Bennett et al., 1965). The highly resistant variant excretes an increased quantity of hypoxanthine into the medium in comparison with wild-type cells (Chan et al., 1973).

4. *8-Azahypoxanthine (AZH)* (Table VI)

An AZH-resistant variant of D98/AG (qv) was selected at a single step for resistance to AZH (Sybalski et al., 1961, 1962). The plating efficiency of D98/AG was 0.1% in the presence of from 1.6×10^{-5} M to 3.6×10^{-3} M AZH. One clone was picked and gave rise to the variant D98/AH, which had lost detectable HGPRT activity and retained resistance after growth for more than one year in the absence of AZH. After growth of either wild-type D98S or D98/AG cells in HAT in an attempt to eliminate preexisting variants, the frequency of variants resistant to AZH was reduced to 0.3 to 1×10^{-6} (Szybalski et al., 1964). The D98/AH variant did not grow in HAT, but revertants, (D98/AHR) were present at a frequency of about 1×10^{-4} after passage of D98S/AH for 2 months in the absence of AZH. A revertant retained an intermediate level of resistance to AZH yet was capable of utilizing hypoxanthine as a purine source. Despite the efficient utilization of exogenously supplied hypoxanthine, the HGPRT activity of

TABLE VI
CELLS SELECTED FOR 8-AZAHYPOXANTHINE (AZH) RESISTANCE

Cell type and reference	Selection level (M)	Frequency of variants	ID_{50} (M)	Reversion rate
Human				
D985/AG (qv) (HeLa) Szybalski et al. (1961, 1962)	Wild type	–	1.4×10^{-6}	–
	D98/AG	–	5×10^{-4}	–
	D98/AH	$0.3–1 \times 10^{-6}$	$>7.3 \times 10^{-3}$	1×10^{-4} (mass)
	D98/AHR	–	1.4×10^{-5}	$<1 \times 10^{-5}$ (clones)
HeLa S3 Vaughan and Steele (1971)	Wild type	–	$<7.3 \times 10^{-7}$	–
	1.8×10^{-4}	–	$>1.8 \times 10^{-4}$	–

cell-free extracts of D98/AHR was only 5% of that of the D98/AG and D98 parental cells. A series of clones of D98S/AH yielded no revertants after plating 10^5 cells in HAT, indicating a low reversion rate despite the high frequency of revertants in the uncloned population. Fetal calf serum was found to contain 1.3×10^{-4} M hypoxanthine, which protected human fibroblasts but not HeLa cells against the toxic effects of AZH (Vaughan and Steele, 1971).

The remaining purine bases that have been used for the selection of variant cells are analogs of adenine. The bases are substrates of the enzyme adenine phosphoribosyltransferase (APRT, EC 2.4.2.7), by which they are converted to their respective nucleotide monophosphates.

5. 2:6-Diaminopurine (DAP) (Table VII)

a. Mouse. Lieberman and Ove (1960) selected L-cell variants resistant to DAP. Twelve days after plating in DAP, surviving cells were transferred to normal growth medium and cloned. After cloning, the variant was resistant to DAP and unable to incorporate adenine; cell-free extracts lacked APRT activity. The variant was capable of growth in HAT and could utilize adenosine and inosine as purine sources.

Blair and Hall (1965) and Blair et al. (1970) selected DAP-resistant variants from the NCTC C1-929 strain of L cells. Resistant cells were passaged for five years in the absence of inhibitor without decreasing their resistance to DAP. Resistant cells incorporated little radioactively labeled DAP or adenine and cell-free extracts had insignificant APRT levels in comparison with wild-type cells.

Atkins and Gartler (1968) obtained DAP-resistant variants of the McCoy monolayer line. After exposure of parental cells to $6.7 \times 10^{-4}\ M$ DAP for 2 weeks, resistant cells were grown up and recloned. They remained resistant to DAP after growth in the absence of the drug. Of eight resistant clones, seven showed less than 1% adenine uptake by intact cells compared to that of the wild-type cells. Cell-free extracts of these variants lacked APRT activity. An eighth clone, though fully resistant to DAP, incorporated adenine at only 8% of the wild-type rate and had a parallel reduction in the APRT activity of cell-free extracts. Selection at $2.7 \times 10^{-4}\ M$ and $4.7 \times 10^{-4}\ M$ DAP led to the production of two classes of clones. The first class consisted of large clones present at a frequency of 4×10^{-3} and were unable to incorporate tritiated adenine (determined by autoradiography). Some of these clones were resistant to $6.7 \times 10^{-4}\ M$ DAP on later testing. After autoradiography of unselected clones of wild-type cells exposed to tritiated adenine, a similar proportion (4×10^{-3}) was unlabeled. The second class comprised smaller clones and had a high or intermediate ability to incorporate tritiated adenine. Variants lacking the ability to incorporate exogenously supplied adenine were therefore present in the population before exposure to DAP and at a similar frequency to the DAP-resistant variants. An estimate of the frequency of reversion of the variants was obtained without selection by autoradiography of clones after exposure to tritiated adenine (Table VII).

b. Human. Rappaport and DeMars (1973) selected DAP-resistant variants of diploid human fibroblasts. Strains were chosen on the basis of survival in 4.1 to $4.9 \times 10^{-5}\ M$ DAP. Of 83 foreskin cultures, 26 survived markedly better than the remainder, possibly being heterozygous for a defective APRT allele. After mutagenesis with MNNG, 16 of the possible heterozygotes were selected in either $7.2 \times 10^{-5}\ M$ or $1.2 \times 10^{-4}\ M$ DAP. Resistant variants were obtained from 10 of the 16 strains at frequencies ranging from 10^{-7} to 10^{-4} and retained resistance after growth in the absence of DAP. The variants obtained fell into three categories. The first contained a single variant with little APRT activity in cell free extracts and was unable to utilize exogenously supplied adenine (APRT⁻). A second group retained APRT activity to a varying degree but had an unimpaired ability to utilize exogenously supplied adenine. Finally there was a third category with a reduced though perceptible ability to use adenine. The loss or partial deletion of chromosome No. 16 was frequently noted in DAP-resistant variants obtained after X-irradiation of parental cultures. The same chromosome was retained selectively in

TABLE VII
CELLS SELECTED FOR RESISTANCE TO PURINE BASE ANALOGS OF ADENINE[a]

Cell type and reference	Selection level (M)	Frequency of variants	ID_{50} (M)	Reversion rate
DAP, mouse				
L				
Lieberman and Ove (1960)	Wild type	—	$<1.2 \times 10^{-8}$	—
	$1.5–3.0 \times 10^{-6}$	$2.5 \times 10^{-6\,b}$	$6 \times 10^{-6}–4.8 \times 10^{-7}$	—
Blair and Hall (1965);	Wild type	—	8×10^{-6}	—
Blair et al. (1970)	Multistep, 6.7×10^{-4}	—	3.3×10^{-4}	
McCoy				
Atkins and Gartler (1968)	4.7×10^{-4}	4×10^{-3}	$<6.7 \times 10^{-4}$	3×10^{-6} or greater
DAP, human				
Diploid fibroblast				
Rappaport and DeMars (1973)	Wild type	—	$<1 \times 10^{-5}$	—
	1.2×10^{-4}	$10^{-4}–10^{-7}$	$<1.6 \times 10^{-4}–12.3 \times 10^{-4}$	—
DAP, pig				
PK15				
Harris and Ruddle (1960)	Wild type	—	6×10^{-5}	—
Harris (1961)	6.7×10^{-4}	$1–3 \times 10^{-5}$	4×10^{-4}	—

		Months after isolation, ID_{50}	
		2	3
	Clone 6.7×10^{-4}	2.7×10^{-4}	3.3×10^{-4}
	Clone 6.7×10^{-4}	1.9×10^{-4}	0.9×10^{-4}
	Clone 6.7×10^{-4}	2.9×10^{-4}	3.9×10^{-4}
	Clone 6.7×10^{-4}	0.5×10^{-4}	0.4×10^{-4}
	Clone 6.7×10^{-4}	2.5×10^{-4}	3.0×10^{-4}
	Clone 6.7×10^{-4}	2.1×10^{-4}	1.7×10^{-4}
	Clone 6.7×10^{-4}	5.6×10^{-4}	1.8×10^{-4}
	Clone 6.7×10^{-4}	4.6×10^{-4}	1.3×10^{-4}
Harris and Ruddle (1961)	6.7×10^{-4}	2.6×10^{-4}	—
FA, human			
HeP No. 2			
Bennett et al. (1966b)	Wild type	3.3×10^{-7}	—
	1st step 1.2–2.5×10^{-5}	—	—
	2nd step 2.6×10^{-4}	$<2.6 \times 10^{-4}$	—
AA, Syrian hamster			
PyY BHK21/C13	Wild type	$<8.1 \times 10^{-5}$	—
Subak-Sharpe	Multistep	6.5×10^{-3}	—

[a] DAP, 2:6-diaminopurine; FA, 2-fluoroadenine; AA, 8-azaadenine.
[b] Rate of appearance of variants determined by a fluctuation test, expressed per cell per generation.

hybrids between APRT⁻ mouse cells and normal human fibroblasts grown under conditions rendering the hybrid auxotrophic for adenine, and thus dependent on the presence of the human APRT for survival. Both lines of evidence suggest that a locus affecting APRT activity is situated on the human chromosome No. 16.

c. *Pig.* Harris and Ruddle (1960) and Harris (1961) selected variants of PK15 cells by exposure to 6.7×10^{-4} M DAP. The frequency of appearance of variants was 1 to 3×10^{-5} at this concentration of DAP, but decreased at higher levels. If lower levels of DAP were used for selection, a greater number of resistant cells were obtained and the distinction between variants and wild-type clones became difficult. Variants were also obtained after three exposures of a mass population to 6.7×10^{-4} M DAP followed by cloning at the same concentration. Clonal sublines were established and passaged for 3 months in the absence of DAP. The ID_{50} of these was tested at 2 and 3 months after isolation (Table VII). One clone had a similar ID_{50} to the wild type in both tests; this clone grew slowly just after isolation and may have been repopulated at that time by a revertant. The ID_{50} of the other seven clones varied by a factor of three being distributed evenly about the ID_{50} of the uncloned parental cells. In five of the clones there was little difference in the ID_{50} between the two tests, but in the remaining pair there was a significant drop between 2 and 3 months after cloning. The rate of growth of these clones, though initially slow, at the time of testing approximated to that of the wild-type cells. The yield of the variants was reduced as the concentration of the serum in the medium used for selection increased, being 1.8×10^{-5}, 4×10^{-4}, and greater than 3×10^{-6} in, respectively, 5%, 15%, and 40% lamb serum. Harris and Ruddle (1961) selected a DAP-resistant variant by growth of a wild-type clone with a marker chromosome induced by X-irradiation in 6.7×10^{-4} M DAP. The marker chromosome was unchanged by the selective procedure.

6. *2-Fluoroadenine (FA)* (Table VII)

Bennet et al. (1966b) isolated variants of H.Ep. No. 2 cells resistant to FA by growth in gradually increasing concentrations of the inhibitor. Intact variant cells failed to incorporate adenine and cell-free extracts had negligible AGPRT activity, but retained adenine kinase and HGPRT activities.

B. PURINE NUCLEOSIDE ANALOGS (Table VIII)

The biochemistry of purine nucleoside analogs has recently been reviewed by Roy-Burman (1970). These are converted to the respec-

TABLE VIII
Cells Selected for Resistance to Purine Nucleoside Analogs[a]

Cell type and reference	Selection level (M)	Frequency of variants	ID_{50} (M)
AGR, human			
D98 (HeLa)			
Szybalski (1959)	D98AG	—	7×10^{-7}
	1×10^{-4}	1.2×10^{-6} [b]	1.6×10^{-4}
TGR, Syrian hamster			
PyY BHK21/13			
Subak-Sharpe (1965, 1969)	Wild type		$<3.3 \times 10^{-7}$
	Multistep TG/TGR		$>3.4 \times 10^{-4}$
	Multistep AA/AAR/TG/TGR		$>3.4 \times 10^{-4}$
MeMPR, mouse			
3T6			
Chan et al. (1973)	Wild type		$<1.6 \times 10^{-7}$
	Multistep		$>3.2 \times 10^{-4}$
Human			
H.Ep. No. 2			
Bennett et al. (1966a)	Wild type		1×10^{-6}
	H.Ep. No.2/MeMPR		$>3.2 \times 10^{-4}$
	H.Ep. No.2/MP/MeMPR		$>3.2 \times 10^{-4}$
Tub, mouse			
3T6			
Chan et al. (1973)	Wild type		$<3.6 \times 10^{-7}$
	3T6/MeMPR		$\simeq 3.6 \times 10^{-6}$
	Multistep		$\simeq 1.4 \times 10^{-4}$
Tub, Syrian hamster			
PyY BHK21/CB			
Subak-Sharpe (1969)	Wild type		7×10^{-6}
	Multistep		$<7 \times 10^{-4}$
FAR, human			
H.Ep. No. 2			
Bennett et al. (1966a)	Wild type		4×10^{-7}
	7×10^{-5}		$<7 \times 10^{-5}$
But2cAMP mouse			
S549.ITB4			
Daniel et al. (1973)	Wild type		$<1.0 \times 10^{-5}$
	Multistep		$>1.0 \times 10^{-3}$

[a] AGR, 8-azaguanosine; TGR, 6-thioguanosine; MeMPR, 6-methylthiopurine ribonucleoside; Tub, tubercidin; FAR, 2-fluoroadenosine; But2cAMP, $N^6,O^{2'}$-dibutyryl adenosine 3':5'-cyclic monophosphate.

[b] Rate of appearance of variants determined by a fluctuation test, expressed per cell per generation.

tive nucleoside monophosphates either directly by a nucleoside kinase or indirectly via the purine base by a nucleoside phosphorylase and HGPRT. No nucleoside phosphorylase activity specific for adenosine has been detected in mammalian cells, but adenosine and some of its analogs may be converted to inosine by adenosine deaminase. Some analogs of adenosine, for example, tubercidin (Tub), are substrates for adenosine kinase (AK) but not for adenosine deaminase.

1. 8-Azaguanosine (AGR)

Szybalski (1959) and Szybalski et al. (1962) isolated an AGR-resistant variant of D98/AG (qv) termed D98/AGR which was 100-fold more resistant to AGR than the original parental cells, D98. The D98/AGR variant had a 50% reduction in the HGPRT activity of cell-free extracts when compared with either D98 or D98/AG. No AGR-resistant variants were obtained at a single step from 10^7 D98 cells, suggesting the requirement for at least two independent events during the development of resistance to AGR.

2. 6-Thioguanosine (TGR)

TGR-resistant variants of PyY Syrian hamster cells were obtained by Subak-Sharpe (1965, 1969) and were unable to incorporate hypoxanthine into intact cells. Cell-free extracts had no detectable HGPRT activity (owing to prior selection for resistance to TG, qv) but possessed normal levels of inosine/guanosine kinase (R. L. Edwards, personal communication). Resistance to TGR was probably the result of a decrease in the rate of entry of the drug into the variant cells.

3. 6-Methylthiopurine Ribonucleoside (MeMPR)

a. *Mouse.* Chan et al. (1973) described the selection of a variant of 3T6 (Todaro and Green, 1963) resistant to MeMPR. The variant retained substantial AK activity and was subsequently selected for tubercidin resistance (qv).

b. *Human.* Bennett et al. (1966a) selected a variant of H.Ep. No. 2 cells resistant to MeMPR by serial passage in gradually increasing concentrations of the drug. A second, doubly resistant variant termed H.Ep. No. 2/MP/MeMPR was selected from a variant already resistant to 2.1×10^{-3} M MP (qv). Cell-free extracts of H.Ep. No. 2/MeMPR and H.Ep. No. 2/MP/MeMPR, unlike parental cells, lacked AK activity and were unable to phosphorylate either adenosine or MeMPR, even after many generations of growth in the absence of the drug. H.Ep. No. 2/MeMPR, unlike H.Ep.

No. 2/MP/MeMPR retained an HGPRT level similar to that of wildtype cells and was capable of incorporating hypoxanthine into intact cells. Both H.Ep. No. 2/MP/MeMPR and H.Ep. No. 2 MeMPR had a reduced capacity to incorporate adenosine compared to wild-type cells. H.Ep. No. 2/MP/MeMPR excreted more hypoxanthine into the medium than either wild-type cells or H.Ep. No. 2/MP cells (Chan et al., 1973).

4. *Tubercidin (7-Deazaadenosine) (Tub)*

a. Mouse. Chan et al. (1973) selected a Tub-resistant variant from a MeMPR-resistant variant of 3T6 (qv). There was no detectable AK activity in cell-free extracts of the variant and clones derived from it. The variant excreted fifteen times more hypoxanthine and xanthine than wild-type cells; the increase ranged from 8- to 20-fold among clones derived from the variant.

b. Syrian Hamster. Subak-Sharpe (1969) selected variants of PyY AA cells (qv) resistant to 8-azaadenosine (AAR) and subsequently to Tub. Cell-free extracts of PyY AA/AAR/Tub had negligible APRT activity but retained AK activity (Edwards, personal communication). The ability of intact cells to incorporate adenine was reduced to 3% of the wild type, but the incorporation of adenosine was not significantly reduced (Clements, 1972). A quadruply resistant variant PyY AA/AAR/TG/TGR (qv) incorporated neither adenine, adenosine, hypoxanthine, nor guanosine into intact cells.

5. *2-Fluoradenosine (FAR)*

Bennett et al. (1966a) isolated a variant of H.Ep. No. 2/FA (qv) resistant to FAR. Cell-free extracts of the variant were unable to phosphorylate adenosine which, however, could be incorporated by intact cells.

6. *$N^6, O^{2'}$-Dibutyryladenosine 3':5'-cyclic Monophosphate (But2cAMP)*

Daniel et al. (1973) isolated a But2cAMP-resistant population of S49.1TB4 cells (Horitaba and Harris, 1970), a murine lymphoma line which undergoes cytolysis 48 hours after treatment with 0.1 to 1.0×10^{-3} M But2cAMP together with 2×10^{-4} M theophylline. Variants were selected by growth in the presence of 2×10^{-4} M theophylline, gradually increasing the But2cAMP concentration from 1×10^{-6} M to 1×10^{-4} M over 30 days. This selection procedure resulted in partially resistant cells, and a completely resistant variant was selected from them by exposure to 10^{-3} M But2cAMP for 1 week. No cytolysis occurred in this variant after exposure to 1×10^{-3} M But2cAMP with 2×10^{-4} M theophylline. Resistance was retained after growth in the absence of But2cAMP for at least 6 months. Resistant cells contained less cytoplasmic cAMP binding activity than parental. The molecular weight of the component having the residual binding activity as determined by filtration on Sephadex G-200 was higher in the resistant variant than the parental cells.

C. THYMIDINE AND ITS ANALOGS

The metabolism of these components has been reviewed recently by Roy-Burman (1970). TK converts FUdR to the deoxyribonucleotide (dFUMP) which specifically inhibits deoxythymidylate synthetase, so preventing synthesis of TMP from dUMP. BUdR and IUdR, after conversion to the deoxyribonucleotides by TK, are phosphorylated further and incorporated into DNA.

1. *5-Fluoro-2'-deoxyuridine (FUdR)* (Table IX)

Morris and Fischer (1960, 1961, 1963) selected an FUdR-resistant variant of the near diploid mast cell neoplasm P815Y. The variant was obtained after growth of the wild-type cells in 1×10^{-7} M FUdR for 7 days followed by cloning in drug-free medium. Resistance to FUdR persisted for at least two years after isolation when passaged in the absence of drug. Intact variant cells incorporated insignificant amounts of exogenously supplied thymidine into their DNA; they were unable to grow in HAT and were not inhibited by high concentrations of thymidine. Cell-free extracts had no detectable thymidine kinase activity. The variant was resistant to high concentrations of TdR, IUdR, and BUdR, but not CAR (Chu and Fischer, 1962).

Roosa *et al.* (1962) isolated P388 cells resistant to FUdR. The initial selection was carried out at 5×10^{-9} M FUdR followed by a second step at 5×10^{-8} M. The latter, while difficult to obtain, was resistant to levels of FUdR much higher than used for selection. The extremely high levels of resistance were lost during growth in the absence of inhibitor, though resistance to 5×10^{-8} M FUdR was retained, but reappeared quickly after reexposure to 5×10^{-8} M FUdR.

2. *5-Bromo-2'-deoxyuridine (BUdR)* (Table IX)

a. Mouse. Hsu and Somers (1962) isolated variants of LM cells (Hsu and Merchant, 1961) by continuous growth in one of three concentrations of BUdR for 43 weeks. Variants were obtained capable of normal growth both in the absence of BUdR and also at their respective levels of the drug for which resistance had been selected. The mean number of chromosomes of the parental and variant lines was 62 to 63, no consistent changes being observed during selection. The variant resistant to 8.0×10^{-5} M BUdR had a 10-fold reduction in BUdR-induced breakage of chromosomes after exposure to 8.0×10^{-5} M BUdR for 10 days compared to the parental cells. Kit and Hsu (1961) examined the DNA of resistant cells after growth for 13 weeks in the presence of BUdR and found it to be "heavy," indicating BUdR incorporation as was the case after growth of wild-type cells in the presence of BUdR. Variants resistant to 1.6×10^{-5} M BUdR and 8.0×10^{-5} M BUdR had, respectively, about 40% and 85% reduction of incorporation of exogenously supplied TdR into intact cells (Humphrey and Hsu, 1965). Kit et al. (1963) and Dubbs and Kit (1964) described the isolation of the definitive LM TK$^-$ cells obtained by growth as a monolayer in 8.0×10^{-5} M BUdR for over 100 weeks, followed by cloning. Retrospective studies showed that all lines derived prior to the 63rd week incorporated BUdR into their DNA while those derived after 81st week were unable to incorporate BUdR into their DNA and had become resistant to BUdR (3.2×10^{-3} M), TdR (8.2×10^{-4} M), and IUdR (5.6×10^{-4} M). Cell-free extracts lacked detectable TK activity. A second line, LM BU25 derived from wild-type cells selected in 8.0×10^{-5} M BUdR for 23 weeks retained the ability to incorporate BUdR, but growth in the presence of the drug was unpredictable and slow. LM TK$^-$ had a modal chromosomal number of 56, a reduction of five or six from that of the parental cells. Substantial amounts of thymidine and BUdR incorporation by the mitochondria of LM TK cells has recently been observed by Attardi and Attardi (1972b) and Clayton and Teplitz (1972).

Littlefield and Sakar (1964) and Littlefield (1964a,b, 1965) isolated BUdR-resistant variants of L cells. Wild-type cells were grown in 1×10^{-5} M BUdR as a suspension culture, and after about 2 weeks a slightly resistant variant grew up with about 45% wild-type TK activity. The level of BUdR was increased to 3.2×10^{-5} M and then to 1×10^{-4} M over a period of weeks, thereby selecting variants resistant to 1×10^{-3} M BUdR with less than 1% of wild-type TK activity in cell-free extracts. Variants obtained during the course of selection could be grouped into two classes, those with intermediate and those with absent TK activity.

In one variant clone, B34, reversion occurred at a frequency of 8×10^{-7} as determined by selection in HAT. The TK activity of the revertants was about 30% of that of the wild-type cells. A second clone, B82, produced no revertants in 4×10^7 cells. It was not pos-

TABLE IX
CELLS SELECTED FOR RESISTANCE TO THYMIDINE ANALOGS[a]

Cell type and references	Selection level (M)	Frequency of variants	ID_{50} (M)	Reversion rate
FUdR, mouse				
P815Y				
Morris and Fischer (1960, 1961, 1963)	Wild type	—	4.2×10^{-9}	—
	1×10^{-7}	—	2.8×10^{-6}	—
P388				
Roosa et al. (1962)	Wild type	—	$2 \times 10^{-10} - 4 \times 10^{-10}$	—
	1st step, 5×10^{-9}	—	$1 \times 10^{-9} - 5 \times 10^{-10}$	—
	2nd step, 5×10^{-8}	—	$2 \times 10^{-6} - 5 \times 10^{-6}$	—
BUdR, mouse				
LM				
Hsu and Somers (1962)	1.6×10^{-5}	—	$> 1.6 \times 10^{-5}$	—
	3.2×10^{-5}	—	$> 3.2 \times 10^{-5}$	—
Kit et al. (1963); Dubbs and Kit (1964)	8.0×10^{-5}	—	$> 8.0 \times 10^{-5}$	—
	8.0×10^{-5}	—	$> 3.2 \times 10^{-3}$	—
L				
Littlefield and Sakar (1964); Littlefield (1964a,b, 1965)	Wild type		3×10^{-6}	—
	1×10^{-5}		—	—
	3.2×10^{-5}	$\leq 1 \times 10^{-3}$	$\leq 1 \times 10^{-5}$	—
	1×10^{-4}	$\leq 1 \times 10^{-10}$	$> 1 \times 10^{-3}$	8×10^{-7}
Ignatova et al. (1968b)	1.6×10^{-5}	—	4.8×10^{-5}	—
Murayama and Okada (1970)	1st step, 1×10^{-4}	—	1×10^{-4}	Grow in HAT
	2nd step, 3.2×10^{-4}	—	3.2×10^{-4}	1×10^{-6}
MKS-B				
Dubbs et al. (1967)	Multistep, 3.2×10^{-4}	—	—	—
MKS-4				
Dubbs and Kit (1970)	3.2×10^{-5}	—	—	—

SELECTION OF BIOCHEMICALLY VARIANT CELLS

Cell line / Reference	Condition			
NCTC 2550 Davidson et al. (1968)	—		$>1 \times 10^{-4}$	Low
3T3 Matsuya and Green (1969)	Wild type			—
Basilico et al. (1969)	1.6×10^{-5}	—	$<1.6 \times 10^{-5}$	—
	1×10^{-4} 3T3-4(E)	—	—	Detectable
	1×10^{-4} 3T3-4(C2)	—	3×10^{-4}	None detected
L5178Y Clive et al. (1972)	Wild type	—	1.5×10^{-5}	—
	Single step, 1.6×10^{-4}	$5 \times 10^{-11\,b}$		$6.0 \times 10^{-9\,b}$
	Revertant → TK⁻	1.9–$0.6 \times 10^{-7\,b}$	—	—
EL4 (Gorer, 1950) Mohit and Fan (1971)	3.2×10^{-4}	—	—	Not grow in HAT
B16 (Hu and Lesney, 1964) Pasztor and Hu (1971, 1972)	Multistep, 1.3×10^{-4}	—	$<1.5 \times 10^{-4}$	—
T1M1 Hyman (1973)	1st step, 1×10^{-2} TdR	—	—	—
	2nd step, 1×10^{-4} BUdR	—	—	1×10^{-7}
A10 Rothschild and Black (1973)	Multistep, 8.2×10^{-5}	—	—	—
BUdR, Chinese hamster B14-FAF28 Humphrey and Hsu (1965)	1st step, 8.0×10^{-5}			
	2nd step, 1.6×10^{-4}			
Don Westerveld et al. (1971)	3.3×10^{-4} (tetraploid)	—	—	Not grow in HAT
	3.3×10^{-4} (hyperdiploid)	—	—	Not grow in HAT

(Continued)

TABLE IX (Continued)

Cell type and references	Selection level (M)	Frequency of variants	ID_{50} (M)	Reversion rate
BUdR, Human				
D98S (HeLa)				
Djordjevic and Szybalski (1960)	Wild type	—	3×10^{-6}–3×10^{-5}	—
	1.6×10^{-5}	—	$>1.6 \times 10^{-4}$	—
HeLa S3				
Tolivar and Simon (1967)	3.2×10^{-5}	—	$>3.2 \times 10^{-5}$	—
Kit et al. (1966)	Wild type	—	$\leqslant 1 \times 10^{-4}$	—
	Multistep to 3.2×10^{-4}	—	$>3.3 \times 10^{-4}$	Not grow in HAT
KB				
Higgins et al. (1969)	Wild type	—	2.6×10^{-7}	—
			$>2.6 \times 10^{-5}$	—
P3HR1				
Hampar et al. (1971)	Multistep, 3.3×10^{-4}	—	—	Not grow in HAT
Raji				
Hampar et al. (1972)	Multistep, 3.3×10^{-4}	—	—	Not grow in HAT
BUdR, Syrian hamster				
BHK21/C13				
Littlefield and Basilico (1966)	Wild type	—	$<3.5 \times 10^{-6}$	—
	1st step, 1×10^{-5}	2×10^{-4}	—	—
	2nd step, 1×10^{-4}	—	$\cong 1 \times 10^{-3}$	1×10^{-7}
BHK PyY 21/C13, (PyYTG/CAR)				
Bürk et al. (1966)	Multistep, 3×10^{-3}	—	—	—

Cell/Reference				
RPM1-3460				
Davidson and Bick (1973)	1×10^{-5}		$\leq 1 \times 10^{-4}$	—	—
	Multistep, 1×10^{-6}	—	—	—
BUdR, Frog				
Mezger-Freed (1972); Freed and Mezger-Freed (1973)				
Haploid ICR2A	Single step, 1×10^{-3}	None detected	—	—
	1st step, 5.0×10^{-5}	3×10^{-8}	$\leq 1 \times 10^{-4}$	—
	2nd step, 1×10^{-3}	9×10^{-7}	$\leq 1 \times 10^{-3}$	—
60% Haploid ICR21	5.0×10^{-5}	1×10^{-7}	—	—
Pseudodiploid ICR132	5.0×10^{-5}	7×10^{-7}	$< 1.6 \times 10^{-6}$	—
IUdR, Mouse				
LM				
Humphrey and Hsu (1965)	7×10^{-5}		—	—
P388F				
Ayad and Fox (1968)	Wild type	—	1×10^{-5}	—
	Multistep, 5.6×10^{-5}	—	5.6×10^{-5}	5.0×10^{-6}
Fox (1971)	Single step, 4×10^{-5}	1.1×10^{-2}–4.2×10^{-3}	—	—
	Single step, 2.8×10^{-5}	2.4×10^{-3}–4.8×10^{-5}	—	—
	Single step, 5.6×10^{-5}	1.5×10^{-4}–5.0×10^{-5}	—	—
	Single step, 2.8×10^{-4}	4.5×10^{-4}–1.1×10^{-5}	—	—
THK-1				
Rothschild and Black (1970)	Multistep, 3.3×10^{-4}	—	$> 8.2 \times 10^{-5}$	2–5×10^{-7}

[a] FUdR, 5-fluoro-2'-deoxyuridine; BUdR, 5-bromo-2'-deoxyuridine; IUdR, 5-iodo-2'-deoxyuridine; TdR, thymidine; TK⁻, TK-deficient cell.

[b] Rate of appearance of variants expressed per cell per generation.

sible to make direct measurements of the frequency with which resistant cells appeared. By extrapolation from the time of appearance of variants, partially resistant cells appeared with a frequency of 1×10^{-3} and fully resistant ones at 1×10^{-10}.

Murayama and Okada (1970) selected clones of L cells resistant to BUdR. The initial selection procedure in 1×10^{-4} M BUdR yielded resistant variants capable of growth in HAT which retained TK activity. Cells grown in medium containing 1×10^{-4} M BUdR were exposed to visible light and subsequently grown in the presence of 3.2×10^{-4} M BUdR. Colonies picked were unable to grow in HAT.

Dubbs et al. (1967) obtained BUdR-resistant variants of an SV40-transformed mouse kidney cell line, MKS-B, by growth in increasing levels of the drug. During selection two critical stages were noted, at 8×10^{-5} M and 1.6×10^{-4} M respectively, but by the 52nd passage a variant was obtained that could be passaged in 3.2×10^{-4} M BUdR. This variant and also a variant isolated at an earlier stage resistant to 8×10^{-5} M BUdR incorporated a reduced amount of exogenously supplied TdR into intact cells and crude extracts contained about 1% of wild-type TK activity. Dubbs and Kit (1970) selected BUdR-resistant variants of MKS-U cells, a line of primary mouse (Swiss) kidney cells transformed by UV-irradiated SV40 (Dubbs and Kit, 1968). Selection was carried out by growth in 3.2×10^{-5} M BUdR. Some cultures passed through a critical phase within the first few passages in BUdR necessitating growth in normal medium for a short time, but after recovery they could be passaged in 3.2×10^{-5} M BUdR. Cell-free extracts of six variants selected in this way had 2% or less of wild-type TK activity in four cases but in the remaining two TK activity was retained. Both the latter variants could grow in HAT unlike the pair of TK⁻ variants tested. Buoyant density measurements of cell DNA after prolonged growth in BUdR confirmed these results, the DNA of variants lacking TK activity maintained a normal density under these conditions.

Matsuya and Green (1969) and Basilico et al. (1969) selected BUdR-resistant variants from a clone of 3T3 (Todaro and Green, 1963) by growth at 1.6×10^{-5} BUdR. Two clones resistant at this level were independently subjected to a second selective step by growth at 1×10^{-4} M BUdR at low cell concentrations and subsequently recloned. One clone 3T3-4 (E) had a low plating efficiency and an appreciable reversion rate. Clonal derivatives of each line grew normally at 1×10^{-4} M BUdR; intact cells failed to incorporate thymidine, and cell-free extracts were deficient in TK activity. No inhibitor of TK activity was present in the variants: extracts of variant cells mixed with extracts of wild-type cells did not inhibit the TK activity present.

Clive et al. (1972) isolated BUdR-resistant variants of L5178Y murine lymphoma cells (Fischer, 1958) grown in suspension culture as an indicator sytem. Selection was effected in medium containing 0.37% agar. Initially a TK+ clone was isolated by the growth of wild-type cells in agar containing HAT and formed the starting point for all subsequent experiments. The standard BUdR concentration for selection was chosen to be 1.6×10^{-4} M at a density of 10^5 cells per milliliter. Under these conditions a single BUdR-resistant variant appeared after plating 4.4×10^8 cells giving an estimated frequency of 5×10^{-11} per cell per generation. Reconstruction experiments eliminated the possibility that BUdR-resistant variants were appearing at a higher frequency but being killed by interaction with wild-type cells. Mixtures of wild-type and variant cells were plated in the presence of BUdR, a decrease in the frequency with which variants appeared only became apparent at cell densities above 10^5 per milliliter. TK activity could not be demonstrated in cell-free extracts of the resistant variant. By selection in HAT nine independent revertants were obtained, the average TK activity of which was 50% of that of the original wild-type cell. It was suggested that the original wild-type cell selected in HAT could be TK+/+, the BUdR-resistant variants TK−/−, and the revertants TK+/−. Hyman (1973) selected variants from a clone of T1M1, a radiation leukemia virus-induced tumor of a C57BL/6, resistant to 1×10^{-4} M BUdR by growing cells in increasing concentrations of thymidine (10^{-4} to 10^{-2} M) followed by selection in BUdR.

b. *Chinese Hamster.* Humphrey and Hsu (1965) selected a BUdR-resistant variant of the Chinese hamster cell line B14-FAF28 by serial culture in concentrations of BUdR increasing from 1.6×10^{-6} M. to 8.0×10^{-5} M. Variants resistant to the latter level were then selected for resistance to either 1.4×10^{-4} M IUdR or 1.6×10^{-4} M BUdR. Highly resistant variants incorporated little or no TdR into intact cells. The IUdR-resistant variant retained the wild-type modal chromosome number, 23, but the variant resistant to 1.6×10^{-4} M BUdR was subtetraploid with a mode at 35 to 36. The population resistant to 8.0×10^{-5} M BUdR from which these variants were selected contained a mixture of both cell types.

c. *Human.* Djordjevic and Szybalski (1960) isolated a BUdR-resistant variant of D98S. Wild-type cells grew normally for long periods, though slowly, at concentrations below 3×10^{-5} M BUdR, and for limited periods at 3×10^{-4} M BUdR. D98/BUdR was selected by growing wild-type cells for 40 generations in $1.6 \times 10^{-5}\,M$ BUdR and had a relative plating efficiency of 59% at $1.6 \times 10^{-4}\,M$ BUdR. The variant remained capable of incorporating exogenously supplied thymidine and BUdR into DNA, though at a reduced rate compared to the wild type.

Kit et al. (1966) isolated variants of HeLa S3 resistant to $3 \times 10^{-4}\,M$ BUdR that were deficient in TK activity. Selection began at $1.6 \times 10^{-5}\,M$, the concentration of BUdR being gradually increased to $3 \times 10^{-4}\,M$ over a period of 50 weeks. Incorporation of thymidine by intact cells was assayed by autoradiography. HeLa/BUdR-15 (resistant to $4.8 \times 10^{-5}\,M$ BUdR) and variants resistant to the inhibition at less than this level showed significant incorporation while variants resistant to higher levels of BUdR incoporated little thymidine. Assays of cell-free extracts confirmed a lack of TK activity measured using deoxyuridine and BUdR as substrates, the activity being reduced to 2.5% of the wild type in HeLa/BU-25, -50, and -100. (Resistant to, respectively, $8.0 \times 10^{-5}\,M$, $1.6 \times 10^{-4}\,M$, and $3.2 \times 10^{-4}\,M$ BUdR). The TK activity of HeLa/BU-100 remained unchanged after growth for 5 weeks in the absence of BUdR. Using UdR as a substrate the TK activity of HeLa/BUdR-10 and BUdR-15 (resistant to $3.2 \times 10^{-4}\,M$ and $4.8 \times 10^{-5}\,M$ BUdR) were, respectively 50% and 8% of that of the wild type. Mixing experiments, assaying the TK activity of mixtures of cell-free extracts from wild-type and HeLa/BU-100 indicated that there was no inhibitor of TK activity present in the extract of the variant. Normal levels of thymidylate synthetase, thymidylate kinase, and uridine kinase were present in all cells. Kit et al. (1972) showed that HeLa/BU-25 incorporated tritiated thymidine and BUdR into superhelical mitochondrial DNA and retained TK activity (more than 80% of all activity present) in the mitochondrial fraction. The TK activity of whole-cell extracts of the variant remained negligible. The soluble HeLa enzyme and the residual BU-25 enzyme have different pH optima and different electrophoretic mobilities during polyacrylamide gel electrophoresis (Kit and Minekawa, 1972; Kit et al., 1973).

Hampar et al. (1971) selected a line of P3HR1 cells (Hinuma et al., 1967) resistant to $3.2 \times 10^{-4}\,M$ BUdR. The TK activity of cell-free extracts was 5–8% of the wild type. Whole cells incorporated less than 1% tritiated BUdR when compared to the wild type except for a subpopulation that correlated with these cells expressing Epstein–Barr virus (EBV) surface antigens. Hampar et al. (1972) selected BUdR-resistant variants of Raji cells, another human lymphoblastoid cell line, by gradually increasing the concentration of BUdR in the medium. At 2.5×10^{-5} M BUdR selection was slow, but once past this level it progressed smoothly. Most of the BUdR-resistant Raji cells were unable to incorporate TdR or BUdR and did not grow in HAT; a minority (5%) also correlated with cells expressing EBV surface antigens, could incorporate thymidine. Cell-free extracts had less than 1% of the wild-type TK activity.

d. *Syrian Hamster.* Littlefield and Basilico (1966) selected BUdR-resistant variants of BHK21/C13 cells. Cells from these colonies were exposed to 3.5×10^{-5} M and subsequently to 1×10^{-4} M BUdR; two of the colonies that grew out were propagated as sublines. Both proved to be highly resistant to BUdR, having plating efficiencies of 30% at 1×10^{-4} M and 1×10^{-3} M BUdR, though at the highest concentration the colony size was reduced. Cell extracts lacked TK activity, and intact cells were incapable of incorporating exogenously supplied thymidine. Selection in HAT yielded revertants at a frequency of approximately 1 per 10^7 cells per generation. These had about 60% of wild-type TK activity.

Bürk *et al.* (1966) and Subak-Sharpe (personal communication) selected BUdR-resistant variants of PyY cells by a multistep procedure. Variants resistant to 3.2×10^{-3} M BUdR were obtained; these were unable to incorporate TdR into intact cells and lacked TK activity in cell-free extracts. BUdR-resistant variants were selected from lines that had previously been selected for resistance to TG and CAR (qv).

Davidson and Bick (1973) derived BUdR-resistant variants from a pigmented clone of Syrian hamster melanoma line RPM1-3460 (Moore, 1964). Cells plated at low densities were exposed to 1×10^{-5} M BUdR. After 3 weeks about 40 large colonies had appeared and were pooled and passaged twice in medium containing 1×10^{-5} M BUdR and then twice in 1×10^{-4} M BUdR. After the last passage several large colonies were picked, which may or may not have been of independent origin. These were subsequently passaged independently; all were unpigmented. The variants were maintained for 6 weeks, and in one case for 6 months (75 generations) in medium containing 1×10^{-4} M BUdR, but cell-free extracts retained wild-type levels of TK activity. In the absence of BUdR seven variants and subclones derived from one of them all flattened, enlarged, and grew poorly. The variants had become dependent on BUdR; a concentration of 1×10^{-4} M being optimal. Neither TdR, bromouracil, uridine, deoxyuridine, bromouridine, nor iodouridine were effective substitutes for BUdR, and a 10-fold excess of thymidine competed with BUdR and inhibited growth. After aminopterin block of *de novo* thymidine synthesis both thymidine and BUdR were necessary to support growth. The density of the DNA of the variant cells after prolonged growth in the presence of BUdR indicated that 50% of the thymidine residues in the DNA were substituted by BUdR and the variant was highly light sensitive. The incorporated BUdR was found to be distributed evenly throughout the whole genome. One revertant was selected that was capable of rapid growth in the absence of BUdR. When reselected for resistance to BUdR the revertant gave rise to a variant capable of growth in both normal medium and medium containing BUdR, and which incorporated BUdR into its DNA. This differed from the original variant in being resistant to, but not dependent on, BUdR.

e. Frog. Mezger-Freed (1972) and Freed and Mezger-Freed (1973) selected BUdR-resistant variants of lines derived from androgenic haploid frog embryos, ICR2A (95–100% haploid), ICR21 (60% haploid), and also ICR132 (93% pseudodiploid) (Freed and Mezger-Freed, 1970). Variants were selected at a single step for resistance to 5×10^{-5} M BUdR, this frequency being increased by prior mutogenesis with a variety of agents in the case of ICR2A. There was no increase in the frequency of variants after mutagenesis of the other two lines used. Variants derived from ICR2A were resistant to BUdR, and intact cells incorporated 7% or less TdR than the wild type into both the acid-soluble and acid-precipitable fractions. The variants were unable to grow in HAT containing 1.6×10^{-5} M. TdR, but in the two cases examined, ICR B20 and ICR B9, there was growth in HAT containing between 1×10^{-4} M and 2×10^{-3} M. TdR. *In vitro* assays indicate the retention of TK activity in these variants, and it was suggested that TdR was unable to enter because of a defective transport system. In a second selective step for resistance to 10^{-3} M BUdR, resistant variants were obtained from ICR-B20; their frequency was increased after mutagenesis. No variant has been obtained resistant to high levels of BUdR at a single step, even after mutagenesis. Cell-free extracts of 24 of the second-step variants had 7% or less TK activity than the wild type while four retained substantial levels. Variants isolate from ICR132, the pseudodiploid line, were not resistant to 1.6×10^{-6} M BUdR on retesting and incorporated significant quantities of TdR into intact cells. Reconstruction experiments using mixtures of TK$^-$ and wild-type cells indicated that selection at high cell density did not depress the recovery of these BUdR-resistant variants. The different phenotypes of BUdR-resistant variants obtained using the haploid and the diploid lines makes comparison and evaluation of the frequencies with which they yield variants hazardous, particularly in view of the heterogeneous ploidies of the populations from which they were derived.

The behavior of these frog cells is analogous to that described using mammalian cells, selection for TK⁻ cells being a multistep procedure. In only one case have TK⁻ cells been obtained using a single-step procedure by selection in BUdR, and then at low frequency (Clive et al., 1972). The alterations allowing the development of the first step resistance may involve modifications to the *de novo* synthetic pathway of thymidine and its deoxyribonucleotide phosphates.

3. *5-Iodo-2'-deoxyuridine (IUdR)* (Table IX)

a. Mouse. Humphrey and Hsu (1965) noted that a line of L cells tolerant to 8.0×10^{-5} M BUdR, LM BU-25 (qv), which normally incorporated BUdR and TdR, ceased to be capable of incorporation of IUdR, BUdR, and TdR after passage in the presence of 7×10^{-5} M IUdR. A variant resistant to 7×10^{-5} M IUdR was selected from a line LM BU-5 that had previously been selected for resistance to 1.6×10^{-5} M BUdR. The TK activity in a population of these cells exposed to 1.6×10^{-5} M IUdR decreased as an exponential function over a period of 60 days with a half-life of 8.5 days. The resulting variant failed to incorporate TdR into intact cells, the ability to incorporate TdR was not regained after passage for one year in normal medium.

Ayad and Fox (1968) using the P388F clone derived from the P388 murine lymphoma (Fox and Gilbert, 1966; Fox and Fox, 1967) selected a variant resistant to IUdR. Wild-type cells were grown in increasing concentrations of IUdR until after 54 days a population was produced with a normal doubling time in 5.6×10^{-5} M IUdR. After growth in this concentration of IUdR, the variant was cloned in agar in the presence of 5.6×10^{-5} M IUdR, wild-type cells had a cloning efficiency of less than 1% in 1.4×10^{-5} M IUdR. Intact variant cells incorporated thymidine and IUdR at less than 5% of the wild type rate. The variant retained resistance to IUdR after growth in drug-free medium for many generations.

Fox (1971) using P388 cells selected for resistance to various concentrations of IUdR (Table IX). The frequency of clones surviving at all concentrations of the drug and also of revertants, was increased by X-irradiation prior to selection. Clones selected for growth in concentrations lower than 2.8×10^{-5} M IUdR did not retain resistance when retested 10 days after isolation. Clones selected in 5.6×10^{-5} M and 2.8×10^{-4} M IUdR retained resistance on later testing. Recloning five times in $2.8 \times 10^{-5}\,M$ IUdR resulted in the gradual development of resistance that was retained in the absence of selection.

4. Thymidine (Table X)

At high concentrations, generally above $1 \times 10^{-4}\,M$, thymidine inhibits cell growth (Hakala and Taylor, 1959). Reichard, Canellakis, and Canellakis (1961) showed that a derivative of thymidine, thymidine triphosphate (TTP), inhibited the conversion of cytidine 5'-monophosphate (CMP) to dCMP by a chick embryo extract. The complicated allosteric regulation of the step affected, conversion of cytidine 5'-diphosphate (CDP) to dCDP by ribonucleotide reductase, has been reviewed by Reichard (1968). The inhibitory effect of thymidine at high concentrations is specifically reversed by deoxycytidine (Morris et al., 1963). Cell variants incapable of phosphorylating thymidine were resistant to high levels of exogenous thymidine (Morris and Fischer, 1963). High levels of thymidine have been used to select variant cells incapable of synthesizing TTP from exogenously supplied thymidine.

a. Mouse. Littlefield (1965) selected a variant of L cells by growth in $2 \times 10^{-4}\,M$ TdR, which was found to be partially resistant to BUdR. Harris and Cohn (1970) using clones of two lymphomas derived from BALB/c mice, SIA and S49 (Horitaba and Harris, 1970), selected variants with increased resistance to high external concentrations of thymidine. Variants were initially selected for resistance

TABLE X
CELLS SELECTED FOR RESISTANCE TO THYMIDINE

Cell type and references	Selection level (M)	Frequency of variants	ID_{50} (M)
Mouse			
L			
Littlefield (1965)	2×10^{-4}	—	—
SIA and S49			
Harris and Cohn (1970)	Wild type	—	2×10^{-5}
	Multistep, 3×10^{-3}	—	—
Chinese hamster			
Don			
Breslow and Goldsby (1969)	Wild type	2.5×10^{-3}	—
	Tritiated TdR	$2.6 \times 10^{-4\,a}$	—
	8×10^{-3}	$2.5 \times 10^{-4\,a}$	—

[a] Rate of appearance of variants determined by a fluctuation test, expressed per cell per generation.

to 3×10^{-5} M and subsequently to 1×10^{-4} M TdR. The latter variants failed to grow in 3×10^{-4} M TdR, but by repetitive stepwise selection in 3-fold increasing concentrations of TdR resistance was increased to 3×10^{-3} M. At any given level, resistance was retained for at least 20 generations of growth in the absence of TdR. The pattern of resistance was similar in variants selected from both parental lines.

b. Chinese Hamster. Breslow and Goldsby (1969) selected variants of Don ATC and also a subline previously selected for the ability to grow at 40°C, Don HHT, by culturing in a medium containing 2–5 µCi of tritiated thymidine per milliliter for several days. The rate of appearance of variant Don ATC cells resistant to both tritiated thymidine and also 8.2×10^{-3} M thymidine were the same (2.5×10^{-4} per cell per generation) by a fluctuation test. Variants were derived from both cell lines by selection in tritiated thymidine and, without cloning, assayed for thymidine incorporation. The TK activity of the HHT cell-free extract was 45% that of the wild-type cells, but autoradiography of intact HHT cells after incubation with tritiated thymidine indicated little thymidine incorporation. Thymidine uptake of the variants at 4°C and 26°C, temperatures at which there is little nucleic acid synthesis, were reduced when compared to that of the wild type, suggesting defective thymidine uptake. Screening wild-type cells by autoradiography indicated that one in 2.5×10^{-3} clones was unable to incorporate tritiated thymidine.

D. DEOXYCYTIDINE ANALOGS

1. *1-β-D-Arabinofuranosylcytosine, Cytosine Arabinoside (CAR)* (Table XI)

The only analog of deoxycytidine that has been used to select variant cells is CAR. It is phosphorylated by deoxycytidine kinase (EC 2.7.1.74) to the monophosphate and subsequently to the triphosphate. The mechanism of inhibition of cell growth by CAR has been controversial and is discussed by Roy-Burman (1970). In mammalian systems it is probable that DNA polymerase is inhibited by the triphosphate of CAR.

a. Mouse. A CAR-resistant variant of L5178Y was isolated by Chu and Fischer (1963, 1965). Selection was achieved by growth of 1×10^8 wild-type cells in 1×10^{-6} M CAR. After 12 days the survivors, 1×10^6 cells, were changed to normal medium, and one variant clone was isolated. The variant retained resistance during growth for three years in CAR-free medium. Cell-free extracts of the variant had a

TABLE XI
Cells Selected for Resistance to Cytosine Arabinoside (CAR)

Cell type and references	Selection level (M)	Frequency of variants	ID_{50} (M)
Mouse			
L5178Y			
Chu and	Wild type	—	1.3×10^{-7}
Fischer (1962, 1965)	1×10^{-6}	—	4.7×10^{-6}
L1210			
Bach (1969)	Wild type	—	2.6×10^{-8}
	1×10^{-7}	1×10^{-3}–1.6×10^{-4} [a]	8.7×10^{-7}
Momparler	Wild type	—	4×10^{-8}
et al. (1968)	2.4×10^{-6}	—	1.9×10^{-7}
Syrian hamster			
PyY BHK21/C13 (PyY/TG)			
Bürk and Subak-	Wild type	—	$>1.8 \times 10^{-6}$
Sharpe (1968)	7.2×10^{-4}	—	7.2×10^{-4}
Chinese hamster			
V79-4/AG (V79/4/BUdR)			
Smith and Chu	Wild type	—	1.5×10^{-7} to 7.8×10^{-8}
(1972)	3.6×10^{-7}	—	$>3.9 \times 10^{-7}$
Harris (1973)	Wild type	—	1×10^{-7}
B14-150	1st step, 3.6×10^{-6}	—	$\simeq 4.0 \times 10^{-6}$
	2nd step, 3.6×10^{-5}	—	$\simeq 1.2 \times 10^{-4}$
V79-129	1st step, 3.6×10^{-6}	—	3.6×10^{-4}
	2nd step, 3.6×10^{-5}	—	3.6×10^{-4}

[a] Rate of appearance of variants determined by a fluctuation test, expressed per cell per generation.

50% reduction in ability to phosphorylate deoxycytidine compared to those of wild-type cells. Deoxycytidine competed with CAR less efficiently for phosphorylation by extracts of variant cells than of wild-type cells indicating that the basis of resistance may have been due to a modification of dCK. The intracellular CAR concentration was the same in both variant and parental cells eliminating the possibility that resistance was due to the variant having a reduced permeability to CAR. Chu and Fischer (1968) refer to the isolation of a variant of L5178Y highly resistant to CAR that did lack detectable dCK activity.

Bach (1969) selected a CAR-resistant variant from L1210 cells by several passages in 1×10^{-7} M CAR. CAR-resistant cells were 4-fold more resistant to FUdR and 30-fold more resistant to TdR (ID_{50} 1×10^{-3} M) than the parental cells. dCK activity of cell-free extracts from variants grown in the absence of CAR were reduced by 40% in comparison to the parental cells, but if the variant had been grown in the presence of Car there was no reduction in dCK activity. The K_m of dCK from parental and variant cells were the same. The presence of CAR did not increase the frequency of appearance of AG resistant variants, ruling out the possibility that CAR was mutagenic in the system.

A second variant of L5178Y cells was isolated by Momparler et al. (1968) using a clone that had been passaged once through $AKDF_1$ mice. Wild-type cells were exposed to 2.4×10^{-6} M CAR for 12 days, after which the survivors were grown up in drug-free medium for 3 days and then cloned by dilution in drug-free medium. When variant cells were compared to parental cells, although variant cells had a 60% increase in the quantity of exogenously supplied cytidine entering the intracellular dCMP pool, there was little difference in the incorporation into nucleic acid. Similar results were obtained using uridine, but when deoxycytidine was supplied there was a 50% reduction in incorporation into the dCMP pool and a 71% reduction in incorporation into nucleic acid by the variant compared to the parental cells. The size of the pool of phosphorylated derivatives of deoxycytidine was increased 4-fold in the variant over that of the parental cells. There was little difference between variant and parental cells in the incorporation of TdR-^{3}H into the thymidine pools and DNA. There was a slight reduction of incorporation of CAR into the acid-soluble material in the variant as compared to the parental cells, and there was no difference in the rate of phosphorylation of CAR by cell-free extracts of the two cell lines, nor was CAR deaminated or cleaved to free cytosine. It was considered that the main mechanism of resistance was competition out of exogenously supplied CAR and deoxycytidine by an increased intracellular pool of phosphorylated derivatives of deoxycytosine.

b. *Chinese Hamster.* Smith and Chu (1972) selected CAR-resistant variants from derivatives of V79-4 cells previously selected for resistance to either BUdR (qv) or TG (qv) by continuous propagation in 3.6×10^{-7} M of inhibitor. The variant previously selected for resistance to BUdR was less sensitive to CAR. Hybrids between CAR-sensitive and CAR-resistant cells were selected in HAT using the preexisting markers and were found to be CAR sensitive in all 15 cases examined. Hybrids between resistant variants retained their resistance in three combinations, but a fourth produced a hybrid sensitive to CAR.

Harris (1973) selected two CAR-resistant variants, one from B14-150 (Humphrey and Hsu, 1965) a BUdR-resistant variant (qv) and the other from 129 (Harris, 1972), a variant of V79 resistant to AG (qv). Mass populations were exposed to the inhibitor at 3.6×10^{-6} M. Resistant colonies appeared and were grown up and then reexposed to 3.6×10^{-5} M CAR. Both variants derived from 129 were highly resistant, being able to grow in a concentration of CAR 10-fold higher than those used for selection. The two variants derived from B14-150 had disparate degrees of resistance. Selection may have taken place in two steps, or alternatively the first low-resistant variant may have been a mixture between low- and high-resistant variants of independent origin, only the latter surviving the second selective procedure. Hybridization between resistant and sensitive cells in every case yielded hybrids that were sensitive to CAR.

E. Uracil and Uridine Analogs (Table XII)

Exogenously supplied uracil is converted to the ribonucleotide uridine by uridine phosphorylase (EC 2.4.2.3) and subsequently

TABLE XII
Mouse Cells Selected for Resistance to Analogs of Uracil and Uridine

Cell type and references	Selection level (M)	Frequency of variants	ID_{50} (M)
5-Fluorouracil			
P388			
Roosa and Herzenberg (1959)	Wild type	—	1×10^{-7}
Roosa et al. (1962)	5×10^{-7}	—	1×10^{-6}–5×10^{-7}
	Multisteps, $\times 10^{-5}$	—	2×10^{-6}
5-Fluorouridine			
P388			
Roosa et al. (1962)	Wild type	—	2–5×10^{-9}
	1×10^{-8}	—	2×10^{-8}
	8×10^{-8}	—	1×10^{-7}
6-Azauridine			
L5178Y			
Pasternak et al. (1961)	Wild type	—	1×10^{-6}
	Variant	—	$\simeq 1 \times 10^{-3}$

phosphorylated to UMP by uridine kinase. The analogs of uracil and uridine that have been used for the selection of variant cells are all converted to the ribonucleotide monophosphate and in some cases to the higher nucleotide phosphates. A detailed description of their metabolism and inhibitory effects is given in Roy-Burman (1970).

1. *5-Fluorouracil (FU)*

Roosa and Herzenberg (1959) and Roosa *et al.* (1962) selected FU-resistant variants from P388. With difficulty two variants were selected for resistance to 5×10^{-7} M FU. These were then cloned and selected for resistance to increasing levels of the drug, resulting in two lines of cells resistant to 1×10^{-6} M FU. Both variants retained resistance after growth in absence of the drug.

2. *5-Fluorouridine (FUR)*

Roosa *et al.* (1962) selected variants of P388 resistant to FUR at two different concentrations, although again with difficulty. Both variants retained their respective levels of resistance after growth in the absence of the drug. Reconstruction experiments using mixtures comprising 1% or 10% variant with wild-type cells yielded the expected number of resistant clones after selection in FUR.

3. *6-Azauridine (6-aza-UR)*

Pasternak *et al.* (1961) selected a variant of L5178Y for resistance to 6-aza-UR as a suspension culture in gradually increasing levels of 6-aza-UR. A resistant clone was then isolated, using a dilution technique, that grew in 1×10^{-3} M 6-aza-UR. After growth in the absence of inhibitor the variant quickly lost resistance. Uridine incorporation into perchloric acid-soluble material was reduced 30-fold in resistant cells, but orotic acid was incorporated at the same rate as in the parental cells. There was also a 30-fold reduction of incorporation of uridine and 6-aza-UR into their respective monophosphates by the intact variant in comparison with the parental cells. The activity of uridine phosphokinase in cell-free extracts from variant cells was reduced to 14% of the parental and to 36% using 6-aza-UR.

F. FOLIC ACID ANALOGS (Table XIII)

1. *Mouse*

Fischer (1959, 1961, 1962, 1971; also review by Fischer and Sartorelli, 1964) selected amethopterin-resistant variants from an adherent near diploid murine lymphoblastoid cell line L5178Y charac-

TABLE XIII
CELLS SELECTED FOR RESISTANCE TO FOLIC ACID ANALOGS

Cell type and references	Selection level (M)	Frequency of variants	ID_{50} (M)	Reversion rate
Amethopterin, mouse				
L5178Y				
Fischer (1961);	Wild type		0.9×10^{-8}	
Fischer and Sartorelli (1964)	2.0×10^{-8}	5×10^{-6}	1.3 to 4.3×10^{-8} (20 lines)	
Fischer (1971)	3.6×10^{-8}	2.4×10^{-4}	—	
	5.2×10^{-8}	4.0×10^{-4}	—	
	7.2×10^{-8}	8×10^{-6}	—	
	1.1×10^{-7}	2.2×10^{-6}		
Robins and Courtenay (1970)	Wild type		$1 \times 10^{-9\,a}$	
Courtenay and Robins (1972)			$4.4 \times 10^{-7\,a}$	
			$2.2 \times 10^{-4\,a}$	5×10^{-2}
			$1.1 \times 10^{-3\,a}$	
L cell, clone 929				
Aronow (1959)	Wild type	—	2–4×10^{-8}	
	Multistep, 1×10^{-7}	—	2–4×10^{-7}	
	Multistep, 1×10^{-6}	—	1–10×10^{-6}	
	Multistep, 1×10^{-5}	—	1×10^{-3}	
P388				
Roosa and Herzenberg (1959)	Wild type	—	$4 \times 10^{-9\,a}$	
Herzenberg (1961); Roosa et al. (1962)	8×10^{-6}	—	$1 \times 10^{-5\,a}$	
S180				
Hakala et al. (1960, 1961)	Wild type	—	5×10^{-8}	
	Multistep, AH 5×10^{-7}	2×10^{-7}	3.6×10^{-6}	
	Multistep, AT 5×10^{-7}	$<2 \times 10^{-7}$	9.4×10^{-6}	
Hakala and Ishihara (1962)	Multistep, 5×10^{-5}	—	1.6×10^{-4}	

Amethopterin, Chinese hamster

CLM-7			
Biedler and Albrecht (1971)	Wild type	—	8×10^{-9}
Biedler et al. (1972)	1.1×10^{-6}	—	2.4×10^{-4}
DC3F			
Biedler and Albrecht (1971)	Wild type	—	1.6×10^{-8}
Biedler et al. (1972)	1.1×10^{-6}	—	1.2×10^{-5}
	5.5×10^{-6}	—	8.0×10^{-6}
	5.5×10^{-5}	—	7.0×10^{-4}
	1.1×10^{-4}	—	1.6×10^{-3}
DC3F8			
Biedler and Albrecht (1971)	Wild type	—	2.4×10^{-8}
Biedler et al. (1972)	2.2×10^{-7}	—	9.0×10^{-6}
	2.2×10^{-5}	—	1.1×10^{-5}
	1.1×10^{-5}	—	1.1×10^{-4}
	5.5×10^{-5}	—	5.0×10^{-4}

Aminopterin, human

HeLa			
Vogt (1959)	Wild type	$<10^{-4}$	1×10^{-8}
	Multistep, 1.1×10^{-6}	—	$1.1 \times 10^{-6\,a}$
DeMars and Hooper (1960)	Wild type	$<10^{-5}$	2×10^{-9}
	1×10^{-8}	—	—

Aminopterin, pig

PK15			
Harris and Ruddle (1960)	2.2×10^{-7}	$1\text{--}10 \times 10^{-6}$	—
Harris (1961)	Wild type	—	3.1×10^{-8}
	2.2×10^{-7}	—	3.1×10^{-7}
PK14			
Harris and Ruddle (1961)	2.2×10^{-7}	—	1.9×10^{-7}

(Continued)

TABLE XIII (Continued)

Cell type and references	Selection level (M)	Frequency of variants	ID_{50} (M)	Reversion rate
Aminopterin, Syrian hamster				
BHK21/C13				
Littlefield (1969)	Wild type	—	—	
	$B_s(TK^-)$			
	3×10^{-8}	—	5×10^{-9}	
Orkin and Littlefield (1971)	1st step, 6×10^{-8}	2×10^{-4}–1×10^{-6}	3×10^{-8a}	
	2nd step, 1×10^{-6}	—	6×10^{-8a}	
	Multistep, 3×10^{-5}	3×10^{-6}	—	
		—	3×10^{-5a}	

[a] Dose tolerated.

terized by a requirement for high levels of folic acid in the growth medium (Fischer, 1958). Selection was accompanied by an increase in the level of folic acid reductase in cell-free extracts and correlated directly with the degree of resistance. The frequency with which resistant variants appeared and the degree of resistance was found to depend on the concentration of methotrexate used for selection (Table XIII). Levels of resistance of up to 10^5-fold above that of the wild type were obtained. Some variants retained resistance after up to 6 months passage in the absence of amethopterin. Resistant cells retained a requirement for a high concentration of folic acid in the growth medium and their folic acid reductase had the same affinity for folic acid as enzyme from wild-type cells. The excess folic acid reductase may bind essentially irreversibly nearly all the amethopterin entering the resistant cell. Since the entry of amethopterin into the cells was found to be slower than the *de novo* synthesis of folic acid reductase, enough active enzyme may remain in the resistant cells in the presence of amethopterin to supply the cell with reduced folic acid. [Resistance may alternatively be due to a reduced rate of entry of amethopterin (Fischer, 1962).] One clone selected in 2×10^{-8} M amethopterin had an ID_{50} of 5.6×10^{-7} M, a 70-fold increase over that of the parental cells. Uptake of folic acid by this variant was 14-fold reduced compared to the wild type, and the folic acid reductase had an unaltered affinity for amethopterin. Variants having defects in transport of amethopterin, unlike those with elevated folic acid reductase levels, are not cross-resistant to pyrimethamine, another antifolate.

Robins and Courtenay (1970) selected variants of L5178Y cells by continuous exposure to amethopterin. Variants resistant to 4.4×10^{-7} M had their uptake of the inhibitor reduced to 25% that of wild-type cells and retained normal activities of folic acid reductase. A variant resistant to 2.2×10^{-4} M amethopterin had a similarly reduced drug uptake but additionally a 30-fold increase in folic acid reductase activity. A radiation-resistant variant (qv) was 20-fold more resistant to amethopterin than wild-type cells. In a second series of experiments, variants were obtained by growth in suspension with increasing levels of aminopterin, starting at 3.3×10^{-9} M; after 83 days of selection, a variant resistant to 1×10^{-3} M was obtained and cloned in agar (Courtenay and Robins, 1972). The modal chromosome number of the variant was 40, the same as that of the wild type. The folic acid reductase levels of resistant clones were initially increased 100-fold or more, but declined to normal levels after about 100 days in the absence of amethopterin, accompanied by a rapid reduction in resistance.

Reexposure of variants to amethopterin after their folate reductase levels had declined led to a rapid increase in the folic acid reductase levels and the reacquisition of high levels of resistance. By cloning in agar an estimate was made of the number of cells within a population selected for resistance to 2.2×10^{-4} M amethopterin and having an elevated folic acid reductase level that retained a high level of resistance during growth in the absence of amethopterin. The data obtained were compatible with a high reversion rate of 5×10^{-2} per cell per generation.

Aronow (1959) selected variants of L cells, clone 929, by growth in amethopterin 3×10^{-8} M for 2 weeks, 6×10^{-8} M for 6 weeks, and finally 1×10^{-7} M. Growth in the absence of the inhibitor for a period of months resulted in the loss of some resistance, though not a return to wild-type sensitivity. Folic acid was a poor antagonist of amethopterin, but N_5-formyltetrahydrofolic acid was an efficient competitive antagonist. Variants were also obtained resistant up to 1×10^{-5} M amethopterin.

Roosa and Herzenberg (1959), Herzenberg (1961), and Roosa et al. (1962) selected amethopterin-resistant variants of a monolayer culture of P388 cells by serial cultivation in increasing concentrations of amethopterin. Initial selection was carried out at 4×10^{-8} M amethopterin, and subsequentially variants were sequentially selected for resistance to 1×10^{-7} M, 2×10^{-7} M, 8×10^{-7} M, and 8×10^{-6} M. Once obtained, these variants were very stable, retaining their resistance over many months of growth in the absence of amethopterin.

Variants of S180 cells (Foley and Drolet, 1956) were derived by Hakala et al. (1960, 1961) that were resistant to amethopterin. Selection was effected by growth as a monolayer in increasing concentrations of amethopterin from 2×10^{-8} M to 5×10^{-7} M. In two selections either 10^{-4} M hypoxanthine (AH) or 3×10^{-5} M thymidine (AT) were added to the medium. Resistant variants were obtained having a 65-fold (AH) and a 155-fold (AT) increase in folic acid reductase activity over the wild type which correlated well with degree of resistance (Table XIII). The K_m and turnover number of folic acid reductase from wild type and variant cells were identical and the increased dihydrofolate reductase activity of the variants was due to the presence of greater amounts of the normal enzyme. Growth of the variants in the absence of amethopterin was associated with a decrease in resistance and a decrease in folic acid reductase activity, a 50% decrease taking place over 30–40 days. Hakala and Ishihara (1962) found no alteration in the karyotypes of the resistant variants when compared to that of the wild type. At low levels of resistance the increase in folic acid reductase was in direct proportion to the increase in resistance to amethopterin. Proportionality was lost, however, at very high levels of resistance to amethopterin; so additional changes were sought to account for the increased resistance. Hakala (1965) detected no alterations of permeability changes to amethopterin in the S180 variants and suggested that at high levels of enzyme intracellular dissociation of enzyme–amethopterin complexes though slight was significant and the cause of the nonlinear relationship between resistance and folic acid reductase levels in highly resistant variants. The dihydrofolate reductase of highly resistant variants has been purified and characterized (Zakrzewski et al., 1966). It had a molecular weight of 21,000 and migrated as a single peak to the anode at pH 8.7 during free-boundary electrophoresis.

2. Chinese Hamster

Biedler and Albrecht (1971) and Biedler et al. (1972) selected amethopterin-resistant variants from diploid CLM-7 (one variant) and DC3F and its sublcone DC3F8 (eight variants) lines derived from normal Chinese hamster bone marrow and lung tissue, respectively (Biedler and Riehm, 1970b). Wild-type cells were grown in increasing concentrations of amethopterin; the higher the level of amethopterin used for selection, the higher in general was the level of resistance (Table XIII). Each subline remained near-diploid and had an individual rearrangement of karyotype. Folic acid reductase of all resistant variants was at least slightly increased over that of the parental cells, the greatest increase being 170-fold in the variant resistant to 1.1×10^{-4} M. Generally speaking, the higher the level of resistance, the greater the folic acid reductase activity, but there was no consistent relationship between folic acid reductase levels and the degree of resistance to amethopterin. Although in some cases it may have been the primary determinant, the increased enzyme activity was insufficient to wholly explain the resistance. Dose-response data for sensitive and resistant lines demonstrated that while the parental lines reponded identically to amethopterin and methaquin, some but not all of the resistant variants had divergent responses indicating that qualitative as well as quantitative alterations in folic acid reductase had taken place. Partial purification and characterization of enzyme from some of the variants provided evidence of two types of adaptation; the production of increased quantity of parental enzyme and the production of another form of the enzyme insensitive to the effects of amethopterin and with a different pH optimum (Albrecht et al., 1971, 1972).

The latter adaptation was present in the group of variants with relatively little increase in enzyme activity and disparate degrees of resistance to amethopterin and methaquin. The preexistence of small quantities of this newly detected dihydrofolate reductase activity in wild-type cells could not be excluded (particularly since multiple forms of the enzyme are known to exist). Sobel et al. (1971) fused a variant resistant to high levels of amethopterin and high levels of dihydrofolate reductase to a variant of DC3F selected for actinomycin D resistance (qv) having normal levels of dihydrofolate reductase. The dihydrofolate reductase levels of the hybrids were intermediate to those of the parental cells.

3. Human

Vogt (1959) isolated variants of HeLa (Gey et al., 1952) resistant to aminopterin commencing selection at 1×10^{-8} M and increasing gradually to in some cases 1.1×10^{-6} M. The plating efficiency of aminopterin-resistant cells in the presence of aminopterin was unaffected by the addition of wild-type cells to the culture. One variant selected for resistance to increasing concentrations of aminopterin was grown without inhibitor for one period of 30 generations during selection and grew both in the presence and absence of aminopterin. Another variant similarly selected apart from the omission of the period of growth in normal medium was aminopterin dependent; the cloning efficiency in the absence of aminopterin was 1% of that in 3.5×10^{-8} M aminopterin.

4. Pig

Harris and Ruddle (1960) selected variants of PK15 cells resistant to aminopterin at a single step. The frequency of appearance of variants varied with the concentration of lamb serum used. Variants were selected capable of growth at 2.2×10^{-7} M aminopterin by three exposures, each for 1 week, to 2.2×10^{-7} M aminopterin; between each selection the population was allowed to grow up (Harris, 1961). Harris and Ruddle (1961), using cells that had been exposed to X-irradiation and were carrying a chromosome marker, selected aminopterin-resistant variants by a single exposure to 2.2×10^{-7} M aminopterin.

5. Syrian Hamster

Littlefield (1969) selected aminopterin-resistant variants of BHK21/C13 cells (TG- and BUdR-resistant variants were used as the parental cell lines, qv) by cloning twice in aminopterin, initially at 3×10^{-8} M and, after growth to a bulk culture, at 3×10^{-7} M. Clones resistant to the latter level had a 2- to 16-fold increase in level of folic acid reductase. Selection was independent of cell density, but the yield was influenced by the growth phase of the culture at the time of selection (Orkin and Littlefield, 1971). Variants resistant to 3×10^{-8} M aminopterin appeared at a frequency of 2×10^{-4} from logarithmically growing cells, 1.5×10^{-5} from early stationary cells and 1×10^{-6} from late stationary phase cells; perhaps a reflection of variations in the level of folic acid reductase with the phase of the cell cycle, a 25–50% decrease in folic acid reductase level having been detected in confluent cultures of the parental cells. Resistance of the variants decreased in the absence of aminopterin and was accompanied by declining levels of folic acid reductase. Reexposure to the drug led to a rapid return of resistance and return to high levels of dihydrofolic acid reductase. One clone selected for resistance to 3×10^{-5} M aminopterin and which had a 125-fold increase in folic acid reductase levels, was the only clone to retain high levels of reductase activity after prolonged growth in the absence of aminopterin. The elevated activity was not due to a diffusible cofactor since extracts of cells containing high and low levels of folic acid reductase always had intermediate reductase activity when mixed. Fusion of aminopterin-resistant variants with sensitive cells, utilizing the preexisting markers to select hybrid cells in HAT, yielded hybrids having folic acid reductase levels intermediate to those of the parents. Variants were derived resistant to aminopterin concentrations of up to 1×10^{-6} M, in some cases using a two-step procedure, after mutagenesis with either EMS or NG (Orkin and Littlefield, 1971). Unlike the spontaneously derived variants the folic acid reductase levels of variants obtained after mutagenesis was the same as the wild type. Folic acid reductase both from wild-type cells, two spontaneously occurring highly resistant variants, and four variants obtained after mutagenesis had grossly similar kinetics of inhibition by aminopterin. No evidence was found for a difference in permeability between the wild-type cells and any of the variants. The biochemical basis of the resistance to aminopterin in the variants obtained after mutagenesis remains to be established.

G. Puromycin (Table XIV)

Puromycin is structurally similar to the adenosine terminal end of an aminoacyl-tRNA and blocks protein synthesis during transpeptidation by substituting for an incoming aminoacyl-tRNA. Several workers have selected variant cells resistant to puromycin.

TABLE XIV
Variants Resistant to Puromycin

Cell types and references	Selection level (M)	Frequency of variants	ID_{50} (M)
Mouse			
L			
Lieberman and Ove (1959a,b)	Wild type 51	—	$<4 \times 10^{-6}$
	Wild type 52	—	$4-8 \times 10^{-6}$
	Multistep R-1, 1.6×10^{-5}	4×10^{-6} [a]	$2.4-3.2 \times 10^{-5}$
	R-2, 8×10^{-5}	1×10^{-4} [a]	$8 \times 10^{-5}-1.6 \times 10^{-4}$
3T3 TK⁻			
Marin and Pugliatti-Crippa (1972)	2×10^{-4}	—	—
Syrian hamster			
PyY BHK21/C13			
Subak-Sharpe (1965)	Wild type	—	6×10^{-6} [b]
	1st step	—	$6-10 \times 10^{-6}$ [b]
	2nd step	—	$8-10 \times 10^{-5}$ [b]
Pig			
PK15			
Harris (1967a)	Wild type	—	5×10^{-7}
	1st step, 1×10^{-6}	—	1.5×10^{-6}
	2nd step, 4×10^{-6}	—	4.6×10^{-6}
Frog			
Mezger-Freed (1971)	Wild type	—	1×10^{-6}
	ICR2A 5×10^{-7}	$1.1-8.5 \times 10^{-5}$	—
	ICR132 5×10^{-7}	$3.9-4.5 \times 10^{-5}$	—
	ICR132 2×10^{-5}	—	$4 \times 10^{-6}-2 \times 10^{-5}$

[a] Rate of appearance of variants determined by a fluctuation test, expressed per cell per generation.
[b] Threshold of inhibition.

1. *Mouse*

Puromycin-resistant mouse cells were selected by Lieberman and Ove (1959a), who exposed subconfluent monolayer cultures to 1.6×10^{-5} M puromycin. Variants resistant to 8×10^{-5} M were selected from this population at a single step, but it was not possible to select variants resistant to higher concentrations. Resistance was stable after growth in the absence of puromycin. Two subpopulations of parental cells could be distinguished after cloning: one, S1, was highly sensitive to puromycin; the other S2 was less sensitive (Table

XIV). It was suggested that there was an obligatory sequence of at least three steps leading from S1 to the highly resistant variant R2 via S2 and R1.

2. Pig

Harris (1967a), using cloned PK cells, found at least two levels of resistance to puromycin. The frequency of appearance of first-step resistant variants to $1 \times 10^{-6}\, M$ puromycin was determined by a fluctuation test and was greatly influenced by the cell density and the ploidy of the wild-type cells. On increasing the population density during exposure to puromycin while maintaining the cell number per dish constant the number of survivors increased. An octaploid line was least influenced by $7 \times 10^{-7}\, M$ puromycin, colonies appearing 50–100 times more frequently than from diploid cells under the same conditions. A tetraploid line behaved in an intermediate fashion, giving rise to colonies 30 or more times more frequently than the diploid cell line.

3. Frog

Mezger-Freed (1971) investigated the resistance to puromycin of the haploid ICR2A and the pseudodiploid ICR132 lines of frog cells. Clones obtained after selection in $5 \times 10^{-7}\, M$ puromycin had increased resistance to puromycin and, unlike wild-type cells, yielded clones when exposed to $6 \times 10^{-6}\, M$ puromycin. No significant increase in the frequency of clones growing in the presence of $2 \times 10^{-6}\, M$ puromycin was observed after mutagenesis with either EMS or MNNG. However the presence of preexisting variants, which could not be eliminated prior to mutagenesis, may have rendered the assay too insensitive to detect an increase in the frequency of variants due to mutagenesis. Two highly resistant variants were obtained. The first from ICR2A by serial selection in increasing concentrations of puromycin was capable of growth in $2 \times 10^{-5}\, M$ of the drug. Resistance was lost after growth in the absence of puromycin. The second variant was isolated at a single step from ICR132 after exposure to $2 \times 10^{-5}\, M$ puromycin and retained resistance even if grown in the absence of puromycin. The ID_{50} of this variant determined by plating efficiency was between 4×10^{-6} and $2 \times 10^{-5}\, M$ puromycin. Clones of increased resistance were derived from both variants by further selection in higher concentrations of puromycin. The reduction in uptake of radioactively labeled puromycin by the highly resistant variants correlated with the degree of resistance.

H. Actinomycin D (Table XV)

Actinomycin D (AcD) binds to DNA and inhibits RNA transcription.

1. *Chinese Hamster*

Biedler and Schwartz (1968) and Biedler and Riehm (1970a,b), using diploid clones of Chinese hamster cells, DC3F (female) and CLM7 (male) growing as monolayer cultures, derived AcD-resistant variants by growth in gradually increasing concentrations of the inhibitor. Growth in the absence of AcD led to a drop in resistance (Sobel et al., 1971). The greater the resistance, the more frequent was the presence of structurally altered chromosomes noted in the variants of DC3F. Autoradiography after exposure to tritiated AcD indicated that uptake of inhibitor was rapidly reduced as resistance increased. AcD-resistant variants were cross resistant to a number of

TABLE XV
Variants Selected for Resistance to Actinomycin D (AcD)

Cell type and references	Selection level (M)	Frequency of variants	ID_{50} (M)
Chinese hamster			
DC3F and CLM7	Wild-type DC3F	—	1.9×10^{-10}
	DC3F, 8×10^{-9}	—	1.6×10^{-8}
	8×10^{-8}	—	7.2×10^{-8}
Biedler and Riehm (1970a,b)	8×10^{-7}	—	4.8×10^{-7}
	Wild type CLM7	—	1.2×10^{-10}
	CLM 7, 8×10^{-9}	—	9.6×10^{-8}
	8×10^{-8}	—	5.0×10^{-8}
Human			
HeLa			
Goldstein et al. (1960, 1966)	Wild type	—	$>8 \times 10^{-9}$
	8×10^{-9}	—	$>8 \times 10^{-9}$
Goldstein and Zeleny (1969)	3.2×10^{-8}	—	$>3.2 \times 10^{-8}$
	1.2×10^{-7}	—	$>1.2 \times 10^{-7}$
Syrian hamster			
PyY BHK21/13			
Subak-Sharpe (1965)	Wild type	—	3.2–$6.4 \times 10^{-10\,a}$
	1st step	3×10^{-6}	0.8–$1.6 \times 10^{-9\,a}$
	2nd step	—	1.6–$3.2 \times 10^{-9\,a}$
Simard and Cassingena (1969)			
$Cl_1\ TSV_5$-S	Stepwise 8×10^{-8}	—	—

[a] Threshold of complete inhibition of colony formation.

inhibitors, including puromycin and daunomycin. Bosman (1971) compared the charge carried on the surface of the DC3F parental cells and the variant resistant to 8×10^{-7} M AcD. The resistant variant had a greater negative charge, probably owing to increased amounts of sialic acid since there was greater glycoprotein synthesis and increased quantities of glycoprotein and glycolipid in the plasma membrane. The variant also had decreased glycosidase activity and increased glycoprotein–glycosyl transferase activity, both of which would be expected to lead to an increase in glycoprotein. After fusion of an AcD-resistant with an amethopterin-resistant variant of DC3F, hybrids retaining their resistance to AcD could be isolated (Sobel et al., 1971); growth in the absence of AcD led to loss of resistance.

2. Human

Goldstein et al. (1960) selected HeLa cells resistant to AcD. A confluent sheet of cells was exposed to 8×10^{-8} M for 48 hours; surviving cells (less than 75%) were subsequently incubated in normal medium until confluent. The selection procedure was repeated several times, resulting in the production of a variant capable of a normal rate of growth in the presence of 3.2×10^{-7} M AcD and characterized morphologically by the presence of small dense nucleoli. Resistance was not retained after growth in normal medium; after 28 weeks in the absence of AcD the variants were as sensitive as wild-type cells. Autoradiography after treatment with tritiated AcD showed grains over the nuclei of sensitive, but not over those of resistant, cells (Goldstein et al., 1966). The level of resistance was increased by prolonged passage in the presence of increasing concentrations of AcD. Wild-type and resistant cells were fused and after exposue to AcD the polykaryons were stained with either acridine orange or fast green (Golstein and Zeleny, 1969). The characteristic loss of nucleolar RNA and alterations to nucleolar structure in the presence of AcD did not occur in the nuclei of the resistant variant even when a second nucleus within the same polykaryon, but originating from a wild-type cell, was markedly affected. It is therefore suggestive that the basis of resistance was not due to permeability changes in the cell membrane, but was a characteristic of individual nuclei.

3. Syrian Hamster

Subak-Sharpe (1965) selected AcD-resistant variants of PyY cells and found them to be cross-resistant to puromycin. Simard and Cassingena (1969) selected AcD-resistant variants of Cl_1TSV_5-S cells (Tournier et al., 1967) by continuous exposure to gradually increasing concentrations of AcD. With the use of electron microscope autoradiography little difference was found between the degree of nuclear labeling of wild-type and variant cells after incubation with tritiated AcD. To achieve enough incorporation, tritiated AcD concentrations were used above those for which resistance had been selected.

I. CARBOHYDRATE ANALOGS

1. *2-Deoxyglucose*

a. *Human.* Barban (1962a) developed a variant of HeLa S3 resistant to 2-deoxyglucose (2DG) an analog of glucose that is converted by hexokinase (EC 2.7.2.1) to 2-deoxyglucose 6-phosphate (2DG6P), which is inhibitory at several steps in glycolysis (Barban and Schultze, 1961). Growth of wild-type cells was inhibited in the presence of equimolar proportions of glucose and 2DG. During selection, wild-type cells were first grown in suspension culture containing 5×10^{-3} M glucose and 0.2 to 0.5×10^{-3} M 2DG. After 2–3 weeks, surviving cells were cloned in medium containing higher proportions of 2DG, and a variant was obtained capable of growth in the presence of medium containing 10 parts of 2DG to one of glucose. For prolonged growth in 2DG, the variant required the addition of 1×10^{-3} M pyruvate. In comparison with wild-type cells, both the rate of entry 2DG into the variants and its rate of phosphorylation were depressed. An inhibitor of hexokinase was present in extracts of the variant, and increased alkaline phosphatase activity was present in cell-free extracts. Induction of alkaline phosphatase activity by preincubation of wild-type cells with prednisolone or dexamethasone conferred some resistance to 2DG (Barban, 1962b, 1966).

Morrow and De Carli (1967), using cell lines having various levels of alkaline phosphatase activity (Maio and De Carli, 1962; De Carli et al., 1964), confirmed the correlation between alkaline phosphatase level and resistance to 2DG. The ability of cells to grow in the presence of 2DG increased with cell density and the presence of resistant cells protected sensitive ones in cell mixtures. The addition of purified alkaline phosphatase produced an apparent reduction of the hexokinase activity of extracts of sensitive and resistant cells and also of purified yeast hexokinase. The inhibition of hexokinase present in the 2DG-resistant variant derived by Barban (1962b) may have been due to the increased hexokinase activity in the crude cell extracts. The most likely mechanism of resistance, on the basis of the above evidence, is the possession of elevated alkaline phosphatase levels that convert the toxic 2DG6P to the nontoxic 2DG.

b. Pig. Bailey and Harris (1968) isolated 2DG-resistant variants of PK15 cells by selection in medium containing 5×10^{-4} M glucose and 5×10^{-5} M 2DG. Higher levels of 2DG6P were present in sensitive than in resistant cells. Phosphorylation of 2DG took place more rapidly in extracts of resistant than sensitive cells, but alkaline phosphatase was not detectable in extracts of either cell. Resistant cells grew faster than sensitive cells in low glucose medium and may be capable of a more efficient utilization of glucose, possibly through a reduction in the leakage of tricarboxylic acid cycle intermediates from the cells.

J. STEROIDS (Table XVI)

1. *Mouse*

Aronow and Gabourel (1961, 1962) selected a hydrocortisone-resistant variant of a mouse lymphoma cell line, ML-388, that was highly sensitive to anti-inflammatory steroids (Gabourel and Aronow, 1962). After wild-type cells were grown in 1×10^{-6} M hydrocortisone for 4 weeks a population of rapidly growing resistant cells emerged which were resistant to 10^{-5} M hydrocortisone; a 100-fold increase over that of wild-type cells. Resistance was retained after prolonged periods of growth in the absence of hydrocortisone. The variant was cross-resistant to other anti-inflammatory steroids, e.g., corticosterone and dexamethasone.

Hackney *et al.* (1970) using L929 cells, developed variants having a more than 100-fold increased resistance to cortisol by growth at 5×10^{-6} M cortisol for 2 months followed by 1×10^{-5} M cortisol for 19 months. The growth rate was not inhibited by triamcinolone at concentrations of 10^{-5} M, more than 100-fold the concentration totally inhibiting the wild-type cells. The resistant cells bound only 14% as much triamcinolone as the wild-type cells. The variant had not been cloned, and the residual binding may have been due to either high binding by a minority of cells or a low level of binding distributed throughout the whole population of cells.

Baxter *et al.* (1971) and Rosenau *et al.* (1972) selected dexamethasone-resistant variants of a mouse lymphoma line, S49 (Horibata and Harris, 1970; Harris, 1970) by growth in concentrations of dexamethasone increasing from 2×10^{-9} M to 1×10^{-5} M over 20 days. The variant remained resistant to 1×10^{-5} M dexamethasone after culture in the absence of steroid for up to 6 months. The bind-

TABLE XVI
VARIANTS SELECTED FOR RESISTANCE TO STEROIDS

Cell type and references	Selection level (M)	Frequency of variants	ID_{50} (M)
Mouse			
P388, *hydrocortisone*			
Aronow and Gabourel (1961, 1962)	Wild type	–	$\simeq 1 \times 10^{-7}$
	1×10^{-6}	–	1×10^{-5}
L, *cortisol*			
Hackney *et al.* (1970)	Two-step, 1×10^{-5}	–	–
S49, *dexamethasone*			
Harris (1970)	Wild type	–	3×10^{-8}
Rosenau *et al.* (1972)	Multistep, 1×10^{-5}	$\simeq 1 \times 10^{-5}$	–
Sibley and Tomkins (1973)	–	$3 \times 10^{-5\,a}$	–
Human			
U12-79, *hydrocortisone, testosterone, progesterone*			
Grosser and Swim (1958)	Wild type	–	$<3.1 \times 10^{-7}$
	7.8×10^{-5}	–	$<1.5 \times 10^{-5}$
HeLa, *progesterone, testosterone, deoxycorticosterone*			
Stone (1962)	Wild type	–	$<6 \times 10^{-6}$
	3×10^{-5}	–	–

[a] Rate of appearance of variants determined by a fluctuation test, expressed per cell per generation.

ing of dexamethasone by cytosol of the variant was less than 10% of the parental cells. From the kinetics of binding, it was deduced that there were a reduced number of receptors of lower binding affinity in the resistant variant. Such a receptor species may be present in wild-type cells but overshadowed by the major component.

2. *Human*

Grosser and Swim (1957, 1958) selected variants of a human myometrium culture, U12-79, for resistance to either hydrocortisone, testosterone, or progesterone at 8×10^{-5} M. A cortisol-resistant variant metabolized cortisol at least twice as fast as the parental cells, but the increased degradation of cortisol was not considered to be the whole basis of resistance (Grosser *et al.*, 1962).

K. MISCELLANEOUS COMPOUNDS (Table XVII)

1. α-*Amanitin*

α-Amanitin is a specific inhibitor of RNA polymerase II. α-Amanitin resistant variants of CHO cells were obtained by Chan *et* al. (1972). Selection was carried out by cloning in the presence of 1.1×10^{-7} M α-amanitin using nonmutagenized and mutagenized cells. RNA polymerase II isolated from some of the variants was completely resistant to 1.1×10^{-8} M α-amanitin, a concentration that abolished the wild-type enzyme activity assayed under identical conditions. This is good evidence that a structural gene mutation is involved.

2. Chloramphenicol

Chloramphenicol is an inhibitor of protein synthesis. Spolsky and Eisenstadt (1972) selected chloramphenicol-resistant variants of a cloned line of HeLa S3 cells. Wild-type cells were exposed to 5×10^{-7} M ethidium bromide and plated in medium containing from 6.2×10^{-5} M to 1.1×10^{-4} M chloramphenicol. Resistant variants appeared 6–12 weeks after the start of selection; they were grown up and cloned. Individual clones differed in their levels of resistance, some being capable of growth in up to 3.2×10^{-4} M chloramphenicol. Protein synthesis by mitochondria isolated from the variant cells when incubated in 3.2×10^{-4} M chloramphenicol was reduced to 36–48% of the control without choloramphenicol, but to 15% of the control when mitochondria from wild-type cells were used. A modification to the mitochondria of the variant has occurred and confers some resistance to chloramphenicol.

3. Colchicine

Ling and Thompson (quoted in Thompson and Baker, 1973) obtained colchicine-resistant variants of CHO cells with differing levels of resistance by selection in 2.5×10^{-7} M concentration of the drug, a mitotic-spindle poison. Resistant variants were obtained after three selective steps, the cells being mutagenized prior to selection (Till et al., 1973). Highly resistant clones were characterized by a 2-fold increase in their doubling times. Resistance of the variants was retained after growth in the absence of colchicine. Although extracts of most, but not all, the resistant variants bound colchicine normally, the rate of accumulation of the inhibitor from the medium by intact variants was decreased in comparison to the wild type.

4. Concanavalin A (Con A)

Con A, a lectin from jackbeans, binds to the cell surface and has been used to select variant cells. Ozanne and Sambrook (1971) selected variants of SV3T3 cells by exposure to 4.2×10^{-6} M Con A for 24 hours. The majority of cells rounded up and lysed, but about 1×10^{-4} survived. Clones obtained by growth of the survivors in

TABLE XVII
VARIANTS RESISTANT TO MISCELLANEOUS COMPOUNDS

Compounds, cells, and references	Selection level (M)	Frequency of variants	ID_{50} (M)
α-AMANITIN			
Chinese hamster			
CHO			
Chan et al. (1972)	1.1×10^{-7}	$>1 \times 10^{-6}$	—
	Mutagenized, 1.1×10^{-7}	1.8 to 3.0×10^{-5}	—
BIS(2-CHLOROETHYL) SULFIDE			
Mouse			
L			
Walker and Reed (1971)	1.5 μg/ml	—	—
CHLORAMPHENICOL			
Human			
HeLa			
Spolsky and Eisenstadt (1972)	6.2×10^{-5}	—	—
	1.1×10^{-4}	—	—
COLCHICINE			
Chinese hamster			
CHO			
Thompson and Baker (1973)	Wild type		
	2.5×10^{-7}	$\simeq 1 \times 10^{-6}$	$<1.2 \times 10^{-7}$
			—

CONCANAVALIN A			
Mouse			
SV3T3			
Ozanne and Sambrook (1971)	4.2×10^{-6}	$\leqq 1 \times 10^{-4}$	$>1.4 \times 10^{-6}$
Chinese hamster			
CHO			
Siminovitch et al. (1972)	5.6×10^{-7}	$\leqq 1 \times 10^{-5}$	
Wright (1973)	Multistep, 1.1×10^{-6}	—	$>1.1 \times 10^{-6}$
DAUNOMYCIN			
Chinese hamster			
DC3F			
Biedler and Riehm (1970 a,b)	Wild type	—	3×10^{-8}
	Multistep, 3.8×10^{-6}	—	1×10^{-5}
	Multistep, 9.5×10^{-6}	(DC3F/AD, qv AcD)	1.2×10^{-5}
Riehm and Biedler (1971)	2.0×10^{-5}	—	—
DDUG[a]			
S100			
Hakala (1971)	Wild type	—	8×10^{-7}
	1×10^{-5}	—	9×10^{-6}
ETHIDIUM BROMIDE			
Hamster			
F5-1			
Klietman et al. (1972)	5×10^{-6}	—	—

(Continued)

TABLE XVII (*Continued*)

Compounds, cells, and references	Selection level (M)	Frequency of variants	ID_{50} (M)
FLUOROACETATE			
Syrian hamster			
Py6			
Subak-Sharpe (1965)	0.1–0.2%[b]	—	—
	0.3%	—	—
FLUORIDE			
Human			
HeLa			
Carlson and Suttie (1967)	Wild type	—	30 ppm
	95 ppm	—	75 ppm
Mouse			
L			
Quissell and Suttie (1972)	Wild type	—	30 ppm
	80 ppm	—	120 ppm
METHYLENE DIMETHANE SULFATE			
Mouse			
Yoshida tumor			
Szenda and Fox (1973)	Wild type	—	≃2.5 µg/ml
	Multistep, 40 µg/ml	—	≃15 µg/ml
OUABAIN			
Mouse			
L			
Baker and Till (1971)	1×10^{-3}	—	
Ehrlich ascites			
Mayhew (1972)	Wild type	—	3×10^{-4}
	1×10^{-3}	—	

Chinese hamster		
CHO	Wild type	—
Thompson and Baker (1973); Till et al. (1973)	3.0×10^{-3}	—
PHYTOHEMAGGLUTININ		
Chinese hamster		
CHO		
Wright (1973)	180 μg/ml	1×10^{-4}
STREPTOMYCIN		
Mouse		
Mox	5.1×10^{-3}	2×10^{-4}
Metzgar and Moskowitz (1963a)	1.5×10^{-2}	1.4×10^{-7} (cloned)
VINBLASTINE		
Chinese hamster		
V79,129	1.2×10^{-6}	—
V79,B150	1.2×10^{-6}	—
Harris (1973)		
VINCRISTINE		
S180	Wild type	—
Hakala (1971)	1×10^{-7}	—

	—	$\approx 2 \times 10^{-5}$
	—	(5×10^{-4} M K$^+$)
		>600 μg/ml
		—
		—
		6×10^{-2}–6×10^{-3}
		2.4×10^{-1}–1.6×10^{-3}
		5×10^{-9}
		1×10^{-7}

[a] 4:4'-Diacetyl-diphenyl-urea-bisguanylhydrazone
[b] Threshold of complete inhibition of colony formation.

normal medium were subjected to a second cycle of selection. Survivors were recloned and were resistant to 1.4×10^{-6} M Con A. The Con A-resistant variants unless treated with trypsin were flattened and less agglutinable by Con A than SV3T3 cells.

Siminovitch et al. (1972) and Wright (1973) selected variants of CHO cells (grown at 34°C) resistant to Con A. After treatment with MNNG, the cells were exposed to gradually increasing concentrations of Con A over a period of weeks until variants were selected that grew in 1.1×10^{-6} M Con A. Variants were also selected without mutagenesis by a single exposure to 5.6×10^{-7} M Con A. The variants were subsequently cloned. The colony-forming efficiency of two out of four clones at 38.5°C was only 5% in comparison with that at 36°C.

5. *Daunomycin*

Biedler and Riehm (1970a,b) selected daunomycin-resistant variants of DC3F and DC3F/AD (resistant to AcD, qv) Chinese hamster cells by growth in gradually increasing concentrations of the drug. Riehm and Biedler (1971) selected a highly resistant variant by continuous exposure to increasing drug concentrations over a period of 6 months, finally obtaining a variant capable of growth at 2×10^{-5} M daunomycin. There was little uptake of tritiated daunomycin into the nucleus of the variant as determined by autoradiography. A variant was independently obtained by a single exposure of wild-type cells to 2×10^{-5} M of the drug for 72 hours (the 97% effective dose in the standard drug-sensitivity assay) followed by growth on drug free medium. An initial increase in resistance was found but declined after about 100 days, owing either to reversion or to overgrowth of the resistant population by wild-type cells that survived exposure to the inhibitor. It was noted that these variants were cross-resistant to AcD.

6. *4:4'-Diacetyl-diphenyl-urea-bisguanylhydrazone (DDUG)*

Hakala (1971) selected DDUG-resistant variants of S100 cells by growth in concentrations of the inhibitor increasing gradually from 2×10^{-6} M to 1×10^{-5} M over a period of 2 months. Resistance of the variants was unchanged after 2 months growing in drug-free medium. The rate of uptake of DDUG by the variants was reduced about 2-fold.

7. *Fluoride*

Quissell and Suttie (1972), using a multistep procedure, selected variants of L cells capable of growth at 80 ppm fluoride. Growth in the absence of fluoride for 60 days had no effect on the level of resistance. The most likely basis of resistance was an active process removing fluoride from the interior of the cells. The intracellular concentration of fluoride of the variants was low in comparison to that of the wild type after incubation at 37°C, but rose when the temperature was reduced to 0°C.

8. Ouabain

Ouabain is an inhibitor of the cell membrane Na^+/K^+ pump. Baker and Till (1971), Siminovitch et al. (1972), Thompson and Baker (1973), and Till et al. (1973) described the production of variants resistant to ouabain from CHO, 3T3, and L cells. Colonies growing in the presence of 3×10^{-3} M ouabain were picked and in all cases grew normally in this concentration of ouabain after growth to mass culture in normal medium. The frequency of appearance of variants decreased with increasing ouabain concentration used for selection and was increased after mutagenesis. Variants were obtained that varied in resistance from 3- to 30-fold (as defined by the minimum toxic dose) and retained resistance for up to 11 months' growth in the absence of ouabain. The ^{42}K uptake and ATPase activity of the resistant L cells were less affected by ouabain than wild-type cells, but the ATPase activities of the two lines were kinetically indistinguishable.

Mayhew (1972) selected ouabain-resistant variants of Ehrlich ascites cells grown in vitro. After exposure to 1×10^{-3} M ouabain for 3 days, surviving cells were washed and allowed to grow up in normal medium. The selection procedure was repeated three more times, eventually developing a variant capable of growth in the presence of 1×10^{-3} M ouabain. At this concentration of ouabain, although wild-type cells lost K^+ and gained Na^+ the movement of these ions was not affected in the variant, indicating that the basis of resistance was an alteration to the Na^+/K^+ pump of the variant cells.

9. Streptomycin

Metzgar and Moskowitz (1963a) selected variants of Mox cells resistant to streptomycin, an inhibitor of protein synthesis. Five variant clones were passaged for over 4 years both in the presence and in the absence of streptomycin without loss of resistance. When 40 wild-type clones were isolated without selection and tested for the ability to grow in streptomycin, 23 had some degree of resistance. One million cells from each of seven sensitive clones were exposed to streptomycin, but they yielded in all only one resistant colony. The uncloned wild-type population was thus heterogeneous with respect to behavior when grown in streptomycin, about half the cells having some resistance while the remainder were sensitive and gave rise variants at very low frequencies. On subsequent testing, variation in behavior was observed depending on the batch of serum used. Interaction between cells also was a factor influencing growth in streptomycin (Metzgar and Moskowitz, 1963b). Resistant cells failed to grow when mixed with sensitive cells in the presence of streptomycin and in some cases independently isolated variants failed to grow as a mixture in the presence of streptomycin.

10. *Vinblastine*

Harris (1972) selected variants of 129 (HGPRT$^-$, qv) and B150 (TK$^-$, qv) for resistance to vinblastine, a mitotic-spindle poison analogous to colchicine. Utilizing the preexisting markers, hybrids between vinblastine-resistant and vinblastine-sensitive cells were derived by selection in HAT. In all cases examined, hybrids between a vinblastine-resistant variant and a vinblastine-sensitive variant retained resistance. The toxicity of vinblastine for both resistant and wild-type cells was affected by the batch of fetal calf serum used.

IV. Variants with Altered Expression of Antigenic Surface Components or Immunoglobulin Production (Table XVIII)

1. *Mouse*

Cann and Herzenberg (1963a,b) using a clone of ML388, 2B2 (Herzenberg and Roosa, 1960; Herzenberg, 1961), a methylcholanthrene-induced lymphoma of a DBA/2 mouse and homozygous for H-2^d, obtained variants resistant to the cytotoxic effects of anti-H-2^d isoantiserum in the presence of guinea pig complement (C'). Wild-type cells were exposed to C57BL/6J(H-2^b) anti-DBA/2J(H-2^d) isoantiserum and C', and the survivors were allowed to grow up in normal medium. After 14 cycles of selection, 50% of the variant cells survived a half-hour exposure to antiserum that killed 99% of the unselected wild-type cells. The variant was cloned; of eight clones, five grew as well or almost as well after treatment with isoantibody as after exposure to normal serum. By retesting three clones at 3 months and again at 5 months after selection, resistance to antiserum plus complement was shown to be stable. Quantitative adsorption tests indicated that there was less H-2^d isoantigen per variant cell than the

TABLE XVIII
VARIANTS SELECTED FOR ALTERED EXPRESSION OF ANTIGENIC
SURFACE COMPONENTS OR IMMUNOGLOBULIN PRODUCTION

Cell type and references	Antigen selected against	Frequency of variants	Reversion rate
Mouse			
ML 388, 2B2			
Cann and Herzenberg (1963a,b)	H-2^d	Multistep	—
DH1			
Papermaster and Herzenberg (1966)	H-2^d	Multistep	—
MPC-11			
Coffino et al. (1970);	Heavy chain	—	—
Scharff et al. (1970);	Heavy chain	$1.1 \times 10^{-3\,a}$	$<2.6 \times 10^{-4}$
Coffino and Scharff (1971)			
MPC-11 heavy chain$^-$			
Coffino et al. (1971)	Light chain	$1.7 \times 10^{-4\,a}$	$<8 \times 10^{-4}$
Baumal et al. (1973)	Light chain	$4.0 \times 10^{-4\,a}$	—
P3			
Baumal et al. (1973)	Heavy chain	$1.0 \times 10^{-3\,a}$	—
C1			
Baumal et al. (1973)	Heavy and light chain	$2.0 \times 10^{-3\,a}$	—
S49.1TB2			
Hyman (1973)	Thy-1.2, XS63 specificity	Multistep	—
Human			
Fibroblast			
Adman and Pious (1969)	Isoantigen	10^{-5}–10^{-7}	—
RPM1 8866			
Pious et al. (1973)	HL-A2	10^{-5}–10^{-6}	—
Rabbit			
Pious (1966, 1967)	Isoantigen	Multistep	—

^{a} Rate of appearance of variants determined by a fluctuation test, expressed per cell per generation.

wild-type, but, since the variants were larger than the wild-type cells, these results were difficult to assess. Differences in absorption could have been due to alteration of the distribution of antigen on the surface of the cell rather than a reduction in the absolute quantity of antigen.

Papermaster and Herzenberg (1966) selected variants of a lymphoma adapted to grow as a monolayer suspension culture (DH1). The lymphoma had been induced in a (C3H × DBA) F_1 hybrid mouse by methylcholanthrene and therefore carried H-2 /H-2^k antigens. Selection was carried out by incubation with C' and a specific anti-H-2^d antiserum. The few cells that survived this procedure were grown up, and the selection was repeated. The population was passaged, and one year after the original isolation, during which no selection pressure was put on either isoantigen, the variant was resistant to the anti-d but not the anti-k (against which there had been no selection). This variant was the same size as the parental cells.

Coffino et al. (1970, 1972) and Scharff et al. (1970) developed a method for detecting rare variants which had lost this ability to produce immunoglobulins. The parental line used was a murine myeloma (MPC-11), which normally produces IgG_{2b} (Laskov et al., 1971). Wild-type cells were cloned in agar over a feeder layer of primary or secondary mouse fibroblasts and after allowing the cells to grow to form small colonies the culture was overlaid with agar containing rabbit antiserum directed against heavy chains. After 1–3 days the majority of colonies were obscured by a precipitate, but rare colonies had no precipitate. Clones were isolated, grown up, and assayed for their immunoglobulin production. Colonies that had not been surrounded by precipitate neither produced nor secreted heavy chains. The loss of heavy-chain production was inherited; no revertants to heavy-chain production were observed in 26,000 colonies producing light chains. Colony growth and cloning efficiency of wild-type cells were not affected by the presence of antiserum. By a fluctuation test Coffino and Scharff (1971) showed that variants lacking the ability to produce heavy chains arose with a frequency of 1.1×10^{-3} per cell per generation. All these variants continued to produce light chains. Plates overlaid simultaneously with antisera to heavy and light chain yielded no colonies lacking precipitate. It was possible, however, to isolate variants producing no immunoglobulin using variants previously selected for loss of heavy-chain production, at a frequency of less than 1.7×10^{-4} per cell per generation. No reversion to light-chain production was observed in 8000 nonproducing colonies derived from a single clone.

The rate of appearance of variants of MPC-11 not producing heavy chains was increased 2- to 3-fold by treatment with MNNG (Coffino and Scharff, 1971), but was critically dose-dependent (Baumal et al., 1973). Neither X-irradiation nor EMS affected the yield of similar variants under the conditions used. After exposure to the acridine half-mustard ICR191, which induces frame-shift mutations in microorganisms, there was a dose-dependent increase in the yield of variants (Baumal et al., 1973). At doses that killed more than 99% of the wild-type MPC-11 cells more than 6% of the survivors were variants producing only light chains. After similar treatment of variants producing only light chains more than 6% of the survivors were nonproducers. Cytoplasmic extracts of 16 variants producing only light chains isolated after mutagenesis were examined in detail on sodium dodecyl sulfate containing acrylamide gels. Twelve variants produced no detectable heavy chains, similarly to the spontaneously occurring variants, but four produced heavy-chain moieties. Of these four variants, one produced a heavy chain of the same size as that of the parental cells, two produced a heavy chain reduced in size, and the fourth produced a heavy chain of increased size. Differences were detected between the heavy chains of the wild type and all the variants by peptide mapping.

Preud'Homme et al. (1973) found an increase in the frequency of variants producing only heavy chain after treatment of MPC-11 cells with Melphalan (p-[di(chloroethyl)amino]-L-phenylalanine). Reconstruction experiments indicated no selective killing of heavy chain producers by Melphalan. Sixteen of twenty variant clones examined produced no detectable heavy-chain moieties, but four contained defective intracellular immunoglobulin that reacted with anti MPC-11 heavy chain antibody but which lacked the antigenic determinants of the parent protein. The heavy chain produced by one of the latter variants was reduced in size as determined by sodium dodecyl sulfate acrylamide gel electrophoresis and differed in peptide map from wild-type cells. Electrophoresis of extracts of the remaining three variants that reacted with the anti MPC-11 heavy-chain antibody confirmed the production of a modified heavy chain. All subclones of the variants retained the altered characteristics. The high incidence of variants exhibiting altered immunoglobulin production was not accompanied by a similar increase in the frequency of drug-resistant variants in the case of MPC-11 cells (Baumal et al., 1973).

Variants of two other IgG-producing lines, C1 derived from the C3H × 5563 tumor-producing IgG_{2a} and the P_3 line derived from the BALB/C MOPC-21 tumor (Horibata and Harris, 1970) were obtained (Coffino et al., 1972; Baumal et al., 1973). Variants of MPC-11 and P3 producing only light chains were shown by starch gel electrophoresis to contain no detectable intracellular heavy chain. C1 differed in simultaneously losing both heavy- and light-chain production in all 18 variants examined. Hyman (1973) isolated a spontaneous variant of T1M1 not expressing Thy-1.2 by cloning in agar. Also selected was a variant of S49.1TB2, already resistant to thymidine and BUdR (qv), that did not express Thy-1.2. Selection was carried out by short exposures (45 minutes) to antiserum (AKR/J anti-C3H/HeJ normal thymocytes) and C' with intervening periods of growth in normal medium. After four cycles of selection, the population was cloned. One clone showing only partial cytotoxicity in the direct cytotoxicity test was subjected to an additional cycle of selection and then recloned in agar. Five clones were picked, grown up and found to be negative for Thy-1.2 in the direct cytotoxicity test. One variant clone was studied further. Absorption tests indicated that there was 0.04% Thy-1.2 and 15% of $H-2^d$ antigen on the surface of the variant in comparison to the wild type and also a reduction in a specificity defined by a serum made in strain A mice against the variant myeloma XS63 (Hyman et al., 1972). Variants of S49 cells were also selected by treatment with C' and an antiserum to A/XS63 (A/J anti-BALB/c myeloma variant XS63.5). They expressed Thy-1.2, 14% of wild-type $H-2^d$ and lacked detectable A anti-XS63 specificity. The variants were fused in several combinations. The hybrid formed between the two different Thy-1.2 negative variants, one spontaneous (from T1M1), the other selected from S49.1TB2 expressed Thy-1.2; complementation by the two variants indicates that they have different defects resulting in the lack of expression of Thy-1.2. Hybrids formed between the two sublines of T1M1 failed to express Thy-1.2, indicating that fusion per se did not activate expression of the antigen in this parent.

2. *Human*

Adman and Pious (1969) in cases of maternal isoimmunization by fetal cells selected variants of fibroblast cultures from the infant resistant to maternal serum. In this situation, the cells of the infant are obligate heterozygotes at the locus concerned, paternal alleles having led to the isoimmunization. A single exposure to maternal antigen and C' killed 90% of the fibroblasts of the infant. After sufficient time to allow the culture to grow up, the selection was repeated, the concentration of the antiserum being increased with developing resistance. After six exposures, a fully resistant variant was obtained. Similar selection was applied to two other sensitive cell strains from unrelated donors; again variants were obtained after 6–8 cycles of selection. Absorption tests using intact cells demonstrated that the resistant variants, unlike the sensitive wild-type cells, failed to remove antibody from the antiserum suggesting that resistance was due to a loss, probably complete, of surface antigenic receptors. The change was stable within the limits of growth remaining after the selection which was about 20 doublings.

Pious et al. (1973) obtained variants of human lymphoblastoid cells, RPM1 8866, by selecting against alleles of the HL-A system. The HL-A system consists of two linked autosomal loci, LA and Four, linked in turn to the phosphoglucomutase polymorphic system PGM3. All three loci are expressed in human lymphoblastoid cells; the line RPM1-8866 being heterozygous at both HL-A loci (LA: HL-A2,HL-A3; Four: HL-A7, unknown) and also heterozygous at the PGM3 locus. The parental subline retained this phenotype unchanged in the absence of selection, stock cultures being maintained in suspension. Cloning was carried out in agar over a feeder layer of human fibroblasts. For selection, cells were briefly exposed first to HL-A2 antiserum and then to C', after which they were cloned in agar. At low levels of antiserum colony formation decreased with increasing antiserum concentration, but above 25% antiserum 1×10^{-5} to 1×10^{-6} wild-type cells survived. Of the clones appearing after a single treatment with above 25% antiserum 1–15% proved to be variants resistant to HL-A antiserum. Three variants were examined in detail by cytotoxicity testing. All were resistant to HL-A2 antiserum but retained sensitivity to HL-A3 and HL-A7 antisera. The resistance to HL-A2 antiserum was stable for up to 100 generations after cessation of selection. The anti HL-A2 antibody-binding capacity of the variants was reduced 1000-fold in comparison to parental cells giving a similar value to Raji, a line not carrying HL-A2. The loss of HL-A2 was specific since the variants carried similar amounts of HL-A3 and HL-A7 as the parental cells. PGM3 remained heterozygous in all three variants, eliminating the possibility that loss of the whole chromosome carrying HL-A2 was the basis of resistance.

3. Rabbit

Pious (1966, 1967) selected isoantigenic variants of strain TC2 rabbit fibroblasts by exposure to 5% isoantiserum (anti-TC168) and C' for 4 days. The selective medium was then replaced with normal growth medium, and surviving cells allowed to grow up. These survivors (5–0.5%) after a single selection had the same dose-response curve to antiserum as the parental cells, but after the selective procedure was repeated five times, there was no dose-dependent killing of the variant culture. A control culture similarly treated, but exposed only to C' retained complete sensitivity. Variants were isolated in a similar fashion from a cloned line of TC2 by six selective cycles. Resistance was retained by both variants after growth for 56 generations in the absence of selection. The variants absorbed less antiserum than parental cells.

V. Variants with Altered Nutritional Requirements

A. AUXOTROPHS

1. *Human*

DeMars and Hooper (1960) using two lines of HeLa cells, one requiring glutamine but also capable of growth on glutamic acid (HeLa 1-11), the other (HeLa S3-1) prototrophic for glutamine, investigated the possibility of using aminopterin for the selection of auxotrophs. After exposure to 1×10^{-8} M aminopterin for 87 hours in normal growth medium only $1:10^5$ to 10^6 HeLa cells survived to resume growth after removal of aminopterin. Supplementation of the medium with adenine, thymidine, and glycine allowed the cells to grow normally in the presence of aminopterin. Omission of either adenine or thymidine prevented growth, but on reversal of the block at 126 hours growth was reinitiated if adenine had been omitted, but not after omission of thymidine. Cells whose growth was halted by deprivation of arginine survived in the presence of aminopterin without supplementation of the medium and were capable of resuming growth after reversal of the aminopterin block at 120 hours. In an analogous fashion HeLa S3-1, survived exposure to aminopterin if glutamic acid was substituted for glutamine and HeLa 1-11 (capable of utilizing either glutamic acid or glutamine) survived if both were eliminated from the medium. The two lines were mixed in the proportions of 200 HeLa 1-11 to 1 HeLa S3-1 and exposed to growth medium containing glutamine but not glutamic acid in the presence of 10^{-8} M aminopterin for 144 hours. The cultures were then washed free of aminopterin, and surviving cells were grown up in medium containing glutamine but no aminopterin. A culture containing HeLa S1-11 alone was treated in a similar manner. There were many surviving cell clumps in the plate initially seeded with the mixture of cells and much fewer from plates seeded just with HeLa S1-11. Some of these clumps were picked, grown up to large populations, and tested for their growth characteristics. Of twenty samples taken from the plate containing the cell mixture, 19 were unable to grow in medium containing glutamic acid but no glutamine indicating that the selective procedure had favored the HeLa S3-1. One of fifteen populations picked from the HeLa 1-11 plate exposed to the selective conditions was auxotrophic for glutamine and was a newly isolated variant.

2. *Chinese Hamster*

Puck and Kao (1967) using Chinese hamster ovary cells (CHO), a variant auxotrophic for proline, which arose spontaneously (CHO/pro⁻) (Kao and Puck, 1967) and Chinese hamster lung cells (CHL) describe a method of selection for nutritionally deficient cells using a basal medium (Ham, 1965). The CHO/pro⁻ cells reverted to proline independence at a frequency of 1×10^{-6}. Before exposure to selective conditions, cells were grown in medium lacking the component for which auxotrophy was desired, for example, proline. Subsequently the culture was exposed to either tritiated thymidine or BUdR and near-visible light which select against cycling cells. BUdR was added to the culture 24 hours after deprivation of proline and left for 12–24 hours. The culture was subsequently exposed to near-visible light and returned to medium containing proline but not BUdR. In medium lacking proline CHO/pro⁻ cells ceased dividing 18 hours after restriction, but 50% of the cells remained viable for up to 2 days. After exposure of CHO/pro⁻ cells alone to the selective conditions, survival was independent of exposure to BUdR and light since the auxotrophs ceased to cycle prior to exposure to BUdR because of the absence of proline. In reconstruction experiments the phenotypes of cells recovered after exposure of mixtures of CHO and CHO/pro⁻ cells to the selective conditions was as expected from the number of CHO/pro⁻ cells plated and unaffected by the presence of CHO cells.

Kao and Puck (1968, 1969) used the BUdR near-visible light method to select auxotrophs from both CHO/pro⁻ and a variant CHO/pro⁻K1 (with only 20 chromosomes) after mutagenesis. The auxotrophs obtained were completely dependent on the specific nutritional supplements for growth. Proline-independent variants of CHO/pro⁻ were obtained spontaneously at a frequency of 1.3×10^{-6} which could be increased 4-fold after mutagenesis. Kao *et al.* 1969a) carried out a complementation analysis on 13 glycine-requiring auxotrophs of CHO/pro⁻K1 [later extended to 20 (Kao and Puck, 1972)]. All combinations were fused in pairs and the hybrids checked for their ability to grow in medium lacking glycine. The variants fell into four biochemically distinguishable groups. Fusion of variants within groups yielded no cells prototrophic for glycine, but fusion of variants belonging to different groups produced hybrids capable of growth in glycine-deficient medium. In every case variants belonging to group A had less than 5% of wild-type serine hydroxymethylase activity, the other variants had wild-type levels of this enzyme activity. Growth of group B variants, but no others, was stimulated by 2×10^{-4} M folinic acid, the same concentration that reversed 10^{-8} M aminopterin block of wild-type cells. Group B variants may have a deficiency of tetrahydrofolate, though their folic acid reductase activity was normal. The last two groups could be distinguished by their behavior in medium containing both folinic acid and 10^{-5} M glycine, the growth of group C being stimulated slightly but that of group D not at all.

In those auxotrophs so far examined, all the phenotypic changes have behaved in a recessive manner after fusion; 1–2% of the plated cells after fusion of a CHO/gly$^-$ and a CHO/hyp(ade)$^-$ were capable of growing in medium lacking hypoxanthine and glycine (Kao et al., 1969b). In addition, hybrids between CHO-K1/pro$^-$, gly$^-$ and CHL/Pro$^+$, gly$^-$, hyp(ade)$^-$, thy$^-$ were wild type for all markers, indicating that the pro$^-$, hyp(ade)$^-$, thy$^-$ were all recessive and the two gly$^-$ defects complemented each other.

Kao and Puck (1972) describe the isolation of fresh variants of CHL. Eleven CHO-K1 clones auxotrophic for adenine (ade$^-$), including some previously referred to as hyp$^-$, were fused in pairs and hybrids were examined for their abilities to grow in the absence of adenine. The auxotrophs fell into two classes, one (ade A$^-$) complementing all the other ten (ade B$^-$) which failed to complement each other. The two groups could not be distinguished by biochemical criteria, in both cases there being evidence that the block was at some point in the *de novo* synthetic pathway of purines. Hypoxanthine, adenine, adenosine, adenylic acid, adenosine triphosphate, inosine, inosinic acid, and 5-aminoimidazole-4-carboxylic acid were all reported to act as purine sources, while guanine, guanosine, guanylic acid, and xanthine among others could not. Two auxotrophs independently derived (GAT$^-$) each having a requirement for glycine, adenine, and thymidine were fused and did not yield hybrids capable of growth in basal medium. However, fusion of auxotrophs with different requirements, gly A$^-$, gly B$^-$, gly C$^-$, gly D$^-$, ade A$^-$, ade B$^-$, ino$^-$ (auxotrophic for inosine), GAT$^-$, and AT$^-$ (auxotrophic for adenine and thymidine) did yield hybrids capable of growth in basal medium. This also indicates that AT$^-$ and GAT$^-$ have no difference in common, nor any with the other auxotrophs. Complementation between gly A$^-$ and gly B$^-$ auxotrophs was confirmed by Chasin (1972).

Jones and Puck (1973) isolated serine-requiring auxotrophs from a gly A$^-$ clone of CHO-K1 cells after mutagenesis first with EMS and subsequently with an acridine mustard ICR191. Four weeks elapsed both between the mutageneses and also between the second mutagenesis and selection by growth in BUdR followed by exposure to near-visible light.

The chromosomes of CHO cells have been examined (Kao and Puck, 1969) and recently by Deaven and Peterson (1973) the latter using G-band, C-band, and autoradiographic techniques. A karyotype of CHO-K1 has been described (Kao and Puck, 1970). On the basis of both DNA content and chromosomal arm length, the CHO cells have lost 3% of the euploid complement and less than half the chromosomes are normal compared to the euploid Chinese hamster karyotype. Deaven and Peterson (1973) found that extensive changes (translocations, deletions, and pericentric inversions) had occurred in 13 of the 21 chromosomes and also a total loss of the late-replicating X chromosome.

Taylor et al. (1971) found sparse cultures of CHO/pro⁻ cells to be auxotrophic for asparagine in addition to proline. Purine requiring auxotrophs were isolated by modification of the method of Kao and Puck (1968) after mutagenesis with NMMG. The six variants isolated were auxotrophic for a purine source, which may be adenine, hypoxanthine, or, unlike the auxotrophs described by Kao and Puck (1972), glycinamide ribotide or aminomidazole 4-carboxamide. Complementation was observed between all six variants after fusion, and they also grew in the absence of a purine source.

Chu et al. (1967, 1969b) selected glutamine auxotrophs of an aneuploid line of Chinese hamster cells, V79-122D1, using aminopterin as described by DeMars and Hooper (1960). From two separate experiments the survival rate was 3×10^{-4} and 3×10^{-3}. Of 68 colonies isolated, 57 showed an absolute requirement for glutamine when tested immediately after isolation. Reversion was observed in two variants analyzed 4 months after selection and fluctuation tests on one indicated that reversion was occurring randomly at a rate of 1.4×10^{-7} per cell per generation. Chu et al. (1972) selected auxotrophs of V79 cells by exposure to BUdR and black light (300–500 nm). Selection essentially under the conditions of Puck and Kao (1967) and Kao and Puck (1968) produced no auxotrophs in 1180 colonies and reconstruction experiments using artificial mixtures of a variant auxotrophic for glycine, hypoxanthine, and thymidine, ght-1, with wild-type cells were carried out. There was very poor recovery of the auxotroph after exposure of the mixtures of cells to the selective conditions. The ght-1 cells did not survive for 3 days in medium deficient for any one of the three components for which they were auxotrophic. Similar results were obtained using a uridine-requiring and various galactose-negative variants. A systematic examination was made to determine optimal conditions for the selection of auxotrophs of V79 cells. The eventual modifications to the conditions used for CHO cells were the use of Eagle's medium, black light instead of an ordinary fluorescent lamp, and allowing 2 days instead of a week between the quenching of mutagen and inoculation into BUdR. One in 2×10^5 wild-type cells survived this selective procedure. Depending on the nutritional supplement, 0.1–10% of the survivors proved to be auxotrophic variants. Variants unable to grow in galactose instead of frucose were frequently obtained, also auxotrophs for either glycine, purine, or uridine and triple auxotrophs for glycine, hypoxanthine, and thymidine. Galactose-negative variants were obtained at frequencies ranging from 1 to 10% of the clones surviving the selection procedure regardless of prior mutagenization and without exposure to selective conditions. No galactose-negative variants were detected from plates not exposed to BUdR/black light treatment. The BUdR/black light treatment was highly mutagenic when tested for the production of TG-resistant variants, increasing the frequency nearly 10^3-fold above background levels and should be regarded as producing auxotrophs rather than selecting preexisting variants.

B. Variants That Can Utilize a Wider Range of Metabolites Than Can Wild-Type Cells

1. *Mouse*

Hsu and Kellogg (1959) isolated variants of L cells capable of growing on galactose as the carbohydrate source.

Chang (1960) isolated variants of HeLa cells capable of growth in dialyzed medium in which the carbohydrate source was either xylose, ribose, arabinose, lactate, or pyruvate. Also reported were variants of conjunctival cells capable of growth using xylose, ribose, or lactate. Some variant phenotypes were retained after prolonged culture in medium containing glucose, but in many cases growth was poor and unpredictable on return to the selective conditions. Variants studied utilized more of their respective sugars and had an increased sensitivity to deoxyglucose.

Bradley and Syverton (1962) selected two clones of human epithelial cells (Min EE 55-12-1) (Syverton and McLaren, 1957) capable of growth in yeast-treated medium with galactose substituted for glucose as the sole carbohydrate source. One variant was studied in detail. It ceased to grow at a lower density than the wild-type cells and failed to markedly lower the pH of the medium. The ability to grow on galactose was retained after eight subcultures in glucose-containing medium. The variant was also capable of growth in medium containing either added xylose or lactose. Bradley and Syverton (1960) reported a variant capable of utilizing fructose.

It was suggested that the variability noted by Chang (1960) may have been due to differences in the amounts of nondialyzable glucose in individual batches of serum (Bradley and Syverton, 1962).

2. *Chinese Hamster*

Shapiro *et al.* (1972) selected variants from a hyperdiploid clone of Chinese hamster cells (431-8) that were capable of growth in low glucose medium. Selection in Eagle's medium without glucose with 30% dialyzed serum (containing 15–20 μg of glucose per milliliter) yielded variants that could grow in medium containing 10 μg of glucose per milliliter.

3. *Human*

Jacoby and Littlefield (1972) after mutagenesis of a human fibroblast line (deficient in arginosuccinase) with EMS obtained clones able to grow using either homocysteine or cystathionine instead of cyst(e)ine. The biochemical nature of the alterations permitting survival of the two independently isolated variants was not elucidated and neither contained increased amounts of cystathionase.

C. Variants with Reduced Requirements (Table XIX)

1. *Mouse*

Summers and Handschumacher (1971) obtained variants of L5178Y lymphoblasts that ceased to require asparagine for growth. Asparagine-independent variants were selected by exposure of wild-type cells suspended in agar containing medium lacking asparagine (Summers and Handschumacher, 1973). When deprived of arginine, wild-type cells began to lyse within 6 hours while the resistant variants grew to form colonies. Variants arose at a frequency of 9×10^{-7} per cell per generation as determined by a fluctuation test.

2. *Rat*

Morrow (1971) investigated the rate at which variants whose growth was independent of asparagine arose from a population of Walker 256 rat carcinosarcoma cells requiring asparagine. Variants

TABLE XIX
VARIANTS SELECTED FOR GROWTH INDEPENDENT OF ASPARAGINE

Cell type and references	Frequency of variants
Mouse	
LS7784	
Summers and Handschumacher (1971)	1×10^{-6}
Summers and Handschumacher (1973)	9.0×10^{-7} [a]
L5178Y/CA55	
(Momparler *et al.*, 1968)	
Summers and Handschumacher (1973)	2.6×10^{-7} [a]
Rat	
Walker 256 carcinosarcoma	
Morrow (1971)	1.4 to 3.5×10^{-6} [a]
Jensen sarcoma	
Vernick and Morrow (1973)	5.1×10^{-6}

[a] Rate of appearance of variants determined by a fluctuation test, expressed per cell per generation.

were selected by growth of wild-type cells in the absence of asparagine. Most cells degenerated within the first few days, but clones of resistant cells arose at a frequency of 1.4×10^{-6} to 3.5×10^{-6} per cell per generation as determined by a fluctuation test. These variants could be passaged for at least a month in the absence of asparagine.

Vernick and Morrow (1973) selected variants of Jensen sarcoma cells for the ability to grow in the absence of asparagine. The incidence of variants was increased after UV-irradiation of the wild-type cells.

VI. Temperature-Sensitive Conditionally Lethal Cells

1. *Mouse*

Siminovitch (1970) and Thompson *et al.* (1970) described the selection of L-60T cell (Till *et al.*, 1963) variants *ts* for colony-forming ability, growth in suspension, and thymidine uptake. Suspension cultures growing at 33°C were mutagenized with MNNG. Three days later the temperature was raised to 39°C (the nonpermissive temperature) and after 1 day the cells were exposed to tritiated thymidine at 2 μCi/ml for 2 days. Only replicating cells incorporated thymidine and were killed by self-irradiation. The thymidine was then removed and surviving cells grown up as a monolayer culture at 33°C (the permissive temperature). Three more cycles of selection were carried out as suspension cultures using tritiated thymidine, the monolayer cultures being converted to suspension 4 days before selection. A final selection was carried out as a monolayer by exposure to 4×10^{-5} M CAR at 38.5°C to eliminate clones possibly resistant to tritiated thymidine due to the lack of TK. A two-step selection procedure exposing monolayer cultures to tritiated thymidine followed by CAR was also used. Clones with ts characteristics were isolated by both techniques (seven from the first, one from the second) as judged by growth rate, cloning efficiency, and incorporation of precursors of DNA, RNA, and protein into acid-insoluble material at the permissive and nonpermissive temperatures. Three clones were also isolated with questionable ts characteristics. The behavior of the ts variants after shift from the permissive to the nonpermissive temperature (temperature shift) differed and suggested their independent origin. It was not possible to eliminate the possibility that some of the clones originated from a common ts ancestor but diverged during later growth. Recloning of one variant produced nine subclones whose behavior was identical to that of the ts parent, but one divergent clone was also found. Thompson et al. (1971) and Siminovitch et al. (1972) describe a simplified procedure for selecting ts variants. After cloning at the nonpermissive temperature to eliminate preexisting ts variants, wild-type cells were mutagenized with MNNG and survivors grown at 34°C for 5 days, after which the culture, now in exponential growth, was shifted to 38.5°C. At 24 hours after the shift up, tritiated thymidine (2 μCi/ml) was added to the culture; after 3 days fresh medium containing both tritiated thymidine (2 μCi/ml) and 4×10^{-4} M CAR was added and left for two more days. Cells remaining at the end of selection were inoculated into normal growth medium and allowed to grow up at 34°C into clones that could then be picked and passaged independently. After the above selection procedure and also when exposure to CAR and thymidine was reversed, 50% of surviving clones were ts for growth. On testing 1310 clones of L cells after treatment with MNNG, but with no selection by growth at 38°C, 8 were ts for growth to some degree.

The behavior of 13 ts variants that were selected by these different procedures were investigated with respect to colony-forming ability, incorporation of tritiated thymidine, uridine, and leucine at the permissive (34°C) and nonpermissive (38.5°C) temperatures. In four cases the plating efficiency at 34°C was less than 10% of the wild type, perhaps for reasons other than those causing the ts phenotype. One of these four variants together with three others having higher plating efficiencies at 34°C had very low plating efficiencies at

38.5°C but grew in suspension culture at this temperature. In most cases there was a 100-fold reduction in the uptake of thymidine into acid-insoluble material within 24 hours after shifting to 38.5°C, but four variants exhibited little change in thymidine incorporation even 4 days after shift up. Differences were noted between the *ts* variants in the uptake of uridine after shift up while the leucine incorporation was either unchanged or slightly reduced. Clones isolated without selection (eight were examined) had generally higher cloning efficiencies at 34°C than those that had passed through a selective procedure. One spontaneous variant that grew at the nonpermissive temperature in suspension culture exhibited a density dependent *ts* reduction in plating efficiency that was expressed when the variant was seeded at low density. Revertant colonies derived from *ts* variants that grew at the nonpermissive temperature were obtained at a frequency of 10^{-4} to 10^{-6}. When grown up and retested at the nonpermissive temperature, they had a 10^3-fold increased plating efficiency over the parental variant.

Wittes and Ozer (1973) isolated a variant of BALB/c 3T3 clone A1 cells that was *ts* for growth. After mutagenesis with NMMG and growth at the permissive temperature (33°C) for 3 days, the culture was shifted to the nonpermissive temperature (38.5°C). Twenty-four hours after the shift 2 μCi of tritiated thymidine per milliliter was added for 48 hours. The culture was then washed, and survivors allowed to grow up at the permissive temperature in the presence of 10^{-5} M cold thymidine. The selection procedure was repeated from one to three times, after which clones were isolated and grown up independently. One out of ten clones derived from a particular selection was *ts* for growth, having a cloning efficiency of 0.75 to 2% at the permissive temperature but less than 0.002% at the nonpermissive temperature; wild-type cells had plating efficiencies of 7% at both temperatures. Incorporation of uridine and thymidine into both DNA and RNA gradually declined after shift to the nonpermissive temperature. There was considerable incorporation of thymidine by variant cells at the nonpermissive temperature, though the total DNA content of the cells was not changing, perhaps owing to turnover. The time of cessation of growth after shift up was dependent on the culture density at the time of the shift, there being more prolonged growth at higher cell densities.

2. Rat

Loomis *et al.* (1973) selected variants with *ts* properties after treatment with MNNG from a clone (L6D) of the rat myoblast line

L6 (Yaffé, 1968, 1969) which after reaching confluence fuses into multinucleated myotubes and concomitantly accumulates several proteins characteristic of muscle tissue. Thirty-four clones were derived having good growth at 37°C, of which 12 were ts in some aspect of their behavior. Four were ts for growth, being unable to grow at 41°C (the nonpermissive temperature); of these only two remained capable of differentiating into myotubes at 37°C. Six clones were ts for differentiation and grew both at 37°C and 41°C. Five differentiated into myotubes only at 37°C; the sixth could differentiate only at 41°C. Also isolated were two variants that grew at both temperatures but did not differentiate at either. Revertants were obtained from several of these variants. Variants of a similar nature were present in the wild-type population at frequencies below 3%.

3. Chinese Hamster

Thompson and Baker (1973) reported the isolation of variants of CHO cells ts for growth as described by Thompson et al. (1971) except that tritiated thymidine alone was used to select against cells replicating DNA at the nonpermissive temperature. One of these variants has been characterized (Thompson et al., 1973). The variant had a similar doubling time to the wild type at the permissive temperature, but degenerated within 24 hours of shift to the nonpermissive temperature. Treatment with EMS increased the yield of revertants 10-fold, though most remained partially temperature sensitive. Detailed analysis of the variant indicated that within 1 hour of shift up there was a dramatic decrease in protein synthesis; RNA and DNA synthesis were little affected at this time. The leucyl-tRNA synthetase activity in cytoplasmic extracts of the variant, unlike those of the wild type, was temperature sensitive. These data are most simply explained by there being a structural alteration in the leucyl-tRNA synthetase of the variant as a result of a mutation in the structural gene.

Smith and Chu (1973) selected variants ts for growth from a clone of V79-426 Chinese hamster cells which had a high plating efficiency at 41°C (nonpermissive temperature) and at 37°C (permissive temperature). Two spontaneous variants were isolated from nonmutagenized cells and 11 after mutagenesis with EMS, which were ts for growth at the nonpermissive temperature. In most cases the ts phenotype was density dependent, being expressed only after plating at low densities.

Scheffler and Buttin (1973) selected variants of the Dede Chinese hamster line (CCL 39 of the American Type Culture Collection) ts for growth. After mutagenesis with EMS and growth at 34°C (permissive temperature) for 72 hours, the culture was trypsinized and replated at low density. One day later the culture was shifted to 39°C (nonpermissive temperature). The cells were grown in 4.8×10^{-5} M BUdR and 9×10^{-7} M FUdR from 6 to 18 hours after shift up and subsequently were exposed to light and then incubated at 34°C in normal medium. Surviving clones were trypsinized off and pooled after growth for 5 days. The whole selective procedure was repeated three times. One variant ts for growth and colony formation has been studied in detail. Incorporation of thymidine into acid-insoluble material was abolished within 1 day of shift up. Uridine, and to a lesser extent amino acid incorporation, were reduced within 24 hours of shift up. The variant has been cultured under permissive conditions for more than a year without any loss of the ts phenotype, and no revertants have been obtained. After release of a hydroxyurea block at the nonpermissive temperature lasting longer than one cell generation none of the variant cells were viable. After a hydroxyurea block at the permissive temperature for a similar time and simultaneous shift up and release of the block the variant cells were capable of one round of DNA synthesis but not more.

4. Syrian Hamster

Meiss and Basilico (1972) isolated variants ts for growth from BHK21/C13 cells after mutagenesis with either MNNG or EMS. The mutagenized cells were grown at the permissive temperature (33.5°C) for three generations, then shifted to the nonpermissive temperature (38.6°–39°C) for 24 hours before addition of 1.7×10^{-4} M FUdR for 38–48 hours. The surviving cells (0.1%) were washed and grown in fresh medium at 33°C for 2 weeks before subculturing, they were finally reexposed to FUdR at the nonpermissive temperature. Reconstruction experiments using mixtures of ts and wild-type cells indicated that a single FUdR exposure enriched the population 10-fold for ts variants. Of those colonies surviving the selection procedure, 90% were ts for growth to a varying degree. Clones having low reversion frequencies, similar plating efficiencies to the wild type at the permissive temperature and plating efficiencies of less than 10^{-5} at the nonpermissive temperature comprised less than 1% of the surviving clones. In some cases the ts phenotype was dependent on the initial seeding density, being expressed only after plating the variant at low density. Two good variants were also derived using the T6a HGPRT-deficient variant (qv). Three of the variants had a 10-fold increased reversion frequency of the ts phenotype after mutagenesis with NTG. Fusion of the variants *ts* for growth in different combinations and analysis of the growth characteristics of the hybrids indicated five complementation groups. One containing three clones, possibly of common origin, the other groups containing only one variant each.

One variant, 422E, stopped growing within 24 hours of shift up to the nonpermissive temperature and lost colony-forming ability with a half-life of 24 hours on continued exposure to the nonpermissive temperature. Two other variants, AF 8 and BCH, had 75–80% survival even after 3 days at the nonpermissive temperature. Clone 422E, has been examined in detail (Toniolo *et al.*, 1973). The rate of incorporation of uridine and amino acids into acid-insoluble material was unaffected by exposure for 48 hours to the nonpermissive temperature and incorporation of thymidine was depressed slightly. Morphological changes were noted at the nonpermissive temperature, both the cells and the nucleoli enlarging. Examination of cell extracts showed that the variant produced cytoplasmic 28 S rRNA and 60 S ribosomal subunits at the permissive, but not at the nonpermissive, temperature. Cytoplasmic 18 S rRNA and 40 S ribosomal subunit production were normal at both temperatures. No 28 S rRNA was present in nuclear fractions from variant cells exposed to the nonpermissive temperature, indicating a block in the production of rRNA at the 32 S RNA level. After shift up the production of cytoplasmic 28 S RNA dropped exponentially with a half-life of 4 hours; recovery after shift down took 24–28 hours, and only after the appearance of newly synthesized cytoplasmic rRNA did growth resume. Additional evidence was obtained linking the defect in rRNA production with the defect of growth. Revertants selected for the ability to grow at the nonpermissive temperature exhibited normal patterns of rRNA production at that temperature.

Smith and Wigglesworth (1973) reported the isolation of BHK21/C13 variants *ts* for cytokinesis. After mutagenization with MNNG and growth for 24 hours at 31°C, the cultures were shifted up to the nonpermissive temperature (39°C); after 6 hours 3.6×10^{-6} M CAR was added, and incubation was continued for 48 hours. The cultures were then washed and incubated with fresh growth medium at 31°C. Surviving cells grew to form clones. Of 60 clones picked, 20 were *ts* for growth at 39°C. One clone was *ts* for growth when seeded at low cell densities and had a *ts* defect in mitosis. Many cells failed to enter mitosis at the nonpermissive temperature; of those that did enter, a majority did not complete mitosis successfully. There was a defect in cytokinesis in many cases.

5. Monkey

Naha (1969) isolated clones of BS-C-1 monkey kidney cells (Meyer et al., 1962) ts for growth. After mutagenesis with MNNG the cells were grown for 5–7 days in the presence of $4\text{--}5 \times 10^{-6} M$ BUdR at the nonpermissive temperature (39°C), before being exposed to visible light. Surviving cells in fresh medium were then shifted to the permissive temperature (35°C) and after 12–15 days clones isolated. One variant, ts-2, had the same plating efficiency as the wild type at 35°C, but formed colonies neither at 37°C nor 39°C. This clone was deficient in tritiated thymidine uptake in the nucleolus at the nonpermissive temperature judged by autoradiography (Naha, 1970). No defect in incorporation of uridine was noted. Ts-2 reverted to wild type both with respect to growth and metabolic activity after the 12th passage. The optical density of the nucleoli of the variant cells was reduced after incubation at the nonpermissive temperature (35°C) and there was a defect in the ability to either synthesize or process 45 S, 28 S, and 18 S rRNA at the nonpermissive temperature (Naha, 1971). It was suggested that there may be a ts defect in the RNA polymerase activity in the variant and a decrease of activity of crude extracts of RNA polymerase of ts-2 was observed at the nonpermissive temperature (Naha, 1973b). Variants with ts defects in uridine metabolism and in both uridine and thymidine metabolism have also been obtained by means of a modified selection procedure (Naha, 1973a).

VII. Variants Resistant to Physical Agents

1. Heat

Harris (1967b) exposed PK15 cells to 47°C for periods of 90 minutes, reducing the plating efficiency by a factor of 10^5. In some cases selection was repeated up to four times with intervening periods of growth at 37°C to allow the population to recover. Variants were obtained with varying degrees of increased thermotolerance. Passage of the variants for 6 months at 37°C was accompanied in some cases by a reduction in thermotolerance but not a return to wild-type levels. These variants were as sensitive as wild-type cells when tested for their ability to grow at 42.5°C (Harris, 1969). By exposure to 42.5°C for 29 days followed by growth at 37°C, Harris (1969) obtained a variant capable of surviving but not proliferating at 42.5°C. The karyotype of the variant exhibited no gross differences from that of the wild type. Further selection of the variant at 42.5°C for periods up to 122 days did not yield cells capable of growth at the elevated temperature. The variant obtained by prolonged exposure to 42.5°C was no more resistant to an acute exposure to 47°C than wild-type cells. These two types of variant selected in different ways for thermotolerance were each resistant only to the conditions under which they themselves were selected, indicating the utilization of different mechanisms of resistance.

Harris (1971b) found that the frequency with which variants of V79-122D1 Chinese hamster cells surviving an acute heat shock (exposure to 44.5°C for 1 hour) arose differed little between diploid, tetraploid, and octaploid cells.

2. *Ultraviolet Irradiation*

Randtke *et al.* (1972) selected variants of Chang liver cells whose progress into DNA synthesis was sensitive to UV irradiation. A modification of the method used by Puck and Kao (1967) was used. A synchronized culture was given a sublethal dose of UV during the later part of the G_1 phase of the cell cycle. The culture was then exposed to BUdR and subsequently to visible light, and then the survivors were grown up in normal medium. Control cultures similarly treated but not UV-irradiated yielded no colonies. Clones were derived from the UV-irradiated cultures which differed from wild-type cells in doubling time and colony morphology, but not in their X-ray sensitivity. One of these variants had an increase in the width of the shoulder of the dose-response curve to UV. These altered properties were retained during passage for 8 months.

Todd and Hellewell (1969) derived a clone of V79-1 Chinese hamster cells from a population whose sensitivity both to X-irradiation and to UV-irradiation was greater than that of wild-type cells. A decrease in unscheduled synthesis of DNA after UV irradiation (Djordjevic and Tolmach, 1967), which is a reflection of repair replication, was observed in the variant (Cleaver, 1969).

3. *β-Irradiation*

Courtenay (1969) obtained variants of L5178 cells resistant to β-irradiation by continuous irradiation at 4.8 rads/hour from tritiated water added to the medium. In 16 independent selections the growth rate of the cultures suddenly increased between the 39th and 85th day of selection, the culture having been overgrown by resistant variants. The resistance of the variants remained unchanged after growth for 2 months without selection. Immediately after isolation the doubling times of the variants varied from 14.5 to 72 hours, but after continuation of selection for up to one year all had doubling times of less than 19 hours. The continued selective pressure for resistant variants selected the more rapidly growing clones. The variants could be placed into two classes on the basis of dose-response curves after acute X-irradiation and their response to chronic X-irradiation. The first contained variants most resistant to chronic irradiation which showed an increase in the width of the shoulder of the dose-response curve, but little increase in the slope of the expontential part of the curve. The second class had little if any change in the shoulder of the dose-response curve, but a decreased slope of the exponential part of the curve and were not as resistant to chronic irradiation. The two classes of variant probably represent changes in two different mechanisms by which damage to DNA is repaired.

4. X-Irradiation

Rhynas and Newcombe (1960) isolated ten lines of L cells with increased resistance to short exposures to X-irradiation. Over a period of 5 months cultures were given three exposures of 100 r and one of 2000 r. The cultures were allowed to recover between exposures. There was no loss of resistance after growth for up to 35 generations without selection.

Whitfield and Rixon (1960) developed variants of L cells with increased resistance to X-irradiation. After 1000 r between 0.4 and 1.0% of wild-type cells formed clones. Some of these clones had an increased ability to form colonies after irradiation, 5.3% surviving 1000 r. Representatives of these were grown up and irradiated with three more doses of 1000 r at intervals of 15 generations. The variant obtained had an increased resistance over wild-type cells at all doses of X-irradiation, the greatest difference being at 1000 r. There was no additional increase in resistance after multiple selections. Resistance was retained after passage for 2 months in the absence of selection.

5. γ-Irradiation

Courtenay (1965) obtained a variant of the L5178Y mouse lymphoma with increased resistance to γ-irradiation after continuous exposure to 3.0 r/hour for 10 months. There was no difference in the doubling time of the variant and wild-type cells under normal growth conditions. During continuous irradiation the doubling time of the variant increased from 9 to 12 hours. The dose-response curve of the variant to acute doses of X-rays showed both a wider shoulder prior to the exponential region of the curve and also a reduction in the slope of the exponential part of the curve. Two distinct mechanisms may be involved in the development of this variant.

VIII. Spontaneous Variants

No extensive discussion can be entered into on the subject of spontaneous variants that have been observed during prolonged passage of established cell lines without selection; several have been noted in the previous discussion—for example, the CHO/pro⁻ (Puck and Kao, 1967). They are variants that have overgrown the parental population. Spontaneous variants may also be isolated by cloning without the requirement for overgrowth of the population (e.g., Coffino et al., 1970; Thompson et al., 1971).

In a particularly notable paper Povey and co-workers (1973) screened a battery of human lymphoblastoid cell lines at 26 isozyme loci for shifts in isozyme expression. Two spontaneous shifts were noted, the loss of peptidase D activity as it is normally assayed for in a line of F137-D (Jensen et al., 1967) and in one line of JIJOYE (Pulvertaft, 1965), a shift from the normal triple band of APRT to a single band. The variant F137-D line was exposed to either UV irradiation (35 "clones" isolated) or MNNG (80 "clones" isolated) and examined at up to 26 loci. Four changes in isozyme pattern were noted. After MNNG treatment, there was in one case a triple-banded phosphogluconate dehydrogenase, the variant band being more heat stable than the wild type. In a second case a band was lost, the variant being peptidase A2 instead of the parental peptidase A 2-1, and probably indicating a structural alteration to the polypeptide chain. In two cases, one after exposure to MNNG and the other after UV-irradiation a normal pattern of peptidase D reappeared. Many more changes may have occurred since only those that altered the electrophoretic mobility or the activity of the enzyme could be detected.

IX. Conclusions

The preceding summary of the characteristics of biochemically variant mammalian cells isolated in culture underlines both their potential and also the patchy nature of our present knowledge of them. A few selective systems have been thoroughly characterized and extensively studied, but very little is known of the remainder. Each individual variant isolated should be regarded as unique, and extrapolation of results from one system to another should be subjected to experimental verification. Detailed investigation of many variants isolated independently under similar conditions indicates the presence of several phenotypes; moreover, those with the same phenotype may have achieved it in different ways. Our understanding of the mechanisms underlying the appearance of variant mammalian cells in culture is increasing. In a few cases there is powerful evidence that mutations in structural genes may have occurred. Other variants will prove to be the result of epigenetic changes and provide material for investigating the regulatory systems controlling the expression of the genetic information by mammalian cells. Methods which may be used for the investigation of variants have been outlined in Section II. As indicated in the preceding pages, there is an extensive range of phenotypes for which selective systems are presently available in culture. Although the analysis of the variants produced by the selective systems presently available is far from exhausted, there is an obvious need for a greater variety of selective systems, particularly those for which there exists a counterselective system for obtaining revertants. This limitation is partially overcome by the use of variants *ts* for growth of which several examples have been obtained recently.

The rate of appearance of variants resistant to a particular set of selective conditions has been summarized in the tables of this review and the important distinction between the rate of appearance and the frequency of the variants has been made. In those cases in which one of several alterations may lead to the development of resistance to the selective conditions the rate of appearance of variants will be the sum of the separate frequencies of these alterations.

The emphasis of the present review has been to assemble the information available concerning the selection and characteristics of biochemically variant mammalian cells that have been selected in culture. The information is presented in a manner that will encourage the comparison of results obtained in different systems yet also emphasize the unique nature of each variant.

References

Adman, R., and Pious, D. A. (1969). *Science* **168**, 370–372.
Adomaitiene, D. (1971). *Tsitologiya* **13**, 368–373.
Adomaitiene, D., Ignatova, R. N., Podgajetskaya, D. Y., and Gershun, V. A. (1970). *Tsitologiya* **12**, 457–464.
Albertini, R. J., and DeMars, R. (1970). *Science* **169**, 482–485.
Albertini, R. J., and DeMars, R. (1973). *Mutat. Res.* **18**, 199–224.
Albrecht, A. M., Biedler, J. L., and Hutchinson, D. J. (1971). *Proc. Amer. Ass. Cancer Res.* **12**, 77.
Albrecht, A. M., Biedler, J. L., and Hutchinson, D. J. (1972). *Cancer Res.* **32**, 1539–1546.
Aronow, L. (1959). *J. Pharmacol. Exp. Ther.* **127**, 116–121.
Aronow, L., and Gabourel, J. D. (1961). *Biochem. Pharmacol.* **8**, 73.
Aronow, L., and Gabourel, J. D.(1962). *Proc. Soc. Exp. Biol. Med.* **111**, 348–349.

Atkins, J. H., and Gartler, S. M. (1968). *Genetics* **60**, 781–792.
Attardi, B., and Attardi, G.(1972a). *Proc. Nat. Acad. Sci. U. S.* **69**, 129–133.
Attardi, B., and Attardi, G. (1972b). *Proc. Nat. Acad. Sci. U. S.* **69**, 2874–2878.
Ayad, S. R., and Fox, M. (1968). *Nature (London)* **220**, 35–38.
Bach, M., K. (1969). *Cancer Res.* **29**, 1036–1044.
Bailey, P. J., and Harris, M. (1968). *J. Cell. Physiol.* **71**, 23–32.
Bakay, B., Croce, C. M., Koprowski, H., and Nyhan, W. L. (1973). *Proc. Nat. Acad. Sci. U. S.* **70**, 1998–2002.
Baker, R. M., and Till, J. E. (1971). *Annu. Meet., 15th, Biophys. Soc., New Orleans* p. 283a. (Abstr.)
Barban, S. (1962a). *J. Biol. Chem.* **237**, 291–295.
Barban, S. (1962b). *Biochim. Biophys. Acta* **65**, 376–377.
Barban, S. (1966). *Biochim. Biophys. Acta* **115**, 197–204.
Barban, S., and Schultze, H. O. (1961). *J. Biol. Chem.* **236**, 1887–1890.
Basilico, C., Matsuya, Y., and Green, H. (1969). *J. Virol.* **3**, 140–145.
Baumal, R., Birshtein, B. K., Coffino, P., and Scharff, M. D. (1973). *Science* **182**, 164–166.
Baxter, J. D., Harris, A. W., Tomkins, G. M., and Cohn, M. (1971). *Science* **171**, 189–191.
Beaudet, A. L., Roufa, D. J., and Caskey, C. T. (1973). *Proc. Nat. Acad. Sci. U. S.* **70**, 320–324.
Bennett, L. L., Brockman, R. W., Schnebli, H. P., Chumley, S., Dixon, G. J., Schabel, F. M., Dulmadge, E. A., Skipper, H., Montgomery, J. A., and Thomas, H. J. (1965). *Nature (London)* **205**, 1276–1279.
Bennett, L. L., Schnebli, M. P., Vail, M. H., Allan, P. W., and Montgomery, J. A. (1966a). *Mol. Pharmacol.* **2**, 432–443.
Bennett, L. L., Vail, M. H., Chumley, S., and Montgomery, J. A. (1966b). *Biochem. Pharmacol.* **15**, 1719–1728.
Berebbi, M., and Barski, G. (1971). *C. R. Acad. Sci., Ser. D* **272**, 351–354.
Biedler, J. L., and Albrecht, A. M. (1971). *Proc. Amer. Ass. Cancer Res.* **12**, 42.
Biedler, J. L., and Riehm, H. (1970a). *Proc. Amer. Ass. Cancer Res.* **11**, 8.
Biedler, J. L., and Riehm, H. (1970b). *Cancer Res.* **30**, 1174–1184.
Biedler, J. L., and Schwartz, H. S. (1968). *In Vitro* **4**, 155.
Biedler, J. L., Albrecht, A. M., Hutchinson, D. J., and Spengler, B. A. (1972). *Cancer Res.* **32**, 153–161.
Blair, D. G. R., and Hall, A. D. (1965). *Can. J. Biochem.* **43**, 1857–1877.
Blair, D. G. R., Peesker, S. J., and Cross, D. C. (1970). *Can. J. Microbiol.* **16**, 775–781.
Bosman, H. B. (1971). *Nature (London)* **233**, 566–569.
Bradley, S. G. (1962). *Approaches Genet. Anal. Mammalian Cells, Mich. Conf. Genet.* pp. 47–54.
Bradley, S. G., and Syverton, J. T. (1960). *Proc. Soc. Exp. Biol. Med.* **103**, 215–221.
Bradley, S. G., and Syverton, J. T. (1962). *Exp. Cell Res.* **27**, 25–30.
Breslow, R. E., and Goldsby, R. A. (1969). *Exp. Cell Res.* **55**, 339–346.
Bridges, B. A., and Huckle, J. (1970). *Mutat. Res.* **10**, 141–151.
Bridges, B. A., Huckle, J., and Ashwood-Smith, M. J. (1970). *Nature (London)* **226**, 184–185.
Brockman, R. W. (1963). *Advan. Cancer Res.* **7**, 129–234.
Brockman, R. W. (1969). *In* "Exploitable Molecular Mechanisms and Cancer." M. D. Anderson Hospital and Tumor Institute, pp. 435–463. Williams & Wilkins, Baltimore, Maryland.

Brockman, R. W., Kelley, G. G., Stutts, P., and Copeland, V. (1961). *Nature (London)* **191**, 469–471.
Brockman, R. W., Roosa, R. A., Law, L. W., and Stutts, P. (1962). *J. Cell. Comp. Physiol.* **60**, 65–84.
Bürk, R. R., and Subak-Sharpe, J. H. (1968). *Heredity* **23**, 162.
Bürk, R. R., Subak-Sharpe, J. H., and Hay, J. (1966). *Heredity* **21**, 343.
Cann, H. M., and Herzenberg, L. A. (1963a). *J. Exp. Med.* **113**, 259–266.
Cann, H. M., and Herzenberg, L. A. (1963b). *J. Exp. Med.* **117**, 267–284.
Carlson, J. R., and Suttie, J. W. (1967). *Exp. Cell Res.* **45**, 415–422.
Chan, T. S., Ishii, K., Long, L., and Green, H. (1973). *J. Cell. Physiol.* **81**, 315–322.
Chan, V. L., Whitmore, G. F., and Siminovitch, L. (1972). *Proc. Nat. Acad. Sci. U. S.* **69**, 3119–3123.
Chang, R. S. (1960). *J. Exp. Med.* **111**, 235–254.
Chasin, L. A. (1972). *Nature (London), New Biol.* **240**, 50–52.
Chasin, L. A. (1973). *J. Cell. Physiol.* **82**, 299–308.
Chu, E. H. Y. (1970). *In* "Chemical Mutagenesis in Mammals and Man" (F. Vogel and G. Röhrborn, eds.), pp. 241–250. Springer-Verlag, Berlin and New York.
Chu, E. H. Y. (1971). *In* "Chemical Mutagens, Principles and Methods for Their Detection" (A. Hollaender, ed.), pp. 411–444. Plenum, New York.
Chu, E. H. Y., and Malling, H. V. (1968a). *Proc. Int. Congr. Genet. 12th,* **1**, 102.
Chu, E. H. Y., and Malling, H. V. (1968b). *Proc. Nat. Acad. Sci. U. S.* **61**, 1306–1312.
Chu, E. H. Y., Merriam, E. V., and Brimer, P. (1967). *Genetics* **56**, 550.
Chu, E. H. Y., Brimer, P., and Malling, H. V. (1969a). *Genetics* **61**, $_s$10.
Chu, E. H. Y., Brimer, P., Jacobson, K. B., and Merriam, E. V. (1969b). *Genetics* **62**, 359–377.
Chu, E. H. Y., Sun, N. C., and Chang, C. C. (1972). *Proc. Nat. Acad. Sci. U. S.* **69**, 3459–3463.
Chu, M. Y., and Fischer, G. A. (1962). *Biochem. Pharmacol.* **11**, 423–430.
Chu, M. Y., and Fischer, G. A. (1965). *Biochem. Pharmacol.* **17**, 333–341.
Clayton, D. A., and Teplitz, R. L. (1972). *J. Cell Sci.* **10**, 487–493.
Cleaver, J. E. (1969). *Int. J. Radiat. Biol.* **16**, 277–285.
Clements, G. B. (1972). Ph.D. Thesis, Univ. of Glasgow, Glasgow.
Clive, D., Flamm, W. G., Machesko, M. R., and Bernheim, N. J. (1972). *Mutat. Res.* **16**, 77–87.
Coffino, P., and Scharff, M. D. (1971). *Proc. Nat. Acad. Sci. U. S.* **68**, 219–223.
Coffino, P., Laskov, R., and Scharff, M. D. (1970). *Science* **167**, 186–188.
Coffino, P., Baumal, R., Laskov, R., and Scharff, M. D. (1972). *J. Cell. Physiol.* **79**, 429–460.
Cohen, E. P., and Eagle, H. (1961). *J. Exp. Med.* **113**, 467.
Courtenay, V. D. (1965). *Int. J. Radiat. Biol.* **9**, 581–592.
Courtenay, V. D. (1969). *Radiat. Res.* **38**, 186–203.
Courtenay, V. D., and Robins, A. B. (1972). *J. Nat. Cancer Inst.* **49**, 45–53.
Croce, C. M., Bakay, B., Nyhan, W. L., and Koprowski, H. (1973a). *Proc. Nat. Acad. Sci. U. S.* **70**, 2590–2594.
Croce, C. M., Litwack, G., and Koprowski, H. (1973b). *Proc. Nat. Acad. Sci. U. S.* **70**, 1268–1272.
Daniel, V., Litwack, G., and Tomkins, G. M. (1973). *Proc. Nat. Acad. Sci. U. S.* **70**, 76–79.
Davidson, E. A. (1964). *Advan. Genet.* **12**, 143–280.

Davidson, J. D., Bradley, T. R., Roosa, R. A., and Law, L. A. (1962). *J. Nat. Cancer Inst.* **29**, 789–800.
Davidson, R. L. (1972). *Proc. Nat. Acad. Sci. U. S.* **69**, 951–955.
Davidson, R. L., and Bick, M. D. (1973). *Proc. Nat. Acad. Sci. U. S.* **70**, 138–142.
Davidson, R. L., Ephrussi, B., and Yamamoto, K.(1966). *Proc. Nat. Acad. Sci. U. S.* **56**, 1437–1440.
Davidson, R. L., Ephrussi, B., and Yamamoto, K. (1968). *J. Cell. Physiol.* **72**, 115–128.
Dawe, C. J., and Potter, M. (1957). *Amer. J. Pathol.* **33**, 603.
Deaven, L. L., and Peterson, D. F. (1973). *Chromosoma* **41**, 129–144.
De Carli, L. L., Maio, J. J., Nuzzo, F., and Benerecetti, A. S. (1964). *Cold Spring Harbor. Symp. Quant. Biol.* **29**, 223–231.
DeMars, R., and Held, K. R. (1972). *Humangenetik* **16**, 87–110.
DeMars, R., and Hooper, J. L. (1960). *J. Exp. Med.* **111**, 559–572.
Djordjevic, B., and Szybalski, W. (1960). *J. Exp. Med.* **112**, 509–531.
Djordjevic, B., and Tolmach, J. E. (1967). *Radiat. Res.* **32**, 327.
Dubbs, D. R., and Kit, S. (1964). *Exp. Cell Res.* **33**, 19–28.
Dubbs, D. R., and Kit, S. (1968). *J. Virol.* **2**, 1272–1282.
Dubbs, D. R., and Kit, S. (1970). *Int. J. Cancer* **6**, 223–233.
Dubbs, D. R., Kit, S., deTorres, R. A., and Anken, M. (1967). *J. Virol.* **1**, 968–969.
Eagle, H. (1959). *Science* **130**, 432.
Eagle, H. (1965). *Science* **148**, 42–51.
Elkind, M. M., and Sutton, H. (1960). *Radiat. Res.* **13**, 556–593.
Fischer, G. A. (1958). *Ann. N. Y. Acad. Sci.* **76**, 673–680.
Fischer, G. A. (1959). *Cancer Res.* **19**, 372–376.
Fischer, G. A. (1961). *Biochem. Pharmacol.* **7**, 75–80.
Fischer, G. A. (1962). *Biochem. Pharmacol.* **11**, 1233–1237.
Fischer, G. A. (1971). *Nat. Cancer Inst., Monogr.* **31**, 131–134.
Fischer, G. A., and Sartorelli, A. C. (1964). *Methods Med. Res.* **10**, 247–262.
Foley, G. E., and Drolet, D. P. (1956). *Proc. Soc. Exp. Biol. Med.* **92**, 347.
Ford, D. K., and Yerganian, G. (1958). *J. Nat. Cancer Inst.* **21**, 393–425.
Fox, M. (1971). *Mutat. Res.* **13**, 403–419.
Fox, M., and Fox, B. W. (1967). *Cancer Res.* **27**, 1805–1812.
Fox, M., and Gilbert, C. W. (1966). *Int. J. Radiat. Biol.* **11**, 339–347.
Freed, J. J., and Mezger-Freed, L. (1970). *Proc. Nat. Acad. Sci. U. S.* **65**, 337–344.
Freed, J. J., and Mezger-Freed, L. (1973). *J. Cell. Physiol.* **82**, 199–212.
Fujimoto, W. Y., Subak-Sharpe, J. H., and Seegmiller, J. E. (1971). *Proc. Nat. Acad. Sci. U. S.* **68**, 1516–1519.
Gabourel, J. D., and Aronow, L. (1962). *J. Pharmacol. Exp. Ther.* **136**, 213.
Gartler, S. M. (1967). *Nat. Cancer Inst. Monogr.* **26**, 167–178.
Gartler, S. M., and Pious, D. A. (1966). *Humangenetik* **2**, 83–114.
Gey, G. O., Coffman, W. D., and Kubicek, M. T. (1952). *Cancer Res.* **12**, 264–265.
Gillin, F. D., Roufa, D. J., Beaudet, A. L., and Caskey, C. T. (1972). *Genetics* **72**, 239–252.
Gilman, A. G., and Minna, J. D. (1973). *J. Biol. Chem.* **248**, 6610–6617.
Goldsby, R. A., and Zipster, E. (1969). *Exp. Cell Res.* **54**, 271–275.
Goldstein, M. N., and Zeleny, V. (1969). *J. Cell Biol.* **43**, 44a.
Goldstein, M. N., Slotnick, I. J., and Journey, L. J. (1960). *Ann. N. Y. Acad. Sci.* **89**, 474–483.
Goldstein, M. N., Hamm, K., and Amrod, E. (1966). *Science* **151**, 1555–1556.

Gorer, P. A. (1950). *Brit. J. Cancer* **4**, 372.
Grosser, B. I., and Swim, H. E. (1957). *J. Lab. Clin. Med.* **50**, 820–821.
Grosser, B. I., and Swim, H. E. (1958). *Proc. Amer. Ass. Cancer Res.* **2**, 304.
Grosser, B. I., Sweat, M. L., Berliner, D. L., and Dougherty, T. F. (1962). *Arch. Biochem. Biophys.* **96**, 259–264.
Hackney, J. F., Gross, S. R., Aronow, L., and Pratt, W. B. (1970). *Mol. Pharmacol.* **6**, 500–512.
Hakala, M. T.(1957). *Science* **126**, 255.
Hakala, M. T. (1965). *Biochim. Biophys. Acta* **102**, 198–209.
Hakala, M. T. (1971). *Biochem. Pharmacol.* **20**, 81–95.
Hakala, M. T., and Ishihara, T. (1962). *Cancer Res.* **22**, 987–992.
Hakala, M. T., and Taylor, E. (1959). *J. Biol. Chem.* **234**, 126–128.
Hakala, M. T., Zakrzewski, S. F., and Nichol, C. A. (1960). *Proc. Amer. Ass. Cancer Res.* **3**, 115.
Hakala, M. T., Zakrzewski, S. F., and Nichol, C. A. (1961). *J. Biol. Chem.* **236**, 952–958.
Ham, R. G. (1965). *Proc. Nat. Acad. Sci. U. S.* **53**, 288–293.
Hamerton, J. L., Douglas, G. R., Gee, P. A., and Richardson, B. J. (1973). *Cytogenet. Cell Genet.* **12**, 128–135.
Hampar, B., Derge, J. G., Martos, L. M., and Walker, J. L. (1971). *Proc. Nat. Acad. Sci. U. S.* **68**, 3185–3189.
Hampar, B., Derge, J. G., Martos, L. M., and Walker, J. L. (1972). *Proc. Nat. Acad. Sci. U. S.* **69**, 78–82.
Harris, A. W. (1970). *Exp. Cell Res.* **60**, 341–353.
Harris, A. W., and Cohn, M. (1970). In "Developmental Aspects of Antibody Formation and Structure" (J. Sterzl and I. Riha, eds.), Vol. 1, pp. 275–279 Academic Press, New York.
Harris, M. (1961). *J. Nat. Cancer Inst.* **26**, 13–18.
Harris, M. (1964). "Cell Culture and Somatic Variation." Holt, New York.
Harris, M. (1967a). *J. Nat. Cancer Inst.* **38**, 185–192.
Harris, M. (1967b). *Exp. Cell Res.* **46**, 301–314.
Harris, M. (1969). *Exp. Cell Res.* **56**, 382–386.
Harris, M. (1971a). *Exp. Cell Res.* **66**, 329–336.
Harris, M. (1971b). *J. Cell. Physiol.* **78**, 177–184.
Harris, M. (1972). *J. Cell. Physiol.* **80**, 119–128.
Harris, M. (1973). *J. Nat. Cancer Inst.* **50**, 423–429.
Harris, M., and Ruddle, F. H. (1960). In "Cell Physiology of Neoplasia," pp. 524–542. Univ. of Texas Press, Austin.
Harris, M., and Ruddle, F. (1961). *J. Nat. Cancer Inst.* **26**, 1405–1411.
Herzenberg, L. A. (1961). *J. Cell. Comp. Physiol.* **60**, Suppl. 1, 145–157.
Herzenberg, L. A., and Roosa, R. A. (1960). *Exp. Cell Res.* **21**, 430–438.
Higgins, M. L., Tillman, C., Leach, K. K., Melnykovych, G., and Leach, F. R. (1969). *Tex. Rep. Biol. Med.* **27**, 1013–1026.
Hinuma, A. Y., Konn, M., Yamaguchi, J., Wudarski, D. J., Blakeslee, J. R., Jr., and Grace, J. T., Jr. (1967). *J. Virol.* **1**, 1045–1051.
Horibata, K., and Harris, A. W. (1970). *Exp. Cell Res.* **60**, 61–77.
Hsu, T. C. (1961). *Int. Rev. Cytol.* **12**, 69–161.
Hsu, T. C., and Kellogg, D. S. (1959). *Symp. Fundam. Cancer Res.* **13**, 183–204.
Hsu, T. C., and Merchant, D. J. (1961). *J. Nat. Cancer Inst.* **26**, 1075–1081.
Hsu, T. C., and Somers, C. E. (1962). *Exp. Cell Res.* **26**, 404–410.

Hu, F., and Lesney, P. F. (1964). *Cancer Res.* **24**, 1634–1643.
Huberman, E., and Heidelberger, C. (1972). *Mutat. Res.* **14**, 130–132.
Huberman, E., Aspiras, L., Heidelberger, C., Grover, P. L., and Sims, P. (1971). *Proc. Nat. Acad. Sci. U. S.* **68**, 3195–3199.
Humphrey, R. M., and Hsu, T. C. (1965). *Tex. Rep. Biol. Med.* **23**, Suppl., 321–336.
Hutchinson, D. J. (1963). *Advan. Cancer Res.* **7**, 235–349.
Hyman, R. (1973). *J. Nat. Cancer Inst.* **50**, 415–422.
Hyman, R., Ralph, P., and Sarkar, S. (1972). *J. Nat. Cancer Inst.* **48**, 173–184.
Ignatova, T. N., Blinova, M. I., and Kislova, N. M. (1968a). *Tsitologiya* **10**, 743–749.
Ignatova, T. N., Blinova, M. I., and Kislova, N. M. (1968b). *Tsitologiya* **10**, 1198–1202.
Jacoby, L. B., and Littlefield, J. W. (1972). *Exp. Cell Res.* **69**, 447–449.
Jensen, E. M., Korol, W., Dittmar, S. L., and Medrek, T. J. (1967). *J. Nat. Cancer Inst.* **39**, 745–752.
Jones, C., and Puck, T. T. (1973). *J. Cell. Physiol.* **81**, 299–304.
Kao, F. T., and Puck, T. T. (1967). *Genetics* **55**, 513–524.
Kao, F. T., and Puck, T. T. (1968). *Proc. Nat. Acad. Sci. U. S.* **60**, 1275–1281.
Kao, F. T., and Puck, T. T. (1969). *J. Cell. Physiol.* **74**, 245–258.
Kao, F. T., and Puck, T. T. (1970). *Nature (London)* **228**, 329–332.
Kao, F. T., and Puck, T. T. (1972). *J. Cell. Physiol.* **80**, 41–50.
Kao, F. T., Chasin, L., and Puck, T. T. (1969a). *Proc. Nat. Acad. Sci. U. S.* **64**, 1284–1291.
Kao, F. T., Johnson, R. T., and Puck, T. T. (1969b). *Science* **164**, 312–314.
Kelley, G. G., Vail, M. H., Adamson, D. J., and Palmer, E. A. (1961). *Amer. J. Hyg.* **73**, 231–235.
Kelly-Garvert, F., and Legator, M. S. (1973). *Mutat. Res.* **17**, 223–229.
Khalizev, A. E., Petrova, O. N., and Shapiro, N. I. (1966). *Genetics (USSR)* N12, 18–24.
Khalizev, A. E., Petrova, O. N., Luss, E. V., Varshaver, N. B., and Shapiro, N. I. (1969). *Genetics (USSR)* N1, 58–65.
Kit, S., and Hsu, T. C. (1961). *Biochem. Biophys. Res. Commun.* **5**, 120–124.
Kit, S., and Minekawa, Y. (1972). *Cancer Res.* **32**, 2277–2288.
Kit, S., Dubbs, D. R., Piekarski, L. J., and Hsu, T. C. (1963). *Exp. Cell Res.* **31**, 297–312.
Kit, S., Dubbs, D. R., and Frearson, P. M. (1966). *Int. J. Cancer* **1**, 19–30.
Kit, S., Kaplan, L. A., Leung, W.-C., and Trukula, D. (1972). *Biochem. Biophys. Res. Commun.* **49**, 1561–1567.
Kit, S., Leung, W. C., and Kaplan, A. (1973). *Eur. J. Biochem.* **39**, 43–48.
Klebe, R. J., Chen, T. R., and Ruddle, F. H. (1970). *J. Cell Biol.* **45**, 74–82.
Klein, G. (1963). *In* "Methodology in Mammalian Genetics" (W. J. Burdette, ed.), pp. 407–468. Holden-Day, San Francisco, California.
Klein, G., Bregula, U., Wiener, F., and Harris, H. (1971). *J. Cell Sci.* **8**, 659–672.
Klietman, W., Kato, K., Sato, N., and Koprowski, H. (1972). *Fed. Proc., Fed. Amer. Soc. Exp. Biol.* **31**, 620. (Abstr.)
Koyama, H., Yatabe, I., and Ono, T. (1970). *Exp. Cell Res.* **62**, 455–463.
Laskov, R., Lanzerotti, R., and Scharff, M. D. (1971). *J. Mol. Biol.* **56**, 327–339.
LePage, G. A. (1963). *Cancer Res.* **23**, 1202–1206.
Levisohn, S. R., and Thompson, E. B. (1973). *J. Cell. Physiol.* **81**, 225–232.
Lieberman, I., and Ove, P. (1959a). *Proc. Nat. Acad. Sci. U. S.* **45**, 867–872.
Lieberman, I., and Ove, P. (1959b). *Proc. Nat. Acad. Sci. U. S.* **45**, 872–877.
Lieberman, I., and Ove, P. (1960). *J. Biol. Chem.* **235**, 1765–1768.
Lin, C. C., Chang, T. D., and Niewczas-Late, V. (1971). *Can. J. Genet. Cytol.* **13**, 9–13.

Littlefield, J. W. (1963). *Proc. Nat. Acad. Sci. U. S.* **50**, 568–576.
Littlefield, J. W. (1964a). *Cold Spring Harbor Symp. Quant. Biol.* **29**, 161–166.
Littlefield, J. W. (1964b). *Nature (London)* **203**, 1142–1144.
Littlefield, J. W. (1965). *Biochim. Biophys. Acta* **95**, 14–22.
Littlefield, J. W. (1969). *Proc. Nat. Acad. Sci. U. S.* **62**, 88–95.
Littlefield, J. W. (1970). *In* "Genetic Concepts and Neoplasia," M. D. Anderson Hospital and Tumor Institute, pp. 439–453. Williams & Wilkins, Baltimore, Maryland.
Littlefield, J. W., and Basilico, C. (1966). *Nature (London)* **211**, 250–252.
Littlefield, J. W., and Sakar, P. S. (1964). *Fed. Proc., Fed. Amer. Soc. Exp. Biol.* **23**, 169.
Long, C., Chan, T., Levytska, V., Kusano, T., and Green, H. (1973). *Biochem. Genet.* **9**, 283–297.
Loomis, W. F., Wahrmann, J. P., and Luzzati, D. (1973). *Proc. Nat. Acad. Sci. U. S.* **70**, 425–429.
Luria, S. E., and Delbrück, M. (1943). *Genetics* **28**, 491–511.
McBride, O. W., and Ozer, A. L. (1973). *Proc. Nat. Acad. Sci. U. S.* **70**, 1258–1262.
Maio, J. J., and De Carli, L. L. (1962). *Nature (London)* **196**, 600–601.
Marin, G., and Littlefield, J. W. (1968). *J. Virol.* **2**, 69–77.
Marin, G., and Pugliatti-Crippa, L. (1972). *Exp. Cell Res.* **70**, 253–256.
Matsuya, Y., and Green, H. (1969). *Science* **163**, 697–698.
Mayhew, E. (1972). *J. Cell. Physiol.* **79**, 441–452.
Meiss, H. K., and Basilico, C. (1972). *Nature (London), New Biol.* **239**, 66–68.
Metzgar, D. P., Jr., and Moskowitz, M. (1963a). *Exp. Cell Res.* **30**, 379–387.
Metzgar, D. P., Jr., and Moskowitz, M. (1963b). *Exp. Cell Res.* **30**, 388–392.
Meyer, H. M., Jr., Hopps, H. E., Rogers, N. G., Brooks, B. E., Bernheim, B. C., Jones, W. P., Nisalak, A., and Douglas, R. D. (1962). *J. Immunol.* **88**, 796–806.
Mezger-Freed, L. (1971). *J. Cell Biol.* **51**, 742–751.
Mezger-Freed, L. (1972). *Nature (London), New Biol.* **235**, 245–246.
Miggiano, V., Nabholz, M., and Bodmer, W. (1969). *Wistar Institute Symp. Monogr.* **7**, 61–76.
Miller, O. J., Miller, D. A., Allderdice, P. W., Dev, V. G., and Grewal, M. S. (1971). *Cytogenetics* **10**, 338–346.
Minna, J., Nelson, P., Peacock, J., Glazer, D., and Nirenberg, M. (1971). *Proc. Nat. Acad. Sci. U. S.* **68**, 234–239.
Mohit, B., and Fan, K. (1971). *Science* **171**, 75–77.
Momparler, R. L., Chu, M. Y., and Fischer, G. A. (1968). *Biochim. Biophys. Acta* **161**, 481–493.
Moore, A. E., Sabachewsky, L., and Toolan, H. W. (1955). *Cancer Res.* **15**, 598–602.
Moore, G. E. (1964). *Exp. Cell Res.* **36**, 422–423.
Morris, N. R., and Fischer, G. A. (1960). *Biochim. Biophys. Acta* **42**, 183–184.
Morris, N. R., and Fischer, G. A. (1961). *Fed. Proc. Fed. Amer. Soc. Exp. Biol.* **20**, 358.
Morris, N. R., and Fischer, G. A. (1963). *Biochim. Biophys. Acta* **68**, 84–92.
Morris, N. R., Reichard, P., and Fischer, G. A. (1963). *Biochim. Biophys. Acta* **68**, 93–99.
Morrow, J. (1964). *Genetics* **50**, 270.
Morrow, J. (1970). *Genetics* **65**, 279–287.
Morrow, J. (1971). *J. Cell. Physiol.* **77**, 423–426.
Morrow, J. (1972). *Genetics* **71**, 429–438.
Morrow, J., and DeCarli, L. (1967). *Exp. Cell Res.* **47**, 1–11.
Morrow, J., Colofiore, J., and Rintoul, L. D. (1973). *J. Cell. Physiol.* **81**, 97–100.

Murayama, F., and Okada, Y. (1970). *Biken J.* **13**, 1–9.
Murayama-Okabayashi, F., Okada, Y., and Tachibana, T. (1971). *Proc. Nat. Acad. Sci. U. S.* **68**, 38–42.
Naha, P. M. (1969). *Nature (London)* **223**, 1380–1381.
Naha, P. M. (1970). *Nature (London)* **228**, 166–168.
Naha, P. M. (1971). *Proc. Int. Conf. Cell Differentiation, Amsterdam, 1st*, pp. 171–176.
Naha, P. M. (1973a). *Nature (London), New Biol.* **241**, 13–14.
Naha, P. M. (1973b). *J. Cell Sci.* **12**, 839–845.
Nakano, N. (1966). *Tohoku J. Exp. Med.* **88**, 69.
Nyormoi, O., Sinclair, J. H., and Klein, G. (1973). *Exp. Cell Res.* **82**, 241–251.
Oda, M., and Puck, T. T. (1961). *J. Exp. Med.* **113**, 599–609.
Ohno, S. (1972). *J. Med. Genet.* **9**, 254–263.
Orkin, S. H., and Littlefield, J. W. (1971). *Exp. Cell Res.* **69**, 174–180.
Ozanne, B., and Sambrook, J. (1971). *In* "The Biology of Oncogenic Viruses" (L. G. Silvestri, ed.), pp. 248–257. North-Holland Publ., Amsterdam.
Papermaster, B. W., and Herzenberg, L. A. (1966). *J. Cell. Physiol.* **67**, 407–420.
Pasternak, C. A., Fischer, G. A., and Handschumacher, R. E. (1961). *Cancer Res.* **21**, 110–117.
Pasztor, L. M., and Hu, F. (1971). *Cytobios* **4**, 145–152.
Pasztor, L. M., and Hu, F. (1972). *Cancer Res.* **32**, 1769–1774.
Pekhov, A. P., Stolyarova, L. G., and Ershikova, Y. E. (1970). *Byull. Eksp. Biol. Med.* **69**, 91.
Peters, R. A. (1951). *Proc. Roy. Soc., Ser. B* **139**, 143–170.
Pious, D. A. (1966). *Fed. Proc., Fed. Amer. Soc. Exp. Biol.* **25**, 372.
Pious, D. A. (1967). *Genetics* **56**, 601–612.
Pious, D., Hawley, P., and Forrest, G. (1973). *Proc. Nat. Acad. Sci. U. S.* **70**, 1397–1400.
Pitot, J. C., Peraino, C., Morse, P. A., and Potter, V. A. (1964). *Nat. Cancer Inst., Monogr.* **12**, 229.
Pitts, J. D. (1971). *Growth Contr. Cell Cult., Ciba Found. Symp.* pp. 89–98.
Pontecorvo, G. (1971). *Nature (London)* **230**, 367–369.
Pontén, J., Jensen, F., and Koprowski, H. (1963). *J. Cell. Comp. Physiol.* **61**, 145–154.
Povey, S., Gardiner, S. E., Watson, B., Mowbray, S., Harris, H., Arthur, E., Steel, C. M., Belenkinsop, C., and Evans, H. J. (1973). *Ann. Hum. Genet.* **36**, 247–266.
Preud'Homme, J-L., Buxbaum, J., and Scharff, M. D. (1973). *Nature (London)* **245**, 320–322.
Puck, T. T. (1960). *Progr. Biophys. Biophys. Chem.* **10**, 237–258.
Puck, T. T., and Fischer, H. W. (1956). *J. Exp. Med.* **104**, 427–434.
Puck, T. T., and Kao, F.-T. (1967). *Proc. Nat. Acad. Sci. U. S.* **58**, 1227–1234.
Pulvertaft, R. J. V. (1964). *Lancet* **i**, 238–240.
Pulvertaft, R. J. V. (1965). *J. Clin. Pathol.* **18**, 261–271.
Quissell, D. O., and Suttie, J. W. (1972). *Amer. J. Physiol.* **223**, 596–603.
Randtke, A. S., Williams, J. R., and Little, J. B. (1972). *Exp. Cell Res.* **70**, 360–364.
Rappaport, H., and DeMars, R. (1973). *Genetics* **75**, 335–345.
Reichard, P. R. (1968). "The Biosynthesis of Deoxyribose," Ciba Lecture. Wiley, New York.
Reichard, P. R., Canellakis, Z. N., and Canellakis, E. J. (1961). *J. Biol. Chem.* **236**, 2514.
Rhynas, P. O. W., and Newcombe, H. B. (1960). *Exp. Cell Res.* **21**, 326–331.
Riehm, H., and Biedler, J. L. (1971). *Cancer Res.* **31**, 409–412.

Robins, A. B., and Courtenay, V. D. (1970). *Biochem.* **118**, 34P.
Roosa, R. A., and Herzenberg, L. A. (1959). *Proc. Amer. Ass. Cancer Res.* **3**, 58.
Roosa, R. A., Brockman, R. W., and Law, L. W. (1961). *Proc. Amer. Ass. Cancer Res.* **3**, 262.
Roosa, R. A., Bradley, T. R., Law, L. W., and Herzenberg, L. A. (1962). *J. Cell. Comp. Physiol.* **60**, 109–126.
Rosenau, W., Baxter, J. D., Rousseau, G. G., and Tomkins, G. M. (1972). *Nature (London), New Biol.* **237**, 20–24.
Rothschild, A., and Black, P. H. (1970). *Proc. Nat. Acad. Sci. U. S.* **67**, 1042–1049.
Rothschild, H., and Black, P. H. (1973). *J. Cell. Physiol.* **81**, 217–224.
Roy-Burman, P. (1970). In "Recent Results Cancer Res." Vol. 25. Springer-Verlag.
Ruddle, F. H. (1972). *Advan. Hum. Genet.* **3**, 173–235.
Ryan, F. J. (1962). *Approaches Genet. Anal. Mammalian Cells, Mich. Conf. Genet.* pp. 1–10.
Sanford, K. K., Earle, W. R., and Likely, G. D. (1948). *J. Nat. Cancer Inst.* **9**, 229–246.
Sato, K., Slesinski, R. S., and Littlefield, J. W. (1972). *Proc. Nat. Acad. Sci. U. S.* **69**, 1244–1248.
Scaletta, L. J., Rushforth, N. B., and Ephrussi, B. (1967). *Genetics* **57**, 107–124.
Scharff, M. D., Bargellesi, A., Baumal, R., Buxbaum, J., Coffino, P., and Laskov, R. (1970). *J. Cell. Physiol.* **76**, 231–348.
Scheffler, I. E., and Buttin, G. (1973). *J. Cell. Physiol.* **81**, 199–216.
Sekiguchi, T., and Sekiguchi, F. (1973). *Exp. Cell Res.* **77**, 391–403.
Shapiro, N. I., Petrova, O. N., and Khalizev, A. E. (1968). *Proc. Int. Congr. Genet., 12th*, **1**, 98.
Shapiro, N. I., Khalizev, A. E., Luss, E. V., Marshak, M. I., Petrova, O. N., and Varshaver, N. B. (1972). *Mutat. Res.* **15**, 203–214.
Sharp, J. D., Capecchi, N. E., and Capecchi, M. R. (1973). *Proc. Nat. Acad. Sci. U. S.* **70**, 3145–3149.
Shin, S., Caneva, R., Schildkraut, C. L., Klinger, H. P., and Siniscalco, M. (1973). *Nature (London), New Biol.* **241**, 194–196.
Shows, T. B. (1970). *Amer. J. Hum. Genet.* **22**, 43a.
Shows, T. B. (1971). *Fed. Proc., Fed. Amer. Soc. Exp. Biol.* **30**, 458.
Shows, T. B. (1972). *Proc. Nat. Acad. Sci. U. S.* **69**, 348–352.
Sibley, C. H., and Tomkins, G. M. (1973). *Proc. Int. Congr. Genet., 13th*, Abstr. p. 253.
Simard, R., and Cassingena, R. (1969). *Cancer Res.* **29**, 1590–1597.
Siminovitch, L. (1970). *Can. Med. Ass. J.* **103**, 875–879.
Siminovitch, L., Thompson, L. H., Mankovitz, R., Baker, R. M., Wright, J. A., Till, J. E., and Whitmore, G. F. (1972). *Proc. Can. Cancer Res. Conf.* **9**, 59–75.
Sinclair, W. K. (1964). *Radiat. Res.* **21**, 584–611.
Sinclair, W. K. (1973). *Radiat. Res.* **55**, 41–57.
Sinclair, W. K., and Morton, R. A. (1963). *Nature (London)* **199**, 1158–1160.
Sinclair, W. K., and Morton, R. A. (1965). *Biophys. J.* **5**, 1–25.
Smith, B. J., and Wigglesworth, N. M. (1973). *J. Cell. Physiol.* **80**, 253–260.
Smith, D. B., and Chu, E. H. Y. (1972). *Cancer Res.* **32**, 1651–1657.
Smith, D. B., and Chu, E. H. Y. (1973). *Mutat. Res.* **17**, 113–120.
Smith, J. D., Barnett, L., Brenner, S., and Russell, R. L. (1970). *J. Mol. Biol.* **54**, 1–14.
Sobel, J. S., Albrecht, A. M., Riehm, H., and Biedler, J. L. (1971). *Cancer Res.* **31**, 297–307.

Spolsky, C. M., and Eisenstadt, J. M. (1972). *FEBS (Fed. Eur. Biochem. Soc.) Lett.* **25**, 319-324.
Spurná, V., and Nebola, M. (1971). *Folia Biol. (Prague)* **17**, 290-298.
Stoker, M., and Macpherson, I. (1964). *Nature (London)* **203**, 1355-1357.
Stone, D. (1962). *Endocrinology* **71**, 233-237.
Subak-Sharpe, J. H. (1965). *Exp. Cell Res.* **38**, 106-119.
Subak-Sharpe, J. H. (1969). *Homeostatic Regulators, Ciba Found. Symp.* pp. 275-288.
Subak-Sharpe, J. H., Bürk, R. R., and Pitts, J. D. (1966). *Heredity* **21**, 342.
Subak-Sharpe, J. H., Bürk, R. R., and Pitts, J. D. (1969). *J. Cell Sci.* **4**, 353-367.
Summers, W. P., and Handschumacher, R. E. (1971). *Biochem. Pharmacol.* **20**, 2213-2220.
Summers, W. P., and Handschumacher, R. E. (1973). *Cancer Res.* **33**, 1775-1779.
Suzuki, F., Kashimoto, M., and Horikawa, M. (1971). *Exp. Cell Res.* **68**, 476-479.
Syverton, J. T., and McLaren, L. C. (1957). *Cancer Res.* **17**, 923.
Szende, B., and Fox, M. (1973). *Chem. Biol. Interactions* **6**, 19-24.
Szybalski, W. (1959). *Exp. Cell Res.* **18**, 588-591.
Szybalski, W., and Smith, M. J. (1959). *Proc. Soc. Exp. Biol. Med.* **101**, 662-666.
Szybalski, W., and Szybalska, E. H. (1962). *Approaches Genet. Anal. Mammalian Cells, Mich. Conf. Genet.* pp. 11-27.
Szybalski, W., Szybalska, E. H., and Brockman, R. W. (1961). *Proc. Amer. Ass. Cancer Res.* **3**, 272.
Szybalski, W., Szybalska, E. H., and Ragni, G. (1962). *Nat. Cancer Inst., Monogr.* **7**, 75-89.
Szybalski, W., Ragni, G., and Cohn, N. K. (1964). In "Cytogenetics of Cells in Culture" (R. J. C. Harris, ed.), Symposia of the International Society for Cell Biology, Vol. 3, pp. 209-221. Academic Press, New York.
Taylor, M. W., Souhrada, M., and McCall, J. (1971). *Science* **172**, 162-163.
Terasima, T., and Tolmach, L. J. (1963). *Science* **140**, 490-492.
Thompson, E. B., Tomkins, G. M., and Curran, J. F. (1966). *Proc. Nat. Acad. Sci. U. S.* **56**, 296-303.
Thompson, L. H., and Baker, R. M. (1973). *Methods Cell Physiol.* **6**, 209-281.
Thompson, L. H., Mankovitz, R., Baker, R. M., Till, J. E., Siminovitch, L., and Whitmore, G. F. (1970). *Proc. Nat. Acad. Sci. U. S.* **66**, 377-384.
Thompson, L. H., Mankovitz, R., Baker, R. M., Wright, J. A., Till, J. E., Siminovitch, L., and Whitmore, G. F. (1971). *J. Cell. Physiol.* **78**, 431-440.
Thompson, L. H., Harkins, J. L., and Stanners, C. R. (1973). *Proc. Nat. Acad. Sci. U. S.* **70**, 3094-3098.
Till, J. E., Whitmore, G. F., and Gulyas, S. (1963). *Biochim. Biophys. Acta* **72**, 277-289.
Till, J. E., Baker, R. M., Brunette, D. M., Ling, V., Thompson, L. H., and Wright, J. A. (1973). *Fed. Proc., Fed. Amer. Soc. Exp. Biol.* **32**, 29-33.
Todaro, G., and Green, H. (1963). *J. Cell Biol.* **17**, 299-313.
Todd, P. W. (1968). *Mutat. Res.* **5**, 173-183.
Todd, P. W., and Hellewell, A. B. (1969). *Mutat. Res.* **7**, 129-132.
Toliver, A., and Simon, E. H. (1967). *Exp. Cell Res.* **45**, 603-617.
Tomizawa, S., and Aronow, L. (1960). *J. Pharmacol. Exp. Ther.* **128**, 107-114.
Toniolo, D., Meiss, H. K., and Basilico, C. (1973). *Proc. Nat. Acad. Sci. U. S.* **70**, 1273-1277.
Tournier, P., Cassingena, R., Wicker, R., Coppey, J., and Suarez, H. (1967). *Int. J. Cancer* **2**, 117-132.

Van Zeeland, A. A., vanDiggelen, M. C. E., and Simons, J. W. I. M. (1972). *Mutat. Res.* **14**, 355–363.
Vaughan, M. H., and Steele, M. W. (1971). *Exp. Cell Res.* **69**, 92–96.
Vernick, D., and Morrow, J. (1973). *Mutat. Res.* **18**, 225–231.
Vogt, M. (1959). *Genetics* **44**, 1257–1270.
Walker, I. G., and Reid, B. D. (1971). *Cancer Res.* **31**, 510–515.
Watson, B., Gormley, I. P., Gardiner, S. E., Evans, H. J., and Harris, H. (1972). *Exp. Cell Res.* **75**, 401–409.
Westerveld, A., Visser, R. P. L. S., and Freeke, M. A. (1971). *Biochem. Genet.* **5**, 591–599.
Whitfield, J. F., and Rixon, R. H. (1960). *Exp. Cell Res.* **19**, 531–538.
Wittes, R. E., and Ozer, H. L. (1973). *Exp. Cell Res.* **80**, 127–136.
Wright, J. A. (1973). *J. Cell Biol.* **56**, 666–675.
Yaffé, D. (1968). *Proc. Nat. Acad. Sci. U. S.* **61**, 477–483.
Yaffé, D. (1969). *Curr. Top. Develop. Biol.* **4**, 37–77.
Zakrzewski, S. F., Hakala, M. T., and Nichol, C. A. (1966). *Mol. Pharmacol.* **2**, 423–431.

THE ROLE OF DNA REPAIR AND SOMATIC MUTATION IN CARCINOGENESIS

James E. Trosko[1] and Ernest H. Y. Chu

Department of Human Development, Michigan State University, East Lansing, Michigan; and Department of Human Genetics, University of Michigan Medical School, Ann Arbor, Michigan

I. Introduction	391
II. Mutagenicity of Chemical Carcinogens	393
III. Molecular Basis for Mutagenesis and Carcinogenesis.	395
A. Genetic and Environmental Predispositions.	395
B. Mutagenesis	397
C. Carcinogenesis.	397
D. Genetic Basis for Mutagenesis and Carcinogenesis	399
IV. DNA Damage and Its Repair.	400
A. Initiation of DNA Damage	400
B. DNA Repair Enzymes in Eukaryotic Cells	402
V. Factors Influencing DNA Repair.	407
A. Developmental Factors	407
B. Environmental Factors	409
C. Biochemical Control of Cell Division	412
D. Developmental Consequences of Differential DNA Repair in Eukaryotic Cells.	415
VI. Evolutionary Perspectives of Somatic Mutagenesis	417
VII. Summary and Conclusion	419
References	420

I. Introduction

The concept that neoplasms arise from mutations in somatic cells was postulated (Boveri, 1929; Bauer, 1928) long before there was a knowledge of either the molecular structure of genetic material, the chemical nature of carcinogens, or interaction between cellular DNA and carcinogenic agents. The idea was originally introduced to account for two striking features of cancerous growth in man—the unlimited variety of tumor types and the fact that, on cell division, the daughter cells maintain their neoplastic properties. For a time, it was thought theoretically impossible to prove or disprove the somatic mutation theory of tumor causation, since the acid test of a mutation, by Mendelian analysis, could not be applied to somatic cells

[1] Recipient of RCDA No. CA 24085-03 from the National Institutes of Health.

(Haldane, 1934). Indirect methods of testing the theory were meanwhile attempted. The first approach is to analyze cancer incidence curves with respect to age so as to determine whether a mathematical formula could be found to fit the data, on the assumption of a sequence of random mutations. The second indirect approach is to seek a correlation between mutagenic and carcinogenic action among chemical compounds that were already known to have one or the other property.

It was found that in the case of experimental carcinogenesis in mice, two consecutive random mutations are needed (Charles and Luce-Clausen, 1942; Iverson and Arley, 1950) and 5–6 mutations for cancer development (Fisher and Hollomon, 1951; Nordling, 1953; De Waard, 1964). Knudson (1971) showed that human retinoblastoma is caused by two mutational events. In the dominantly inherited form, one mutation is inherited via germinal cells and the second occurs in somatic cells. In the nonhereditary form, both mutations occur in somatic cells. The data collected by Knudson fit very well with theoretical expectations. However, this only means that the theory of multiple random mutations for cancer development is consistent with the mathematical expression; it does not afford proof that the theory is correct.

In the early 1950s, several thousand chemical compounds had already been tested for carcinogenic activities in animals, of which more than 300 had been found to be carcinogenic (cf. Hartwell, 1951; Shubik and Hartwell, 1959, 1969). Among these, only a dozen or so had been tested for mutagenic action in bacteria, fruit flies, and higher plants. Burdette (1955) reviewed the evidence and concluded that there was no correlation between the mutagenic and carcinogenic activities of those chemicals which had been assayed for both types of activities. In 1955, very little was known with regard to the structure of ultimate reactive forms of chemical carcinogens *in vivo*, but Burdette recognized that lack of correlation could have been due, among other factors, to differences in the metabolic fates of the chemicals in different test organisms.

Since that time, considerable progress has been made in a number of areas of experimental biology, so that a reevaluation of the possible role of somatic mutation in carcinogenesis appears pertinent. These developments include (a) technical improvements in mammalian cytogenetics, (b) modern understanding of repair of DNA damage and the chemical basis of mutagenesis, (c) knowledge of the active forms of chemical carcinogens *in vivo*, and (d) refined systems for testing carcinogenicity and mutagenicity. In this review, we shall attempt to summarize the progress in some of these areas as they may bear directly or indirectly on the role of somatic mutations in carcinogenesis. The possible relationship between chromosome abnormalities and carcinogenesis has been ably treated in recent reviews (Levan, 1969; Koller, 1972) and will not be discussed here. The reader is also referred to a recent excellent paper by Comings (1973), who proposed a general genetic theory of carcinogenesis.

II. Mutagenicity of Chemical Carcinogens

Experimental mutagenesis by a pure chemical agent was first reported in 1944 by Auerbach and Robson, and a variety of such agents are now known. Their mechanism of action is fairly well understood as consisting of expressible, heritable changes in the genetic material (Drake, 1969, 1970). The understanding of the chemical basis of mutation has enhanced the acceptance of the somatic mutation theory of carcinogenesis as an intellectually satisfying theory for the mechanisms of chemical carcinogenesis (Clayson, 1962).

A mutational model system for the study of carcinogenesis is based on the assumption that certain types of mutations in a somatic cell increase the probability that this cell will transform into a neoplastic cell. This increase in susceptibility is the result of a direct reaction of the carcinogen with a biological target molecule, probably DNA. The problem may be approached by at least two types of studies: (1) studies to explore the nature of interaction between the carcinogen and biological molecules, and (2) studies to use biological test systems for assaying the mutagenicity of carcinogens.

In the past decade, considerable progress has been made leading to the recognition that many chemical carcinogens are not active as such but require conversion *in vivo* to metabolites, which are the ultimate carcinogenic forms. Furthermore, in a number of cases, positive correlations have been obtained between the level of protein — or nucleic acid — carcinogen interreaction and the likelihood of tumor development. Mainly through the work of J. A. Miller and E. C. Miller (see reviews, 1969, 1971), it was concluded that most, if not all, chemical carcinogens either are strong electrophilic (i.e., containing relatively electron-deficient forms) reactants as administered, or are converted to potent electrophilic reactants *in vivo*. This generalization not only provides a unified view for the action of structurally diverse chemical carcinogens, but also predicts some uniformity in the sites on the cellular macromolecules susceptible to their attack.

As electrophiles or potential electrophiles, the carcinogens have common nucleophilic targets, which include the guanine, adenine, and cytosine bases and tertiary phosphate group of the nucleic acids, as well as methionine, cysteine, tyrosine, and histidine in proteins. This broad spectrum of chemical reactivity between electrophilic carcinogens and biological macromolecules has been demonstrated both *in vitro* and *in vivo*. Nevertheless, the knowledge of chemical reactions does not necessarily lead to an understanding of the ensuing biological processes, such as mutation induction or tumor formation and development. At best, it might be possible to establish some correlation between the chemical reactivity of a carcinogen, its carcinogenicity, and mutagenicity. It should be noted, however, that such a correlation cannot be expected to be complete. As pointed out by Malling and Chu (1974), the following factors could conceivably affect any attempted correlation between carcinogenicity and mutagenicity of chemical compounds. First, a number of carcinogens or procarcinogens are almost water-insoluble and may not penetrate into the individual cell or organism. Second, mutagenicity tests may have to be done in test systems both remote from the site and different from the type of cells in which tumors occur. Third, promoters may change intracellular or intracellular condition permitting preneoplastic cells to develop into tumors, but may not be mutagenic by themselves. Fourth, many carcinogens require metabolic activation in the mammals to become reactive electrophiles. Hence, tests without the proper activation may not reveal their mutagenicity. Finally, lack of demonstrable mutagenicity could also result from an efficient repair of altered DNA.

Despite these uncertainties and limitations, it is remarkable that considerable inroads have been made in the past several years to establish the mutagenic properties of a host of known chemical carcinogens. This is due largely to the development of biological test systems for this purpose (Hollaender, 1971, 1973; Vogel and Rohrborn, 1970; Fishbein *et al.*, 1970). The biological materials employed have ranged from bacteriophage, bacteria, fungi, higher plants, insects, mammalian cells in tissue culture to intact laboratory mammals. When structurally related chemical potent carcinogens, weak carcinogens, and noncarcinogens were tested in these systems, it became abundantly clear that there is a positive correlation between carcinogenicity and mutagenicity of most chemical compounds tested. Furthermore, these studies have led to the conclusion that certain chemical carcinogens must be metabolically activated before their biological function becomes manifest (cf. Miller and

Miller, 1971; Malling and Chu, 1974). Metabolic activation of procarcinogens or potential mutagens can be achieved experimentally either (a) chemically by Udenfriend's oxidation system, (b) metabolically by liver microsomes, or (c) in host-mediated assays (Malling and Chu, 1974; Legator and Malling, 1971).

In summary, it appears that many, and perhaps all, chemical carcinogens are potential mutagens. Similarly, many but possibly not all mutagens are potential carcinogens (Miller and Miller, 1971). In many instances, reactivity and metabolic and permeability factors appear to have obscured correlations of mutagenic and carcinogenic activities. These potentialities and complications are consequences of the electrophilic nature of many ultimate carcinogenic and mutagenic chemicals. The Millers felt that the ability of these electrophiles to react with nucleophiles in many cell constituents other than DNA makes it impossible to support a somatic mutation theory of carcinogenesis by a chemical. Only a gross correlation between carcinogenesis and mutagenesis could be made at present. We feel, however, there may be alternative and perhaps more crucial assessments of the somatic mutation theory. One of such alternatives is to examine the changes of DNA in response to extrinsic factors and the biological consequences, as will be discussed in detail in the following sections.

III. Molecular Basis for Mutagenesis and Carcinogenesis

A. GENETIC AND ENVIRONMENTAL PREDISPOSITIONS

In any attempt to unravel the many factors that influence complex biological phenomena such as mutagenesis and carcinogenesis, we must recall that every biological trait or phenotype ("normal" or "abnormal") is the result of an interaction of genetic and environmental factors (nature and nurture, not nature versus nurture). The diagram in Fig. 1 illustrates that the genetic information locked in the DNA molecules of the zygote must constantly interact with various environmental factors throughout development. Development will be "normal" or "abnormal" depending on either or both genetic and environmental predispositions. DNA molecules, which are able to code genetically for functional structural or metabolic needs of organisms, might be found in unfavorable environments which inhibit the genetic expression. Alternatively, some genes are unable to code for normal functioning structures or metabolic needs in the prevailing environment (mutated genes).

In the subsequent discussion of a model of carcinogenesis, it will

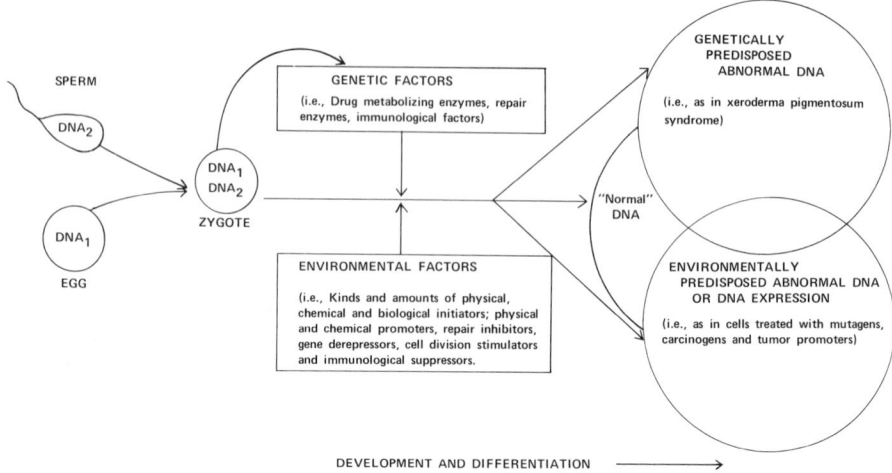

FIG. 1. The "nature and nurture" model for genetic and environmental predispositions to cancer.

become clear that there might be at least three general classes of genetic predisposition to cancer (e.g., genes involved in carcinogenic initiation, in the repair of DNA and in tumor promotion). Within this conceptual framework, genetic diseases, such as xeroderma pigmentosum, which predisposes the individual to cancer in "normal" environments of some chemicals and ultraviolet light (Cleaver, 1973), could shed light on the mechanisms by which abnormal environments (excess amounts of certain agents such as croton oil or radiation) predispose "normal" individuals to cancer. Genetic deficiencies in immunological mechanisms, which also predispose individuals to cancer (Coleman et al., 1961; Good et al., 1962; Kersey et al., 1973), can conceivably aid in understanding why normal biological processes, such as aging, or some environmental conditions, such as immunological suppressant drugs, also predispose individuals to cancer (Penn and Starzl, 1972). Moreover, understanding the influence of genetic variation in certain drug-metabolizing enzymes on carcinogenic predisposition (Conney, 1973), might provide means to predict the consequence on carcinogenesis of environmental stimulators or inhibitors of normal drug-metabolizing enzymes. In any attempt to provide a unified conceptual model between molecular phenomena in DNA molecules (genes and chromosomes) and carcinogenesis, a relationship between permanent or temporary shifts in genetic information and carcinogenesis must be established, possibly including relationships between DNA repair mechanisms and carcinogenesis.

B. MUTAGENESIS

Gene mutation by definition is the alteration of information locked in the nucleotide composition and sequence in DNA. The types of mutation include substitution, insertion, or deletion of nucleic acid bases, which lead either to a change of information (missense mutation) or to incomplete or no information (nonsense mutation). It is possible to account for the mutagenic effect of many physical and chemical agents on the basis of their *in vitro* reactions with DNA (Freese, 1963). Moreover, studies in bacteria indicate that mutagenesis is a complex enzymic process, involving several genes and enzyme systems (*Genetics*, Vol. 73, Suppl., 1973). However, complete analysis of the effect of physical or chemical treatments of DNA will require knowledge of the developmental influences on the metabolic response of an organism to the potential alteration of the DNA molecules, as well as its ability to respond to such alteration.

C. CARCINOGENESIS

Carcinogenesis is believed to be at least a two-staged process (Mottram, 1944; Berenblum, 1954; Boutwell, 1964; Van Duuren, 1969), involving (1) the *initiation* of a normal cell to a potential cancer cell (precancerous cell) and (2) the *promotion* or proliferation of these precancerous cells (Fig. 2). On the molecular level, carcinogenic initiation is thought to involve the stable alteration of DNA molecules by carcinogens (physical, chemical, or viral), either permanently through mutations or temporarily through derepression or repression of DNA molecules of the affected cell. Most, if not all, carcinogens interact with DNA molecules, directly or indirectly, and most physical and chemical carcinogens are mutagens (Miller and Miller, 1971). Restricting our discussion of the molecular basis for the permanent alteration of DNA during the initiation phase of carcinogenesis, initiation would then be viewed as the interaction of a physical or chemical agent with DNA molecules. If the interaction leads to a structural alteration in the DNA molecule which signals the response of one of several repair mechanisms, the DNA is either restituted to its original condition or it is permanently altered during the "repair" process ("mutation-fixation").

Several hypotheses have been advanced for the promotion phase of carcinogenesis on the molecular, biochemical, and cellular levels. Cell proliferation and epidermal hyperplasia are among the more conspicuous effects of promoters (Ryser, 1971), as well as induction of inflammation and influx of leukocytes (Iversen and Evensen, 1962;

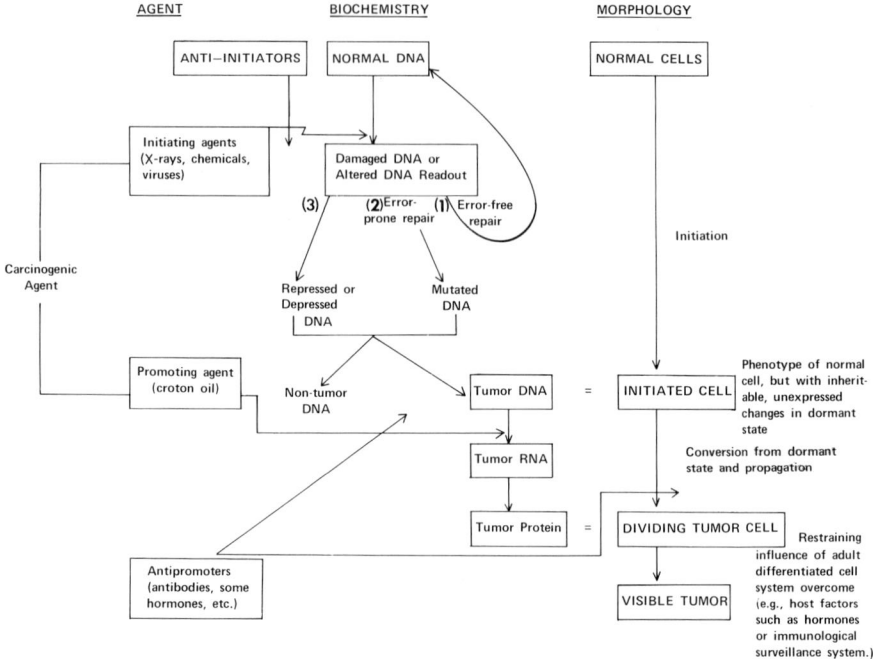

FIG. 2. A heuristic model of carcinogenesis. Carcinogenesis is conceived as a two-stage process involving initiation (altering DNA information) and promotion (proliferation of cells with altered DNA information). Genetic factors can influence carcinogenesis on the level of anti-initiation (drug-metabolizing enzymes), on the level of DNA repair or replication, and on the level of antipromoters (e.g., genetic deficiencies of the immunosurveillance system). Modified after Boutwell (1974).

Frei and Stephens, 1968). However, not all agents which stimulate cell proliferation have tumor-promoting activity (Raick, 1973). Some promoters have been demonstrated to stimulate DNA, RNA, protein, and phospholipid synthesis (Paul and Hecker, 1969; Raick and Ritchie, 1970; Baird et al., 1971; Rohrschneider et al., 1972). Raick (1973) has advanced a hypothesis, based on the observation that promoter-treated cells appear to develop to a less differentiated phenotype, that the tumor-promoter acts by altering the phenotype expression of variant, but quiescent or repressed, initiated cells which are present in the cell population.

On the molecular level, some tumor promoters have been shown to interact with cell membranes (Sivak and Van Duuren, 1971). Gaudin et al. (1972), and Teebor et al. (1973) have demonstrated that tumor promoters tested in their studies can inhibit the excision repair of carcinogen-induced DNA damage. They have advanced the hypothesis that the tumor promotion could be due to the direct inhibition of the excision repair process. Two important observations which are not accounted for in their hypothesis are (1) the tumor-promoting potential of many chemicals exists many months after the application of short half-lived carcinogens (Peraino et al., 1973; Boutwell, 1974), and (2) most of the repair that is going to occur in any given cell (far less than 100% in most mammalian cells tested) takes place within 24 hours (Regan et al., 1968; Edenberg and Hanawalt, 1973). An attempt to resolve these discrepancies is discussed later.

In summary, although it is by no means explicitly known what the exact molecular events are which lead to the initiation and promotion phases of carcinogenesis, it does seem that (1) since most carcinogens, if not all, interact with DNA and (2) since many of these altered DNA molecules are substrates of various types of DNA repair, tumor promoters might be those agents or conditions which alter the repair and/or expression of cells whose repressed DNA, which was not repaired accurately, is now derepressed.

D. Genetic Basis for Mutagenesis and Carcinogenesis

Within the past few years, a number of systems have been found which modify damaged DNA in biologically significant ways. For example, (1) microorganisms separated by a single mutational step differ in their radiation sensitivity (Witkin, 1947; Hill, 1958); (2) it is also possible to demonstrate definite chemical changes in DNA after doses of ultraviolet light, within the biological dose range, and to show that the resulting photoproducts are important in producing certain biological effects associated with irradiation (Wacker, 1963; Setlow and Carrier, 1964); (3) furthermore, nonsensitive wild-type organisms are able to remove UV-produced lesions from their DNA, and this removal can permit the growth of the organism which would otherwise be inactivated (Setlow and Carrier, 1964; Boyce and Howard-Flanders, 1964). Mutant strains for several of the different repair enzymes found in bacteria have led to the concept of genetic control of "error-free" versus "error-prone" DNA repair mechanisms (Witkin, 1969a).

In mammalian systems, several clinical syndromes, among which are xeroderma pigmentosum, dyskeratosis congenita, Fanconi's anemia, ataxia telangiectasia, Werner's, Bloom's, Chediak-Higashi, and Down's syndromes, have genetic predispositions to cancer, as well as to other specific syndrome anomalies. In the case of the xeroderma pigmentosum syndrome, which is characterized by hypersensitivity of the skin to solar radiation and high incidence of multiple carcinomas, the cells from these individuals, in vitro, are more sensitive to ultraviolet radiation than are normal cells (Cleaver, 1970) and lack the ability to excise pyrimidine dimers (Cleaver, 1969a; Setlow et al., 1969; Cleaver and Trosko, 1970) or some other types of base damage (Setlow and Regan, 1972; Stich et al., 1972). Several hypotheses have been advanced to explain the mechanism of carcinogenesis in xeroderma pigmentosum (Xp) individuals: (1) increased mutation rates (both point and chromosomal); (2) induction of oncogenic viruses by low UV doses; and (3) increased malignant transformation of UV-damaged cells by oncogenic viruses (Cleaver, 1973). As pointed out by Cleaver, these might not be mutually exclusive hypotheses. The defect of excision repair in Xp cells is similar to that in UVr⁻hcr⁻ bacterial mutants, which have an elevated UV-induced mutation rate (Witkin, 1969b; Bridges, 1969). Preliminary studies have been reported that indicate chemical carcinogen-induced mutation frequencies in Xp cells are not higher than those found in normal human fibroblasts (Maher et al., 1974). However, studies with 4-nitroquinoline 1-oxide (4-NQO), which induced nonrepairable lesions in the DNA of Xp cells, indicate that this chemical induces many chromosome aberrations in Xp cells. Xp cells, treated with methyl methanesulfonate (MMS), can repair the MMS-damaged DNA without manifesting significant chromosome damage (Sasaki, 1973).

Recent reports indicate that Fanconi's anemia, a genetic syndrome which is characterized by a high incidence of neoplasms and high frequency of spontaneous and chemically induced chromosome breaks in their cells, might be associated with a defect in the exonuclease step of excision repair (Poon et al., 1974). Moreover, according to a report of a study of the repair of induced single-strand breaks in DNA of Hutchinson–Gilford progeria cells, the clinical manifestation of premature aging in this syndrome might be related to the inability of these cells to repair these breaks as well as do normal cells.

These aforementioned genetic syndromes, as well as those associated with immunological deficiencies, indicate that the ultimate appearance of a tumor is the end result of many genetic regulatory mechanisms on the molecular, biochemical, and cellular levels having been overcome.

IV. DNA Damage and Its Repair

A. INITIATION OF DNA DAMAGE

It is important that we understand the nature of the damage incurred in DNA molecules after organisms have been exposed to various environmental mutagens and carcinogens. There is ample evidence indicating that the nature of the DNA lesion determines the nature of the enzymic mechanism(s) responsible for the repair. For example, xeroderma pigmentosum cells, which are unable to repair ultraviolet light (UV)-induced (Cleaver, 1968) or N-acetoxy-2-acetylaminofluorene (N-acetoxy-AAF)-induced (Setlow and Regan, 1972), or 4-NQO-induced (Stich et al., 1971) base damage in DNA, are apparently able to repair X-ray or N-methyl-N-nitro-N-nitrosoguanidine (MNNG)-induced single-strand breaks (Cleaver, 1971).

In eukaryotic systems, the role of DNA repair in mutagenesis and carcinogenesis is complicated by many genetic factors, such as the species, tissue, cell, stage of cell cycle, or developmental stage in which both the DNA is damaged and repaired. Genetic factors influencing detoxifying or metabolizing enzyme activities will influence the level of initial chemical-induced DNA damage, as well as determine both the types and rates of DNA repair enzymes on all lesions. In a recent review article (Conney, 1973), based on observations that high and low levels of aryl hydrocarbon hydroxylase inducibility in human lymphocytes were correlated with high and low incidences of lung cancer in cigarette smokers (Kellermann et al., 1973), Conney (1973) hypothesizes that genetic variation in this drug-metabolizing enzyme will determine the level of potential carcinogen-induced DNA damage. If this is supported by further testing, such as that by Kouri et al. (1974), other such genetic variations could influence the initiation phase of carcinogenesis.

Conceptually, one ought to be able to increase or decrease the ability of a potential mutagen or carcinogen to damage DNA by environmentally inhibiting or stimulating drug-metabolizing enzymes or by adding agents that selectively compete with DNA as a substrate for these mutagens and carcinogens. Apparently this is possible, since it has been demonstrated that antioxidants, such as butylated hydroxytoluene and butylated hydroxyanisole, can reduce the potential of a carcinogen to induce chromosome breaks (Shamberger et al., 1973) and to induce tumor formation (Wattenberg, 1973). Although the molecular basis of the antimutagenic and anticarcinogenic properties of these compounds are not yet known, it has been implied that they act on an anti-initiation level by inducing drug-metabolizing enzymes (Commings and Walton, 1973).

The interaction of mutagens and most, if not all, carcinogens with DNA leads to alterations in the structure of the DNA molecule. If these alterations of structure lead to impairment of function, the cell must repair the lesion or suffer the consequences of impaired function. In general, the lesions which have been identified are those that (1) are associated with altered bases, such as UV-induced pyrimidine dimers (Setlow and Setlow, 1972) or X-ray-induced thymine damage (Cerutti, 1974); (2) are identified as single- or double-strand breaks in the DNA helix (Lett et al., 1970; Corry and Cole, 1968); (3) lead to depurination of DNA (Verly et al., 1973); (4) comprise DNA–protein cross-links (Habazin and Han, 1970); and (5) form cross-links within the DNA molecule (Smith, 1966). The particular lesion somehow signals the specific enzyme system responsible for its repair.

B. DNA Repair Enzymes in Eukaryotic Cells

Although there is a plethora of studies on DNA repair in a wide variety of eukaryotic cells derived from yeasts, higher plants, insects, rodents, birds, fish, and human beings, few, if any, as yet have been analyzed with the precision afforded to microbial systems. Since one can assume that no species or individual organism has DNA molecules that are refractory to deleterious environmental agents, one or more DNA repair systems must be available for the maintenance of the genetic integrity during development. Moreover, several DNA repair mechanisms have been extensively characterized in microbiological systems with the aid of mutant strains, yet the explicit understanding of any one, let alone all, of the repair systems in any one microorganism is far from complete. Although several repair mechanisms have been detected in mammalian systems for a number of years (Rasmussen and Painter, 1964; Regan et al., 1968), the state of the science and art lags far behind that found in microbial systems.

1. *Photoreactivating Repair Enzymes*

The biological phenomenon of photoreactivation has been demonstrated in many plant and animal phyla (Jagger, 1958; Cook, 1971). Photoreactivation may be defined as the amelioration in the response of a biological system to ultraviolet irradiation with wavelengths between 220 and 300 nm by posttreatment with radiation at 310–440 nm. The molecular basis for photoreactivation of UV-induced cell killing, mutagenesis in bacteria (Setlow and Setlow, 1972), and tumor formation in fish (Hart and Setlow, 1973) appears to be associated with the *in situ* photomonomerization of UV-induced pyrimidine dimers by photoreactivating enzymes.

Although the photoreactivating enzyme activity has been demonstrated in many eukaryotic systems, reports have indicated that the enzymic and biological aspects of photoreactivation did not exist in several mammalian *in vitro* cell systems, including those derived from human tissues (Trosko et al., 1965; Cleaver, 1966; Trosko and Isoun, 1970). Recent reports have suggested, however, that at least in some human cells, e.g., leukocytes, the enzyme activity does exist (Sutherland, 1974). What biological role, if any, this repair mechanism plays in the possible amelioration of mutagenesis or carcinogenesis needs to be determined.

With the technological developments of somatic cell hybridization, *in vitro* mutagenesis and *in vitro* transformation studies, using eukaryotic cells known to have the photoreactivating enzyme (Regan and Cook, 1967; Krishman and Painter, 1973; Lohman and Paterson, 1974) should shed light on the molecular basis and the role of DNA repair mechanisms in UV-induced mutagenesis and carcinogenesis in human cells.

2. Dark Repair-Excision Enzymes

Clearly, several mammalian cells have repair enzymes which, ostensibly, resemble dark-repair, excision enzymes in bacterial cells (Regan et al., 1968; Edenberg and Hanawalt, 1972). The "cut-patch" model of an enzyme complex which recognizes, makes initial incisions of the DNA strand, excises the lesion plus variable amounts of undamaged nucleotides, repolymerizes the removed oligonucleotide region, and ligases the new strand to the old, has been demonstrated by various techniques in several eukaryotic cells.

Techniques of varying sensitivity have been developed to measure the actual removal of certain lesions and the replacement of the bases, as well as the completion of the ligation (Carrier and Setlow, 1971; Painter and Cleaver, 1969; Regan et al., 1971; Lucas, 1972; Goodman and Potter, 1972; Paterson et al., 1973; Cox et al., 1973; Wilkins, 1973; Saffhill et al., 1974; Cleaver, 1974; Trosko and Yager, 1974). Demonstration of "unscheduled" DNA repair synthesis (autoradiographic or biochemical measurement of nonsemiconservative nucleotide insertion into DNA during the repression of semiconservative DNA replication), or of repair replication (cesium chloride density gradient technique, which can detect repair in parental strands of DNA), has been generally assumed to reflect the ability of a cell to carry out the direct excision of lesions (Painter and Cleaver, 1969). To put it another way, if a cell does excise its lesions, one would expect to be able to detect its repair capacity by demonstrating that, indeed, new bases are inserted and the original strand-continuity is regained.

Although there are some studies that attempt to characterize the nature of the excision enzyme in mammalian systems (Lindahl, 1972;

Bacchetti et al., 1972; Duncan et al., 1974), our understanding, at the time of this review, is still in its infancy. However, several interesting observations can be noted with regard to the "excision" repair system in mammalian cells. Chemicals, such as caffeine, which inhibit excision repair in bacteria (Sideropoulos and Shankel, 1968; Setlow and Carrier, 1968; Lumb et al., 1968) do not appear to inhibit excision, unscheduled DNA synthesis, or repair replication in the mammalian cells tested (Regan et al., 1968; Cleaver, 1969b). Also, there is a wide variation in the levels of excision and unscheduled DNA repair between cell lines and strains of various species, in vitro (Bootsma et al., 1970; Setlow et al., 1972). The extent and rates of repair are very different in mammalian cells tested, compared to those in bacterial cells. The life-span of the repair enzymes needed for "unscheduled" DNA repair synthesis in several mammalian cells appears to be relatively long (Gautschi et al., 1973).

Recent studies by Lohman and Paterson (1974) have complicated the usual interpretation that "unscheduled" DNA synthesis after UV-irradiation always reflects the ability of a cell to recognize and to excise the UV-induced pyrimidine dimers as lesions. In Lohman's studies, chick embryo cells, in vitro, exhibited UV-induced "unscheduled" DNA repair synthesis even after the UV-irradiated cells photoreactivated the UV-induced pyrimidine dimers. This implies that UV-irradiation induced other, unphotoreactivable lesions which were recognized as repair substrates in the DNA molecules.

Although the excision repair system in bacterial cells appears to function in an "error-free" manner with regard to mutation-fixation (Setlow, 1968; Witkin, 1969b), it has yet to be demonstrated, directly, whether such is the case for excision repair in mammalian cells.

3. Postreplication Repair

Since the demonstration of postreplication or recombinational repair in *Escherichia coli* (Rupp and Howard-Flanders, 1968), many investigators have demonstrated some form of postreplication repair in several mammalian cell lines (Cleaver and Thomas, 1969; Fujiwara and Kondo, 1972; Lehmann, 1972; Trosko and Chu, 1973; Buhl et al., 1972; Trosko et al., 1973). For example, when Chinese hamster cells are exposed to UV or N-acetoxy-AAF, then allowed to synthesize DNA in the presence or in the absence of nontoxic levels of caffeine, the DNA profiles, as measured on alkaline-sucrose gradients, have been interpreted by some to indicate that gaps, which are induced by unrepaired lesions in the template DNA, are not filled or "repaired" in the presence of caffeine. Although the observation of a caffeine inhibition of chain elongation has been repeatedly demonstrated, there is some question as to the most appropriate interpretation (Painter, 1974).

The concept of postreplication repair in mammalian cells originated in the observation that some mutagen-treated mammalian cells, given a posttreatment of nontoxic levels of caffeine, synergistically demonstrated a sensitization in terms of colony-forming ability (Rauth, 1967). Initially, it was thought that caffeine inhibited excision repair as it does in bacterial systems. However, caffeine has been shown not to inhibit excision repair, unscheduled DNA synthesis, or repair replication in these cells (Regan et al., 1968; Cleaver, 1969b). When the DNA is newly synthesized in several mutagen and carcinogen-treated nonhuman cells in the presence of caffeine, it appears that caffeine blocks the chain-lengthening process. The operational measurement of chain elongation of nascent DNA off of damaged template has been referred to as "postreplication" repair. Apparently the process is dissimilar to the postreplication or recombination repair mechanism in bacterial systems, since, unlike the bacterial mechanism, in several mammalian cells tested, there is no detectable exchange or recombination of genetic material (Lehmann, 1972; Buhl and Regan, 1973). Rather, as Lehmann has claimed, the chain elongation is due to "*de novo*" DNA synthesis or gap-filling.

Although the molecular mechanism of this type of postreplication repair is very scant at this moment, there are some interesting observations that are associated with the operational concept of postreplication repair. First, several rodent cell lines *in vitro* have been shown to exhibit both biological and molecular synergism between mutagens and caffeine, whereas several nontransformed and transformed human cell lines do not exhibit this synergism (Wilkinson *et al.*, 1970; Roberts and Ward, 1973). Moreover, in a variant of xeroderma pigmentosum, which demonstrates "normal" excision repair capacities, a caffeine synergism on both biological and molecular levels has been reported (Lehmann, 1974).

If, indeed, the postreplication repair mechanism which has been postulated is not an artifact of the technique to measure the repair, then the exact biological role will have to be delineated. The general interpretation of the demonstration of lowered molecular weight DNA made off of damaged DNA is that, when lesions cannot be removed via excision repair because of structural or time constraints, the lesion prohibits the normal replication of DNA. Unless cells possess genetic means to "bypass" these lesions (Chiu and Rauth, 1972), or to rectify the potentially lethal effects of inducing gaps in the nascent DNA, the viability of cells will be limited to the extent and efficiency of the other mechanisms to repair lesions prior to DNA synthesis and cell division.

4. *Other DNA Repair Mechanisms in Mammalian Cells*

Recent reports have demonstrated that a wide range of DNA repair mechanisms appear to be operative in various cell types. Verly et al. (1973) have shown that several mammalian tissues contain the enzymic function to repair apurinic sites in DNA. Apparently, these apurinic sites can be formed spontaneously by the depurination of DNA, as well as by certain chemical interactions with the DNA. The biological role and consequence of this type of repair have yet to be specified. Cerutti (1974) has also demonstrated the presence of repair mechanisms related to the excision of bases damaged by ionizing radiation. Repair of alkylation-induced cross-linked DNA also occurs in mammalian cells (Roberts et al., 1968).

Single-strand breaks, induced by a variety of physical or chemical mutagens have been shown to be repaired in mammalian cells (Lett et al., 1967; Painter and Cleaver, 1967; Sawada and Okawa, 1970; Horikawa et al., 1970). Repair of double-strand breaks in mammalian DNA also appears to occur (Sawada and Okada, 1972; Corry and Cole, 1973). The techniques used to measure the repair of both double- and single-strand breaks have not yet led to unequivocal interpretations on the characterization of the *in situ* single- or double-strand breaks, or on the significance of the disappearance or repair of the single- and double-strand breaks.

DNA–protein cross-links have been demonstrated as potential lesions in both prokaryotes (Smith, 1964) and eukaryotes (Habazin and Han, 1970). The actual role, if any, of these DNA–protein cross-links as lesions, or the repair of these lesions, is not known. One might speculate that since eukaryotic chromosomes have much of the DNA sequestered by various proteins, and since the differentiation of cells depends on a dynamic ability to derepress or repress certain regions of DNA, the role of these DNA–protein cross-links would be significant.

Recent work by Radman (1974) and by Witkin and George (1973) with *E. coli* indicates that, at least in bacteria, not only are there normal constitutive repair enzymes, but also there is a postulated inducible or "SOS" repair system. Whether an analogous inducible repair system occurs in mammalian cells has yet to be ascertained.

In general, the state of knowledge on the genetics and the molecular or biological roles of DNA repair mechanisms is at a primitive level in eukaryotic systems. Without the genetic mutants to enable investigators to examine the biochemistry and the biological consequences in the same system, interpretations of the role of DNA repair in mutagenesis and carcinogenesis will remain highly speculative.

V. Factors Influencing DNA Repair

A. DEVELOPMENTAL FACTORS

1. *Chromatin*

Clearly, there is ample evidence that the chemistry of eukaryotic chromosomes (e.g., nucleic acid–nuclear protein complexes) which influence DNA transcription and DNA replication during the cell cycle and during development and aging will influence the nature of DNA repair and, by inference, mutagenesis and carcinogenesis. Since the eukaryotic chromosome is distinguished from the bacterial chromosome by the nuclear protein complexes it contains (e.g., histones and acidic "residual" proteins), and since it is known that, at any given moment in time, the chromosome has two distinct but variable regions (euchromatic and heterochromatic regions), it stands to reason that the initiation of DNA damage and the repair of that damage might be different. Recent evidence by Hewish and Burgoyne (1973) indicates that nuclear proteins can regulate the sites of endonuclease activity in rat liver nuclei. Also, Silverman and Mirsky (1973) have shown that nuclear proteins can limit the accessibility of DNA polymerase. More directly, Wilkins and Hart (1974) have shown that chromatin does inhibit excision repair in human cells. It remains to be shown, however, what the implications of differential production and repair of lesions in euchromatic and heterochromatic regions of the chromosomes with mutagens are on the mutagenic and carcinogenic processes.

2. *Differentiation*

Since it is assumed that the process of differentiation involves not only the appearance of new structures and functions in the developing eukaryote, but also the physical repression and derepression of DNA via the nuclear protein mediator, DNA repair studies in differentiating systems might give us a picture of the possible complex relationship between DNA repair and mutagenesis. For example, Darzynkiewicz (1971) has shown that phytohemagglutinin stimulation of lymphocytes, which involves the stimulation of RNA and DNA synthesis and cell division, increased the rate of unscheduled DNA repair synthesis. Darzynkiewicz and Chelmicha-Szorc (1972) have also shown that during avian erythropoiesis, repression of DNA synthesis in red blood cells is accompanied by a depression of unscheduled DNA synthesis. Cell fusion of dormant and active erythrocytes leads to active semiconservative DNA synthesis and unscheduled DNA repair synthesis. Furthermore, Gledhill and Darzynkiewicz (1973) have demonstrated unscheduled DNA repair synthesis decreases as cells progress through spermatogenesis in rats.

Hahn and his co-workers (1971) and Stockdale (1971) have demonstrated quantitative changes in unscheduled DNA repair synthesis in rat and chick embryo muscle cells, respectively. As the cells differentiate from the myeloblast to fully developed muscle fibers, there was a reduction (up to 50% of the nondifferentiated levels) in unscheduled DNA synthesis. In the sense that some cancer cells are characterized by a marked change in the state of differentiation from the tissue of origin, the observation of Huang et al. (1972), that cells from patients suffering chronic lymphocytic leukemia have increased excision repair compared to lymphocytes from normal patients, might not be surprising. Satoh and Yamamoto (1972) have observed that HeLa cells carrying Sendai virus were more resistant than HeLa cells to several chemical carcinogens, and they interpreted their data as indicating that Sendai-carrying HeLa cells have more effective, nonexcision type of DNA repair. Obviously, more work needs to be done to study what effect transformation of cells might have on the repair mechanisms of mammalian cells and to examine the biological significance of any change.

3. Development and Aging

A corollary to the role of differentiation and of "chromatization" on reduced unscheduled or excision repair in eukaryotic systems is the effect of normal development on DNA repair. The very first reports on excision repair in rodent cells (Trosko et al., 1965; Klímek, 1966; Steward and Humphrey, 1966; Horikawa et al., 1968) suggested very little, if any, excision repair in Chinese hamster cells, mouse L cells, and other rodent cells. These studies were performed with transformed cells grown in vitro. Recently, Ruth Ben-Ishai (1974) reported excision repair in mouse embryo cells and its repression in established mouse cell lines. Moreover, although excision repair could be detected in early passages of these primary cell lines from mouse embryos, excision repair gradually disappeared within a few later passages. No excision of DNA damage could be detected in early passages of primary cells derived from "old" embryos.

Goldstein (1971) has observed that very late-passage human fibroblasts had a slightly reduced amount of unscheduled DNA synthesis than did early or intermediate passage cells. A similar observation (e.g., a slight decrease of repair replication) was made by Painter et al. (1973) in late-passage WI-38 cells. Hart and Setlow (1974) have recently demonstrated an interesting correlation between the initial rate and the maximum level of unscheduled DNA synthesis in several types of fibroblasts in vitro and the life-span of the species. They have offered a hypothesis that different species have more or less efficient repair mechanisms which excise lesions from DNA. If a given species accumulates more damage per unit DNA, they speculate that there would be a rapid deterioration of the fidelity of transcription and translation which could, together with other molecular, cellular, and physiological factors, account for the shortened life-span of organisms which have lower levels of excision repair.

There are experiments that relate the existence and efficiency of DNA repair and the accumulations of damage in DNA of older cells. Price et al. (1971) and Modak and Price (1971) observed that old tissues from mice acted as better primers for DNA synthesis than young tissues. They interpreted the observations as being the result of DNA from old cells having larger numbers of strand breaks which act as initiation sites than DNA from younger cells. Karran and Ormerod (1973) have reported that DNA of young red cells had fewer alkali-labile bonds (single-strand breaks) than DNA from old ones. Furthermore, old rat muscle cells did not repair single-strand breaks as did young ones. Wheeler et al. (1973) and Wheeler and Lett (1972), however, have shown that in nondividing cells, such as rabbit retinal and dog neuronal cells, ionizing radiation-induced DNA breaks were repaired, as they were also in fibroblasts.

Cells from individuals suffering from Hutchinson-Gilford syndrome (progeria or premature aging) appeared to be defective in the ability to rejoin DNA strand breaks, but were able to perform normal repair replication after UV irradiation (Epstein et al., 1973). A causal relationship between the lack of any DNA repair and aging has yet to be strictly demonstrated. Furthermore, if such a causal relationship between the loss of DNA repair and some component of aging is shown, the mechanism by which the nonrepair of DNA manifests itself in cellular, physiological, or organism aging will have to be determined.

B. ENVIRONMENTAL FACTORS

Although it goes without saying that environmental factors influence mutagenesis and carcinogenesis, the specific molecular mechanisms have not been delineated for mammalian cells. Along with the genetic tools to measure DNA repair mechanisms and their possible relationship to mutagenesis, we can utilize the fact that genetic information, in order to be functional, must be modulated by proper environmental factors (in this case, either in the synthesis or the functioning of DNA repair enzymes). If we assume for the moment that DNA repair is responsible for some, if not most of the mutation fixation in eukaryotic cells, it should be obvious that environmental agents that cause the initiation and repair of DNA damage, as well as those which stimulate or inhibit drug-metabolizing and DNA repair enzymes, are those which influence mutagenesis and, by inference, carcinogenesis. Consequently, there are two broad approaches to study the influence of DNA repair on mutagenesis, using environmental means. First, the use, as biological end points, of mutations, of cell survival, or of accelerated aging or cancer, a variety of external conditions or chemicals which either sensitize or act synergistically with known mutagens would be candidates for potential inhibitors of DNA repair mechanisms. Alternatively, chemicals suspected or known to inhibit enzymic functions needed for DNA repair or replication (e.g., endonuclease or DNA polymerase inhibitors) should be examined for the mutation-modifying potential.

To illustrate the first of these approaches, both caffeine and the phorbol esters (active factors in croton oil) will be discussed. Caffeine has been known to increase the killing of UV-irradiated bacteria and to modify the frequency of mutations recovered (Witkin, 1969a). The mechanism of caffeine sensitization of UV damage in bacteria has been attributed to the inhibition of the excision of pyrimidine dimers (Sideropoulos and Shankel, 1968; Setlow and Carrier, 1968; Lumb et al., 1968). In mutagen-treated mouse L cells and Chinese hamster cells, but not in human cells, caffeine decreases the colony-forming ability (Rauth, 1967; Walker and Reid, 1971; Wilkinson et al., 1970). Kihlman et al. (1973) have demonstrated the potentiating effect of posttreatment of caffeine on chromosome aberrations induced by UV and chemical mutagens in plants and several mammalian cells. However, as was pointed out earlier, caffeine does not inhibit excision repair, unscheduled DNA synthesis, or repair replication (Regan et al., 1968; Cleaver, 1969b), but it does inhibit a postreplication type of repair in several nonhuman mammalian cell lines (Cleaver and Thomas, 1969; Fujiwara and Kondo, 1972; Lehmann, 1972; Trosko and Chu, 1973).

Although caffeine induces chromosome aberrations in mammalian cells at high concentrations (Kuhlmann et al., 1968), it appears to be ineffective in the induction of auxotrophic mutants (Kao and Puck, 1969). Using the quantitative method for the selection of forward mutations to 8-azaguanine resistance, Trosko and Chu (1973) have found that a nontoxic concentration of caffeine lowers the frequency of mutations in UV-irradiated Chinese hamster cells under the same conditions which inhibit postreplication repair. Arlett and Harcourt (1972), using a similar protocol, found that caffeine reduced the UV-induced mutation frequency only if it was present during the entire postirradiation period. Roberts and Sturrock (1973), using N-methyl-N-nitrosourea to initiate DNA damage have, however, found that although caffeine potentiates the loss of colony-forming ability, it raises, rather than lowers, the mutation frequency of the survivors. They interpret their results as indicating that caffeine inhibits a postreplication repair. Although at first glance both the results and inferred mechanisms seem contradictory, it might be that these two mutagens induce lesions which are repaired by different repair mechanisms. Consequently, the caffeine effect on each might lead to different biological consequences.

To emphasize the possible relationship between DNA repair and biological consequences (e.g., chromosome aberrations, mutagenesis, and carcinogenesis), the observations that caffeine inhibits the postreplication repair of UV damage but not excision repair in rodent cells, and that it lowered UV-induced mutation frequencies, allow one to predict that caffeine would act as an anticarcinogen, if mutagenesis is responsible for some carcinogenic events. Recently, Zajdela and Latarjet (1973) have shown that caffeine posttreatment indeed reduces the frequency of UV-induced skin tumors in mice.

Moreover, since there is reason to believe that lesions in DNA can lead to chromosome aberrations, one would expect that interference with the DNA repair of these lesions would modify the frequency of chromosome aberrations. For example, Griggs and Bender (1973) have shown that *Xenopus* cells, which have the ability to photoreactivate UV-induced pyrimidine dimers, have lower UV-induced chromatid-type aberrations after photoreactivation posttreatment than do nonphotoreactivated cells. If the pyrimidine dimers are at least one of the UV-induced molecular lesions responsible for the appearance of chromosome aberrations, then one would predict that, in cells which cannot repair these lesions via photoreactivation, these lesions could lead somehow to the manifestation of chromosome aberrations. Several reports have been interpreted to indicate that lesions in DNA, or that the excision repair of DNA lesions, were not responsible for chromosome aberrations (Painter and Wolff, 1973;

Wolff and Cleaver, 1973). Recently, Kato (1973) has shown that caffeine, given as a posttreatment to UV-irradiated Chinese hamster cells, significantly decreased the frequency of sister chromatid exchanges, while the frequency of chromatid aberrations of the deletion type strikingly increased after the same treatment. He postulated that there is a relationship between postreplication repair of DNA lesions and the induction of sister chromatid exchanges. However, since caffeine has many effects on the cell [e.g., inhibits adenosine 3′,5′-monophosphate (AMP) phosphodiesterase (Sutherland and Rall, 1958), membrane permeability (Weber, 1968), and induces G_1 arrest in exponentially growing cells (Walters et al., 1974)], it might be quite fortuitous at this time to suggest that the caffeine effect acts at the DNA repair level.

Another class of chemicals, the tumor promoters, also appears to modify the biological consequences of known mutagens and carcinogens. For example, croton oil and the phorbol ester, phorbol myristate acetate, which are not carcinogens alone but which are powerful tumor promoters, have been shown to inhibit carcinogen-induced unscheduled DNA synthesis (Gaudin et al., 1972), as well as to inhibit the excision of UV-induced pyrimidine dimers at relatively high doses (Teebor et al., 1973). As one would predict, the phorbol ester, as an inhibitor to excision repair, would decrease survival as has been shown by Teebor et al. (1973) at high doses in their studies. If one assumes that DNA repair mechanisms are responsible for mutagenesis, and that excision repair is an "error"-free mechanism, then the inhibition of excision repair ought to lead to either no repair or "error-prone" DNA repair and the associated biological consequences of increased mutation frequencies and, by inference again, increased carcinogenic frequencies.

However, as in the caffeine example, the phorbol esters have many effects on several levels. As will be noted in the following, it might be the combination of the multieffects of phorbol ester treatment which is responsible for the tumor-promoting activity. Until the identification of specific DNA repair enzyme inhibitors, the interpretation of the mechanisms by which environmental agents alter mutagenic and carcinogenic frequencies will have to be qualified.

C. BIOCHEMICAL CONTROL OF CELL DIVISION

In an attempt to make sense of all the complex molecular, cellular, and physiological events that ultimately lead to the appearance of a tumor in an organism, several important observations must be the focus of the unifying hypothesis. In recent years, several unifying hypotheses have been offered which encompass two or more levels (e.g., molecular and cellular or cellular and physiological). The observations of many fetal cell characteristics in cancer cells have established a relationship between the biochemistry of cancer cells and that of the undifferentiated fetal tissue cell (Walker and Potter, 1972). For example, the slow-growing, highly differentiated hepatomas contain many biochemical characteristics of the adult liver together with some of the characteristics of fetal tissue, whereas the rapidly growing, poorly differentiated hepatomas retain fewer adult characteristics and more closely resemble fetal liver cells. The concepts of "oncogeny as blocked ontogeny" has been proposed by Potter (1969) as a mechanism to explain these observations. In essence, carcinogenesis appears to be a process by which there is a stable alteration of some genes at various stages of differentiation, such that a wide variety of "fetal" genes, including some of those responsible for cell division, are expressed. In this "blocked ontogeny" hypothesis there would be a persistent formation of certain fetal enzyme systems needed for cell replication, due to a failure to respond to the signals that call for their repression. It seems reasonable, although unsubstantiated, to assume that the failure could be due to a mutation or repression of a gene that is unable to respond to the signals or in a gene product that causes interference with signal transmission.

Holley (1972) recently has proposed that the most crucial changes in a malignant cell is an alteration in the cell surface membrane that results in increased internal concentrations of nutrients that regulate cell growth. Since a tumor is characterized by cells that do not seem to respond to those signals that regulate normal cell division and tissue differentiation, it seems reasonable that there are genes that contribute to the regulation of cell division and that an agent or condition that causes permanent alterations in DNA (mutations) or in gene expression (repression or derepression of genes) could lead to uncontrolled cell division.

On the biochemical level, several observations concerning cyclic nucleotide levels in cells and cell division have been linked together (Clarkson and Baserga, 1974). In general, it appears that intracellular levels of cAMP show an inverse relationship to mitotic rate in normal mouse epidermis (Marks and Grimm, 1972), as well as in pathological human skin (Voorhees et al., 1972). In cultured cells, the relationship also appears to hold. It has been shown that in 3T3 and other mouse fibroblast lines, rapid growth rates are associated with low levels of endogenous levels of cAMP (Otten et al., 1971; Sheppard, 1972). The enzymes responsible for regulating the levels of cAMP, adenylate cyclase, and cAMP phosphodiesterase, as well as the elevated cAMP, are thought to be involved in the regulation of cellular growth rate and the mediation of contact inhibition of growth (Anderson et al., 1973; Millis et al., 1974). Others have contended that it is the interaction of guanosine 3′,5′-monophosphate (c-GMP) and cAMP which may be responsible for the regulatory processes that control mitosis and differentiation (Goldberg et al., 1974).

If one assumes for the moment that the initiation of mitosis is somehow regulated by cyclic nucleotide balance, then conditions that alter this balance ought either to stimulate or repress cell division, and to foster or repress cell differentiation (Voorhees et al., 1974). In the case of tumors, cells within the tumor have somehow lost the ability to respond to those signals that keep mitosis in check. Cho-Chung and Gullino (1974) have demonstrated that the in vivo growth of hormone-dependent mammary tumors could be inhibited by treatment with dibutyryl cAMP. Moreover, tumors, initiated by 7,12-dimethylbenz[a]anthracene, which normally are promoted with croton oil, could be inhibited by steroid hormones (Belman and Troll, 1972). The hormones apparently had both anti-inflammatory and antimitotic effects. The active ingredient of croton oil, the phorbol esters, have been shown to increase cGMP levels (Estensen et al., 1974). These observations all seem to have a common interface.

Although the molecular basis for the regulatory processes that control the cell division, growth, differentiation, and hormonal responses of cells are poorly understood, intracellular concentrations of cyclic nucleotides can influence these processes. Hormones apparently have tissue-specific target sites on cytoplasmic organelles, especially on cell membranes and nuclear chromatin. Phorbol esters also are known to interact with cell membranes (Sivak and Van Duuren, 1971) as well as nuclear chromatin (Slaga et al., 1974). Cyclic nucleotide levels might be expected to be altered as these affected membranes stimulate the production of the cyclic nucleotides, which then, in turn, can affect pleiotropic biochemical reactions (e.g., activation of protein kinase which influences several physiological reactions). The observations that phorbol esters can stimulate protein, RNA, phospholipid and ultimately DNA synthesis as a prelude to mitotic stimulation, as well as an increase in cGMP levels, suggests a complex relationship between the metabolic state of the chromatin, cyclic nucleotide levels, mitosis, the ability of a cell to repair its DNA and mutagenesis.

D. Developmental Consequences of Differential DNA Repair in Eukaryotic Cells

To put all these observations into perspective, a speculative hypothesis linking DNA repair, mutagenesis, and carcinogenesis is proposed. First, the eukaryotic chromosome can be functionally viewed as containing 3 units (Fig. 3): (1) those derepressed regions being expressed or transcribed, (2) those repressed regions capable of being derepressed in an adaptive response of the cell to some stimulus, and (3) those repressed regions of the chromosome that, in a particular cell type will never, under normal conditions, be transcribed. Since there is evidence that chromosomal proteins can inhibit repair (Wilkins and Hart, 1974) and that phytohemagglutinin stimulation (presumably causing derepression) enhances repair (Darzynkiewicz, 1971), one would surmise that the DNA in the dere-

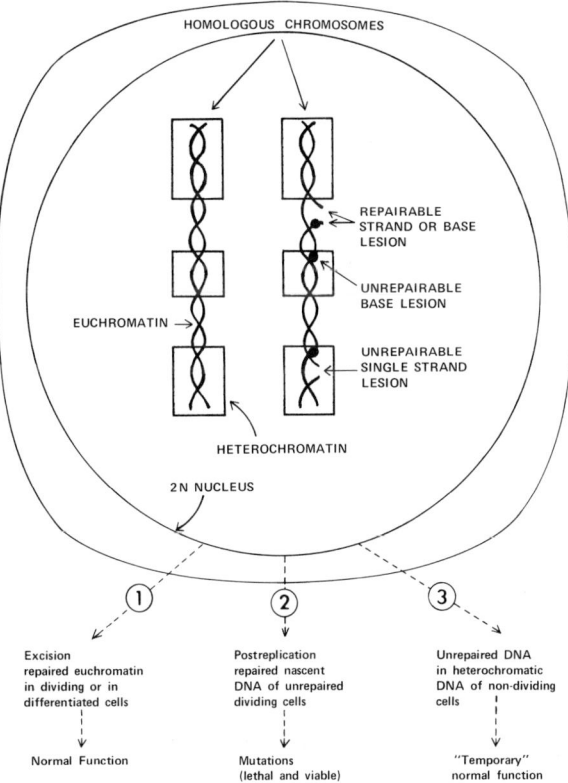

FIG. 3. Diagrammatic representation of the speculated role of chromosomal protein on differential damage and repair in the DNA of eukaryotic chromosomes.

pressed regions (region 1) might be readily accessible to the repair enzymes while the DNA in region 2 would be less accessible but eventually repairable. The permanently repressed regions might be completely inaccessible to the repair enzymes, and it is here that damaged DNA may persist or even accumulate. A model for aging based on the differential repair of damaged DNA has been proposed by Yielding (1974). Support for such a hypothesis can be inferred from the work of Hart and Setlow (1974). There is also evidence that both UV- and X-ray-induced chromosome breaks in human chromosomes are not randomly dispersed throughout the chromosomes (Roman and Bobrow, 1973; Holmberg and Jonasson, 1973). If X-ray-induced DNA breaks are responsible for chromosome breaks, then differential repair, rather than differential damage, apparently would be responsible (Lett and Sun, 1970). One possible interpretation is that these lesions are inaccessible to repair.

In any given nondividing cell, only those regions of DNA responsible for providing information to maintain the developmental and metabolic state of that cell would be repaired by a relatively error-free excision-type repair enzyme. Many of the lesions in the depressed regions, if not repaired, will not interfere with the functioning of this nondividing cell. After treatment with carcinogenic agents (those that damage DNA), different cell types with quantitatively different excision repair capacities (Bootsma et al., 1970; Setlow and Regan, 1972) repair the DNA accessible to repair enzymes to different extents. However, no matter how high a cell's repair capacity, unrepaired lesions will still exist in chromatin inaccessible to repair enzymes. Upon promotion, which might occur minutes or months after initiation of damage, DNA synthesis and concomitant derepression of DNA are stimulated, whereupon nascent DNA is made off of an unrepaired or incompletely repaired template. One would predict that lethal mutagenic and carcinogenic frequencies would be higher in cells that enter DNA synthesis shortly after DNA damage than in those that have more time to repair damage. Such evidence does exist (Hennings et al., 1973). Nascent DNA would be made with gaps occurring adjacent to the unrepaired lesions. These gaps might subsequently be repaired by an error-prone, gap-filling process misnamed *postreplication repair*. In this context, repair only means that the gap was filled, for the cell is certainly not *repaired* or rendered normal. The errors produced (e.g., point mutations or chromosome aberrations) could result in either no adverse effect on the cell, death, or a mutated expression that could, among other things, ultimately give rise to a cancer.

VI. Evolutionary Perspectives of Somatic Mutagenesis

The human being, like most eukaryotic organisms, can be viewed as consisting of somatic and germinal tissues. Mutations on the germ level are the grist for evolution's mill. Organisms live in a constantly changing environment, consequently every species must be able to produce mutant variants that would be adaptable to a new environment that is hostile to the "nonmutant." In this sense, limited mutation on the germ level is of selective advantage. If mutagenesis is the result of genetically controlled repair enzymes (see *Genetics*, Vol. 73, Suppl., 1973), then obviously repair enzymes, which have a degree of "error-proneness" associated with their function, would be of selective advantage to the species.

However, since genes and chromosomes in the somatic tissue are not refractory to environmental damage, repair also must take place. Since mutations can be induced in human somatic cells (Albertini and De Mars, 1973), we have no reason to doubt that they are the result of an "error-prone" repair mechanism. Both cancer and aging might be the "price" individual organisms have to pay for the survival of the species (De Grouchy, 1973).

This hypothesis might help explain, among other things, two observations linking carcinogenesis with the aging process. The first observation is that normal cells, grown in cell cultures as fibroblasts have a finite life-span (Hayflick and Moorehead, 1961), whereas transformed or cancer cells, *in vitro*, can proliferate indefinitely. Normal cells are "mortal," whereas cancer cells are, in essence, "immortal." Therefore, one might surmise that to understand the theoretical mechanism for the transformation of a normal cell to a cancer cell might lead to our understanding of the normal aging process of normal cells. The second observation is that as one gets older, the probability of cancer increases (Dorn and Cutler, 1959).

As an explanation for the increase of tumor frequency with aging, as well as the high frequencies of tumors in genetically deficient individuals, or in individuals with drug-depressed immune systems, the concept of immunological surveillance has been advanced (Wolford, 1969; Burnet, 1970). This hypothesis suggests that growth of neoplasms (promotion of initiated, but latent precancerous cells) is prevented by a complex combination of factors preventing the mitosis of initiated cells and the immunological destruction of some of those that do divide (Fig. 4). In this sense, the immunological surveillance system can be viewed as one of several "antipromoters" (Fig. 2). Other antipromoters might be hormones which repress mi-

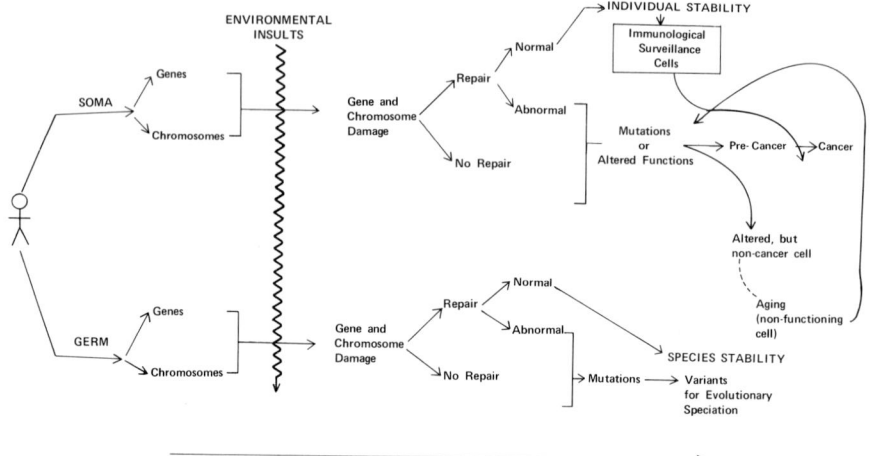

FIG. 4. A speculative model relating faulty DNA repair on the germ and soma levels with evolution, cancer, and aging. Thus, mutated cells, resulting from DNA damage, which have a tumor potential, are held in check only as long as cells of the immunological surveillance system function properly. In time, nonrepaired lesions accumulate in all cells, including those of the immunological surveillance system. Thus, the "aging" of the surveillance cells, due to the nonrepair of DNA lesions, allows mutated somatic cells, on stimulation, to develop into tumors.

tosis. Further, it suggests that the cellular immune response should decline with age. Evidence does exist which supports the prediction that the immune surveillance cells are not "immune" to the aging process. Immunological competence, measured several ways, of lymphocytes from old persons were shown to be depressed compared with the response of lymphocytes from young persons (Weksler and Hutteroth, 1974).

Barnhill and Yielding (1974) have proposed a model for antibody diversity based on somatic mutations. Since the cells of immunological surveillance systems, themselves, are not "immune" to the aging process, one might predict the decline of the immunological competency of cells is positively related to some kind of DNA repair competency during development. Supporting this idea are the series of reports which demonstrate that DNA repair is modulated by genetic factors influencing development and differentiation in eukaryotic organisms (Darzynkiewicz, 1971; Hahn et al., 1971; Stockdale, 1971; Wilkins and Hart, 1974). One would also predict that not only would more tumors appear due to the nonfunctioning (aging) of the immunological surveillance cells, but also to the increased mutations. Assuming that mutagenesis is responsible for some carcinogenic events, Ebbesen (1974) has produced data that support the preceding hypothesis. He was able to show that aging increases susceptibility of mouse skin to chemical carcinogenesis, independent of the general immune status.

VII. Summary and Conclusion

A highly speculative and heuristic scheme has been developed to account for a wide range of observations which make it appear that the carcinogenic process has several heritable components. Based on the assumptions (1) that germ-line mutations on several levels could influence carcinogenesis and (2) that DNA repair and somatic mutagenesis are related in mammalian systems in a manner similar to bacteriological systems, a model was presented that linked various genetic and environmental factors influencing DNA repair with observations on the initiation and promotion of tumors.

Within this model, genes which influence (1) the level of genetic damage, (2) the level and efficiency of the repair of DNA damage, and (3) the proliferation of the altered cells, are those that are subject to wide variation in expression owing to individual genetic or environmental predispositions. At this time, only circumstantial evidence links DNA repair to carcinogenesis in human beings. A critical component of the somatic mutation theory of cancer will be an elaboration of the role of the repair of carcinogen-induced DNA damage to mutagenesis in eukaryotic systems.

Within the framework of the model presented, it would appear that the goal of a total prevention of cancer and the development of a universal therapy for the cure of cancer will be extremely difficult, if not impossible, to attain. Even if the amount of potential carcinogens (initiators) in the human environment could be prevented from increasing, it could never be reduced to zero levels. From the standpoint of the genetic influence on carcinogenesis, one can see from the model presented in Fig. 2 that there are many steps at which genetic variability could lead to the genetic predisposition to cancer, as well as many levels by which certain environmental factors can enhance the carcinogenic and aging processes.

Last, a highly speculative hypothesis was offered which linked somatic mutagenesis, due to faulty DNA repair, to carcinogenesis and aging. Genetic instability, due to faulty DNA repair (or replication) on the gene or chromosomal level in the germ cells, has selective advantage because it can contribute to sources of variation needed for the evolution of the species. At the same time, it was hypothesized that gene and chromosome instability in the soma could manifest themselves in both the carcinogenic and aging process.

In essence, a cybernetic-feedback type of model was advanced which linked germ-line mutations, which favor the initiation and promotion of somatic mutations, to those somatic mutations that alter a cell's ability to respond to cell division regulators.

ACKNOWLEDGMENTS

J. E. T. wishes to acknowledge the stimulating discussion with Dr. James Yager and Dr. June Goodfield on the integrative aspects of carcinogenesis. The authors wish to express their appreciation to Mrs. Pamela Watkins for her cooperation on the typing of this review.

REFERENCES

Albertini, R. J., and De Mars, R. (1973). *Mutat. Res.* **18**, 199–224.
Anderson, W. B., Russell, T. R., Carchman, R. A., and Pastan, I. (1973). *Proc. Nat. Acad. Sci. U. S.* **70**, 3802–3805.
Arlett, C., and Harcourt, S. (1972). *Mutat. Res.* **61**, 301–306.
Auerbach, C., and Robson, J. M. (1944). *Nature (London)* **154**, 81.
Bacchetti, S., van der Plas, A., and Veldhuisen, G. (1972). *Biochem. Biophys. Res. Commun.* **48**, 662–669.
Baird, W. M., Sedgwick, J. A., and Boutwell, R. K. (1971). *Cancer Res.* **31**, 1434–1439.
Barnhill, C. W., and Yielding, K. L. (1974). *J. Theor. Biol.* **43**, 197–209.
Bauer, H. K. (1928). "Mutationstheorie der Geschwulst-Entstehung." Springer-Verlag, Berlin and New York.
Belman, S., and Troll, W. (1972). *Cancer Res.* **32**, 450–454.
Ben-Ishai, R. (1974). *ICN-UCLA Winter Conf. Mol. Biol., Squaw Valley, Calif.* (Abstr.)
Berenblum, I. (1954). *Cancer Res.* **14**, 471–477.
Bootsma, D., Mulder, M. P., Pot, F., and Cohen, J. A. (1970). *Mutat. Res.* **9**, 507–516.
Boutwell, R. K. (1964). *Progr. Exp. Tumor Res.* **4**, 207–250.
Boutwell, R. K. (1974). "Critical Reviews on Toxicology," pp. 244–419. Chem. Rubber Publ. Co., Cleveland, Ohio.
Boveri, T. (1929). "The Origin of Malignant Tumors." Williams & Wilkins, Baltimore, Maryland.
Boyce, R., and Howard-Flanders, P. (1964). *Proc. Nat. Acad. Sci. U. S.* **51**, 293–300.
Bridges, B. A. (1969). *Annu. Rev. Nucl. Sci.* **19**, 139–178.
Buhl, S. N., and Regan, J. D. (1973). *Nature (London)* **246**, 484.
Buhl, S. N., Stillman, R. M., Setlow, R. B., and Regan, J. D. (1972). *Biophys. J.* **12**, 1183–1191.
Burdette, W. J. (1955). *Cancer Res.* **15**, 201–226.
Burnet, F. M. (1970). "Immunological Surveillance." Pergamon, Oxford.
Carrier, W. L., and Setlow, R. B. (1971). *In* "Methods in Nucleic Acids," Part D (L. Grossman and K. Moldave, eds.), Methods in Enzymology, Vol. 21, pp. 330–337. Academic Press, N. Y.
Cerutti, P. A. (1974). *Naturwissenschaften* **61**, 51–59.
Charles, D. R., and Luce-Clausen, E. M. (1942). *Cancer Res.* **2**, 261–263.
Chiu, S. F. H., and Rauth, A. M. (1972). *Biochim. Biophys. Acta* **259**, 164–174.
Cho-Chung, Y. S., and Gullino, P. M. (1974). *Science* **183**, 87–88.

Clarkson, B., and Baserga, R., eds. (1974). "Control of Proliferation in Animal Cells." Cold Spring Harbor Lab., Cold Spring Harbor, New York.
Clayson, D. B. (1962). "Chemical Carcinogens." Little, Brown, Boston, Massachusetts.
Cleaver, J. E. (1966). *Biochem. Biophys. Res. Commun.* **24**, 569–576.
Cleaver, J. E. (1968). *Nature (London)* **218**, 652–656.
Cleaver, J. E. (1969a). *Proc. Nat. Acad. Sci. U. S.* **63**, 428–435.
Cleaver, J. E. (1969b). *Radiat. Res.* **37**, 334–348.
Cleaver, J. E. (1970). *Int. J. Radiat. Biol.* **18**, 557–565.
Cleaver, J. E. (1971). *Mutat. Res.* **12**, 453–462.
Cleaver, J. E. (1973). *In* "Current Research in Oncology" (C. B. Anfinsen and M. Potter, eds.), pp. 15–43. Academic Press, New York.
Cleaver, J. E. (1974). *Radiat. Res.* **57**, 207–227.
Cleaver, J. E., and Thomas, G. H. (1969). *Biochem. Biophys. Res. Commun.* **36**, 203–208.
Cleaver, J. E., and Trosko, J. E. (1970). *Photochem. Photobiol.* **11**, 547–550.
Coleman, A., Leikin, S., and Guin, G. H. (1961). *Clin. Proc. Child. Hosp. Wash.* **17**, 22–27.
Comings, D. E. (1973). *Proc. Nat. Acad. Sci. U. S.* **70**, 3324–3328.
Commings, R. B., and Walton, M. F. (1973). *Food Cosmet. Toxicol.* **11**, 547–553.
Conney, A. H. (1973). *New Engl. J. Med.* **289**, 971–973.
Cook, J. S. (1971). *In* "Photophysiology" (A. C. Giese, ed.), Vol. 5, pp. 191–233. Academic Press, New York.
Corry, P. M., and Cole, A. (1968). *Radiat. Res.* **36**, 528–543.
Corry, P. M., and Cole, A. (1973). *Nature (London), New Biol.* **245**, 100–101.
Cox, R., Damjanov, I., Abanobi, S. E., and Sarma, D. S. R. (1973). *Cancer Res.* **33**, 2114–2121.
Darzynkiewicz, Z. (1971). *Exp. Cell Res.* **69**, 356–360.
Darzynkiewicz, Z., and Chelmicha-Szorc, E. (1972). *Exp. Cell Res.* **74**, 131–139.
De Grouchy, J. (1973). *Biomedicine* **18**, 6–8.
De Waard, R. H. (1964). *Int. J. Radiat. Biol.* **8**, 381–387.
Domon, M., and Rauth, A. M. (1969). *Radiat. Res.* **39**, 207–221.
Dorn, H. F., and Cutler, S. J. (1959). *U. S. Pub. Health Serv., Publ. Health Monogr.* No. 56, 1.
Drake, J. W. (1969). *Annu. Rev. Genet.* **3**, 247–268.
Drake, J. W. (1970). "The Molecular Basis of Mutation." Holden-Day, San Francisco, California.
Duncan, J., Slor, H., Cook, K., and Friedberg, E. C. (1974). *ICN-UCLA Winter Conf. Mol. Biol. Squaw Valley, Calif.* (Abstr.)
Ebbesen, P. (1974). *Science* **183**, 217–218.
Edenberg, H., and Hanawalt, P. (1972). *Biochim. Biophys. Acta* **272**, 361–372.
Edenberg, H., and Hanawalt, P. (1973). *Biochim. Biophys. Acta* **324**, 206–217.
Epstein, J., Williams, J. R., and Little, J. (1973). *Proc. Nat. Acad. Sci. U. S.* **170**, 977–981.
Estensen, R. D., Hadden, J. W., Hadden, E. M., Touraine, F., Touraine, J. L., Haddox, M. K., and Goldberg, N. D. (1974). *In* "Control of Proliferation in Animal Cells" (B. Clarkson and R. Baserga, eds.), pp. 627–634. Cold Spring Harbor Lab., Cold Spring Harbor, New York.
Fishbein, L., Flamm, W. G., and Falk, H. L. (1970). "Chemical Mutagens." Academic Press, New York.
Fisher, J. C., and Hollomon, J. H. (1951). *Cancer (Philadelphia)* **4**, 916–918.

Freese, E. (1963). In "Molecular Genetics" (J. H. Taylor, ed.), Part 1, pp. 207–269. Academic Press, New York.
Frei, J. V., and Stephens, P. (1968). Brit. J. Cancer 22, 83–92.
Fujiwara, Y., and Kondo, T. (1972). Biochem. Biophys. Res. Commun. 47, 557–564.
Gaudin, D., Gregg, R., and Yielding, K. (1972). Biochem. Biophys. Res. Commun. 48, 945–949.
Gautschi, J. R., Young, B. R., and Cleaver, J. E. (1973). Exp. Cell Res. 76, 87–94.
Gledhill, B., and Darzynkiewicz, Z. (1973). J. Exp. Zool. 183, 375–382.
Goldberg, N. D., Haddox, M. K., Dunham, E., Lopey, C., and Hadden, J. W. (1974). In "Control of Proliferation in Animal Cells" (B. Clarkson and R. Baserga, eds.), pp. 609–625. Cold Spring Harbor Lab., Cold Spring Harbor, New York.
Goldstein, S. (1971). Proc. Soc. Exp. Biol. Med. 137, 730–734.
Good, R. A., Dalmasso, A. P., Martinez, C., Archer, O. K., Pierce, J. C., and Papermaster, B. W. (1962). J. Exp. Med. 116, 773–795.
Goodman, J. I., and Potter, V. R. (1972). Cancer Res. 32, 766–775.
Griggs, H., and Bender, M. A. (1973). Science 179, 86–88.
Habazin, V., and Han, A. (1970). Int. J. Radiat. Biol. 17, 569–575.
Hahn, G., King, D., and Young, S. (1971). Nature (London), New Biol. 230, 242–244.
Haldane, J. B. S. (1934). J. Pathol. Bacteriol. 38, 507–508.
Hart, R. W., and Setlow, R. B. (1973). Annu. Meet. Amer. Soc. Photobiol., 1st Sarasota, Fla. p. 120 (Abstr.)
Hart, R. W., and Setlow, R. B. (1974). Proc. Nat. Acad. Sci. U. S. 71, 2169–2173.
Hartwell, J. L. (1951). U. S. Pub. Health Serv. Publ. No. 149.
Hayflick, L., and Moorehead, P. S. (1961). Exp. Cell Res. 25, 585–621.
Hennings, H., Michael, D., and Patterson, E. (1973). Cancer Res. 33, 3130–3134.
Hewish, D., and Burgoyne, L. (1973). Biochem. Biophys. Res. Commun. 52, 504–510.
Hill, R. (1958). Biochim. Biophys. Acta 30, 636–637.
Hollaender, A., ed. (1971). "Chemical Mutagens," Vols. 1 and 2. Plenum, New York.
Hollaender, A., ed (1973). "Chemical Mutagens," Vol. 3. Plenum, New York.
Holley, R. W. (1972). Proc. Nat. Acad. Sci. U. S. 69, 2840–2841.
Holmberg, M., and Jonasson, J. (1973). Hereditas 74, 57–68.
Horikawa, M., Nikaido, O., and Sugahara, T. (1968). Nature (London) 218, 489–491.
Horikawa, M., Nikaido, O., Tanaka, T., Nagata, H., and Sugahara, T. (1970). Exp. Cell Res. 63, 325–332.
Huang, A., Kremer, W., Laszlo, J., and Setlow, R. B. (1972). Nature (London), New Biol. 240, 114–115.
Iversen, O. H., and Evensen, A. (1962). Acta Pathol. Microbiol. Scand., Suppl. 156, 95–143.
Iverson, S., and Arley, N. (1950). Acta Pathol. Microbiol. Scand. 27, 773–803.
Jagger, J. (1958). Bacteriol. Rev. 22, 99–142.
Kao, F. T., and Puck, T. T. (1969). J. Cell. Physiol. 74, 245–258.
Karran, P., and Ormerod, M. G. (1973). Biochim. Biophys. Acta 299, 54–64.
Kato, H. (1973). Exp. Cell Res. 82, 383–390.
Kellermann, G., Luyten-Kellermann, M., and Shaw, C. R. (1973). Amer. J. Hum. Genet. 25, 327–331.
Kersey, J. H., Spector, B. D., and Good, R. A. (1973). Int. J. Cancer 12, 333–347.
Kihlman, B. A., Sturelid, S., Hartley-Asp, B., and Nilsson, K. (1973). Mutat. Res. 17, 271–275.
Klímek, M. (1966). Photochem. Photobiol. 5, 603–607.
Knudson, A. G., Jr. (1971). Proc. Nat. Acad. Sci. U. S. 68, 820–823.

Koller, P. C. (1972). "The Role of Chromosomes in Cancer Biology." Springer-Verlag, Berlin and New York.
Kouri, R. E., Ratrie, H., and Whitmire, C. E. (1974). *Int. J. Cancer* **13**, 714-720.
Krishman, D., and Painter, R. B. (1973). *Mutat. Res.* **717**, 213-222.
Kuhlmann, W., Fromme, H. G., Heege, E. M., and Ostertag, W. (1968). *Cancer Res.* **28**, 2375-2389.
Legator, M. S., and Malling, H. V. (1971). *In* "Chemical Mutagens" (A. Hollaender, ed.), Vol. 2, pp. 569-589. Plenum, New York.
Lehmann, A. R. (1972). *J. Mol. Biol.* **66**, 319-337.
Lehmann, A. R. (1974). *ICN-UCLA Winter Conf. Mol. Biol., Squaw Valley, Calif.* (Abstr.)
Lett, J. T., and Sun, C. (1970). *Radiat. Res.* **44**, 771-787.
Lett, J. T., Caldwell, I., Dean, C. J., and Alexander, P. (1967). *Nature (London)* **214**, 790-792.
Lett, J. T., Klucis, E. S., and Sun, C. (1970). *Biophys. J.* **10**, 277-292.
Levan, A. (1969). *In* "Handbook of Molecular Cytology" (A. Lima-de-Faria, ed.), pp. 717-731. North-Holland Publ., Amsterdam.
Lindahl, T. (1972). *In* "Molecular and Cellular Repair Processes" (R. F. Beers, R. M. Herriott, and R. C. Tilghman, eds.), pp. 3-13. Johns Hopkins Press, Baltimore, Maryland.
Lohman, P. H. M., and Paterson, M. C. (1974). *ICN-UCLA Winter Conf. Mol. Biol., Squaw Valley, Calif.* (Abstr.)
Lucas, C. J. (1972). *Exp. Cell Res.* **74**, 480-486.
Lumb, J. R., Sideropoulos, A. S., and Shankel, D. M. (1968). *Mol. Gen. Genet.* **102**, 108-111.
Maher, V. M., Birch, N., and McCormick, J. J. (1974). *Proc. 65th Amer. Ass. Cancer Res.* **15**, 140 (Abstr.)
Malling, H. V., and Chu, E. H. Y. (1974). *In* "Model Studies in Chemical Carcinogenesis" (P. O. P. T'so and J. A. Di Poalo, eds.), pp. 554-563. Marcel Dekker, New York.
Marks, F., and Grimm, W. (1972). *Nature (London), New Biol.* **240**, 178-179.
Miller, E. C., and Miller, J. A. (1971). *In* "Chemical Mutagens – Principles and Methods for Their Detection" (A. Hollaender, ed.), Vol. 1, pp. 83-119. Plenum, New York.
Miller, J. A., and Miller, E. C. (1969). *Progr. Exp. Tumor Res.* **11**, 273-301.
Millis, A. J. T., Forrest, G. A., and Pious, D. A. (1974). *Exp. Cell Res.* **83**, 335-343.
Modak, S. P., and Price, G. B. (1971). *Exp. Cell Res.* **65**, 289-298.
Mottram, J. C. (1944). *J. Pathol. Bacteriol.* **50**, 181-187.
Nordling, C. O. (1953). *Brit. J. Cancer* **7**, 68-72.
Otten, J., Johnson, G. S., and Pastan, I. (1971). *Biochem. Biophys. Res. Commun.* **44**, 1192-1198.
Painter, R. B. (1974). *Genetics* **78**, 139-148.
Painter, R. B., and Cleaver, J. E. (1967). *Nature (London)* **216**, 369-370.
Painter, R. B., and Cleaver, J. E. (1969). *Radiat. Res.* **37**, 451-466.
Painter, R. B., and Wolff, S. (1973). *Mutat. Res.* **19**, 133-136.
Painter, R. B., Clarkson, J. M., and Young, B. R. (1973). *Radiat. Res.* **56**, 560-564.
Paterson, M. C., Lohman, P. H. M., and Sluyter, M. L. (1973). *Mutat. Res.* **19**, 245-256.
Paul, D., and Hecker, E. (1969). *Z. Krebsforsch.* **73**, 149-163.
Penn, I., and Starzl, T. E. (1972). *Transplantation* **14**, 407-417.
Peraino, C., Fry, R. J. M., Staffeldt, E., and Kisieleski, W. E. (1973). *Cancer Res.* **33**, 2701-2705.

Poon, P. K., Parker, J. W., and O'Brien, R. L. (1974). *Proc. 65th Amer. Ass. Cancer Res.* **15,** 19. (Abstr.)
Potter, V. R. (1969). *Proc. Can Cancer Res. Conf.* **8,** 9–30.
Price, G. B., Modak, S. P., and Makinodan, T. (1971). *Science* **171,** 917–920.
Radman, M. (1974). *In* "Molecular and Environmental Aspects of Mutagenesis" (M. Miller, ed.). Thomas, Springfield, Illinois.
Raick, A. N. (1973). *Cancer Res.* **33,** 269–286.
Raick, A. N., and Ritchie, A. C. (1970). *Proc. Amer. Ass. Cancer Res.* **11,** 65.
Rasmussen, R. E., and Painter, R. B. (1964). *Nature (London)* **203,** 1360–1362.
Rauth, A. M. (1967). *Radiat. Res.* **31,** 121–128.
Regan, J. D., and Cook, J. S. (1967). *Proc. Nat. Acad. Sci. U. S.* **58,** 2274–2279.
Regan, J. D., Trosko, J. E., and Carrier, W. L. (1968). *Biophys. J.* **8,** 319–325.
Regan, J. D., Setlow, R. B., and Ley, R. D. (1971). *Proc. Nat. Acad. Sci. U. S.* **68,** 708–712.
Roberts, J. J., and Sturrock, J. (1973). *Mutat. Res.* **20,** 243–255.
Roberts, J. J., and Ward, K. N. (1973). *Chem.-Biol. Interactions* **7,** 241–264.
Roberts, J. J., Crathorn, A. R., and Brent, T. P. (1968). *Nature (London)* **218,** 970–972.
Rohrschneider, L. R., O'Brien, D. H., and Boutwell, R. K. (1972). *Biochim. Biophys. Acta* **280,** 57–70.
Roman, C. S., and Bobrow, M. (1973). *Mutat. Res.* **18,** 325–331.
Rupp, W. D., and Howard-Flanders, P. (1968). *J. Mol. Biol.* **31,** 291–304.
Ryser, H. J. P. (1971). *New Engl. J. Med.* **285,** 721–734.
Saffhill, R., Cooper, H. K., and Hzhaki, R. F. (1974). *Nature (London)* **248,** 153–156.
Sasaki, M. S. (1973). *Mutat. Res.* **20,** 291–293.
Satoh, T., and Yamamoto, N. (1972). *Cancer Res.* **32,** 440–443.
Sawada, S., and Okada, S. (1970). *Radiat. Res.* **41,** 145–162.
Sawada, S., and Okada, S. (1972). *Int. J. Radiat. Biol.* **21,** 599–602.
Setlow, R. B. (1968). *Progr. Nucl. Acid Res. Mol. Biol.* **8,** 257–295.
Setlow, R. B., and Carrier, W. L. (1964). *Proc. Nat. Acad. Sci. U. S.* **51,** 226–231.
Setlow, R. B., and Carrier, W. L. (1968). *In* "International Conference on Replication and Recombination of Genetic Material" (W. J. Peacock and R. D. Broch, eds.), pp. 134–141. Aust. Acad. Sci., Canberra.
Setlow, R. B., and Regan, J. D. (1972). *Biochem. Biophys. Res. Commun.* **46,** 1019–1024.
Setlow, R. B., and Setlow, J. K. (1972). *Annu. Rev. Biophys. Bioeng.* **1,** 293–346.
Setlow, R. B., Regan, J. D., German, J., and Carrier, W. L. (1969). *Proc. Nat. Acad. Sci. U. S.* **64,** 1035–1041.
Setlow, R. B., Regan, J. D., and Carrier, W. L. (1972). *Annu. Meet. Biophys. Soc. 16th, Toronto.* (Abstr.).
Shamberger, R., Baughman, F. F., Kalchert, S. L., Willis, C. E., and Hoffman, G. C. (1973). *Proc. Nat. Acad. Sci. U. S.* **70,** 1461–1463.
Sheppard, J. R. (1972). *Nature (London), New Biol.* **236,** 14–16.
Shubik, P., and Hartwell, J. L. (1959). *U. S. Pub. Health Serv. Publ., Suppl.* **1.**
Shubik, P., and Hartwell, J. L. (1969). *U. S. Pub. Health Serv. Publ., Suppl.* **2.**
Sideropoulos, A. S., and Shankel, D. M. (1968). *J. Bacteriol.* **96,** 198–204.
Silverman, B., and Mirsky, A. (1973). *Proc. Nat. Acad. Sci. U. S.* **70,** 1326–1330.
Sivak, A., and Van Durren, B. L. (1971). *Chem.-Biol. Interactions* **3,** 401–411.
Slaga, T. J., Rice, J. N., Das, S. B., and Thompson, S. (1974). *Proc. 65th Amer. Ass. Cancer Res.* **15,** 62. (Abstr.)
Smith, K. C. (1964). *Photochem. Photobiol.* **3,** 415–427.

Smith, K. C. (1966). *Radiat. Res., Suppl.* **6**, 54–79.
Steward, D. L., and Humphrey, R. M. (1966). *Nature (London)* **212**, 298–300.
Stich, H. F., San, R. H. C., and Kawazoe, Y. (1971). *Nature (London)* **229**, 416–419.
Stich, H. F., San, R. H. C., Miller, J. A., and Miller, E. C. (1972). *Nature (London), New Biol.* **238**, 9–10.
Stockdale, F. (1971). *Science* **171**, 1145–1147.
Sutherland, B. M. (1974). *Nature (London)* **248**, 109–112.
Sutherland, E. W., and Rall, T. W. (1958). *J. Biol. Chem.* **232**, 1077–1091.
Teebor, G., Duker, N., Ruacan, S., and Zachary, K. (1973). *Biochem. Biophys. Res Commun.* **50**, 66–70.
Trosko, J. E., and Chu, E. H. Y. (1973). *Chem.-Biol. Interactions* **6**, 317–332.
Trosko, J. E., and Isoun, M. (1970). *Int. J. Radiat. Biol.* **18**, 271–275.
Trosko, J. E., and Yager, J. D. (1974). *Exp. Cell Res.* **88**, 47–55.
Trosko, J., Chu, E. H. Y., and Carrier, W. L. (1965). *Radiat. Res.* **24**, 667–672.
Trosko, J. E., Frank, P., Chu, E. H. Y., and Becker, J. E. (1973). *Cancer Res.* **33**, 2444–2449.
Van Duuren, B. L. V. (1969). *Progr. Exp. Tumor Res.* **11**, 31–68.
Verly, W., Paquette, Y., and Thibodeau, L. (1973). *Nature (London), New Biol.* **244**, 67–69.
Vogel, F., and Rohrborn, G. (1970). "Chemical Mutagenesis in Mammals and Man." Springer-Verlag, Berlin and New York.
Voorhees, J. J., Duell, E. A., Bass, J. L., Powell, J. A., and Harrell, E. R. (1972). *Arch. Dermatol.* **105**, 695–701.
Voorhees, J. J., Colburn, N. H., Stawiski, M., Duell, E. A., Haddox, M., and Goldberg, N. D. (1974). *In* "Control of Proliferation in Animal Cells" (B. Carkson and R. Baserga, eds.), pp. 635–648. Cold Spring Harbor Lab., Cold Spring Harbor, New York.
Wacker, A. (1963). *Progr. Nucl. Acid Res.* **1**, 369–399.
Walker, I. G., and Reid, B. D. (1971). *Mutat. Res.* **12**, 101–104.
Walker, P. R., and Potter, V. R. (1972). *Advan. Enzyme Regul.* **10**, 339–364.
Walters, R. A., Gurley, L. R., and Tobey, R. A. (1974). *Biophys. J.* **14**, 99–118.
Wattenberg, L. W. (1973). *J. Nat. Cancer Inst.* **50**, 1541–1544.
Weber, A. (1968). *J. Gen. Physiol.* **52**, 760–772.
Weksler, M. E., and Hutteroth, T. H. (1974). *J. Clin. Invest.* **53**, 99–104.
Wheeler, K. T., and Lett, J. T. (1972). *Radiat. Res.* **52**, 59–67.
Wheeler, K. T., Sheridan, R. E., Pantler, E. L., and Lett, J. T. (1973). *Radiat. Res.* **53**, 414–427.
Wilkins, R. J. (1973). *Int. J. Radiat. Biol.* **24**, 609–613.
Wilkins, R. J., and Hart, R. (1974). *Nature (London)* **247**, 35–36.
Wilkinson, R., Kiefer, J., and Nias, A. H. W. (1970). *Mutat. Res.* **10**, 67–72.
Witkin, E. M. (1947). *Cold Spring Harbor Symp. Quant. Biol.* **12**, 256–269.
Witkin, E. M. (1969a). *Annu. Rev. Microbiol.* **23**, 487–514.
Witkin, E. M. (1969b). *Annu. Rev. Genet.* **3**, 525–552.
Witkin, E., and George, D. (1973). *Genetics* **73**, 91–108.
Wolff, S., and Cleaver, J. E. (1973). *Mutat. Res.* **20**, 71–76.
Wolford, K. L. (1969). "The Immunologic Theory of Aging." Munksgaard, Copenhagen.
Yielding, K. L. (1974). *Perspect. Biol. Med.* **17**, 201–208.
Zajdela, F., and Latarjet, R. (1973). *C. R. Acad. Sci., Ser. D* **277**, 1073–1076.

SUBJECT INDEX

A

A-particles, in lung tumors, 24
Actinomycin, variant-cell selection by, 346–348
Aging
  DNA repair and, 408–409
  epithelial cells and, 251–261
Air pollutants, lung tumor induction by, 37–38
Alkylating agents, lung tumor induction by, 28
α-Amanitin, variant cell resistance to, 350–351
Aminoazo compounds, lung tumor induction by, 33–34
β-D-Arabinofuranosylcytosine, variant-cell selection by, 331–334
Autolysis, tumor cell death and, 90–93
Auxotrophs, as variant cells, 364–368
8-Azaguanine, variant-cell selection by, 289–304
8-Azaguanosine, variant-cell selection by, 316
8-Azahypoxanthine, variant-cell selection by, 309–310
6-Azauridine, variant-cell selection by, 335
Aziridines, lung tumor induction by, 27–28

B

Benzpyrene hydroxylase, lung tumors and, 22–23, 25
Bioassay, of carcinogenesis, mice tumor use in, 1–58
5-Bromo-2'-deoxyuridine, variant-cell selection by, 318–329
Butylated hydroxyanisole (BHA), effect on mouse lung tumors, 23

C

C-particles, in lung tumors, 24
Cancer. (*See also* Malignant tissue; Tumors)
  cells, immune elimination of, 82–90
  tissue, cell death in 59–120
Candida parapsilosis, lung tumors and, 38
Carbamates, lung tumor induction by, 27–28
Carbohydrate analogs, variant-cell selection by, 348–349
Carcinogenesis
  bioassay of, using lung tumors, 1–58
  DNA repair in, 391–425
  genetic aspects of, 395–396
  molecular basis for, 395–400
  somatic mutation in, 391–425
Carcinoma cells, culture of, 259–260
Cats, oncornaviruses in, 175–248
Cell(s)
  cycle of, mathematical models of, 108–110
  mammalian, variant and mutant, in culture, 273–390
    with altered nutritional requirements, 279, 364–370
    antigenic surface variations, 278–279, 358–364
    characterization, 286–289
    drug-resistant, 276–278, 289–358
    resistance to physical agents, 376–378
    selection of, 282–286
    spontaneous, 379
    steroid resistance of, 349–350
    temperature-sensitive, 280, 370–376
  senescence of, theory, 252–253
Cell death, 59–120
  cell identification of, *in vitro*, 77–78
  chromosome aberrations as cause of, 74–77
  continuous labeling data on, 112–113
  by differentiation, 93–96
  in embryogenesis, 61–64
  in experimental tumors, 96–100
  in human tumors, 100–106
  lymphoid infiltration into tumors and, 88–90
  microcinematography of, 68–71

in normal and malignant tissue, 59–120
in tumors
assessment *in vivo*, 78–79
mathematical studies, 108–114
modes, 113–114
phagocytosis and autolysis in, 90–93
scanning electron microscopy of, 71–73
transmission electron microscopy of, 65–68
tumor therapy and, 106–108
Cell division, biochemical control of, 412–414
Chemical carcinogens, as mutagens, 393–395
Chemicals
effect on lung tumors, 22–23
lung tumor induction by, 25–35
Chemotherapy, lung-tumor response to, 35
Chloramphenicol, variant cell resistance to, 351
Chromatin, in DNA repair, 407
Chromosome, aberrations, cell death and, 74–77
Colchicine, variant cell resistance to, 351
Concanavalin A, variant cell resistance to, 351, 356
Cycasin, lung tumor induction by, 34

D

Daunomycin, variant cell resistance to, 356
Deoxycytidine analogs, variant-cell selection by, 331–334
2-Deoxyglucose, variant-cell selection by, 348–349
4,4'-Diacetyl-diphenyl-urea-bisguanyl-hydrazone, variant cell resistance to, 356
2:6-Diaminopurine, variant-cell selection by, 310–314
Dibutyryladenosine, variant-cell selection by, 317–318
Differentiation, tumor cell death by, 93–96
Disease, histocompatibility-linked *Ir* genes in, 168–170

DNA
damage to, 400–407
initiation, 400–402
repair of, 400–407
in carcinogenesis, 391–425
enzymes for, 402–403
in eukaryotic cells, 415–416
factors influencing, 407–416
Drugs, lung tumor response to, 34–35
Dye exclusion test, for cell death, 77–78
Dyes, lung tumor induction by, 33–34

E

Embryogenesis, cell loss in, 61–64
Embryos, of mice, lung tumor studies on, 44–46
Environment, DNA damage and, 409–412
Epithelial cells, 249–271
aging and, 251–261
culture of, 249–271
cell contamination, 249–250
neoplastic, 259–260
normal, 256–259
permanent, 256–257
division potential of, 261–268
intestinal, division of, 267–268
normal and neoplastic, 250–251
squamous, division of, 263–267
Explants, pulmonary, tumor studies on, 44–46

F

Feline leukemia virus (FeLV)
immune response to, 203–205
replication in cultured cells, 186–188
transmission of, 205–230
Feline oncornaviruses, 175–248
antigenic structure of, 181–186
biochemical and biophysical properties of, 180–181
cell-surface antigens induced by, 191–194
characteristics of, 178–181
comparison to other oncogenic viruses, 230–233
core antigens of, 181–184
endogenous, 189–191
envelope antigens of, 184–186
host-cell relationships with, 186–191
human exposure to, 233–235

SUBJECT INDEX

immune response to infections of, 199–205
infection by, in various diseases, 226–230
in laboratory and field cats, 220–223
morphology of, 178–179
public health significance of, 233–235
serologic detection of, 181–186
serologic studies on, 223–226
transmission of, 205–230
  horizontal, 208–216
  vertical, 216–220
tumor induction by, 194–199
Feline sarcoma viruses (FeSV)
  immune response to, 199–203
  transformation by, 188–189
Fibroblasts, culture of, 254–255
Fibrosarcoma, feline, virus induction of, 197–199
2-Fluoroadenine, variant-cell selection by, 314
2-Fluoradenosine, variant-cell selection by, 317
Fluoride, variant cell resistance to, 356–357
5-Fluorouracil, variant-cell selection by, 335
5-Fluorouridine, variant-cell selection by, 335
Folic acid analogs, variant-cell selection by, 335–343
Food additives, lung tumor induction by, 34
Fungi, lung tumors and, 38

G

Genes, histocompatibility-linked immune response type, 121–173
Guinea pig, histocompatibility-linked immune response genes in, 122–124

H

Heat, variant cell resistance to, 376–377
Histocompatibility-linked immune response genes, 121–173
  cell types expressed by, 135–140
  in disease, 168–170
  function, 165–168
  immunoglobulin structural genes and, 133–135

mapping of, 130–133
products of
  identification, 153–162
  interrelationships, 162–165
  role in T-B interactions, 143–159
  species distribution of, 121–130
Hormones, effect on mouse lung tumors, 23
Humans, exposure to feline oncornaviruses, 233–235
Hydrazine derivatives, lung tumor induction by, 32–33
Hydrocarbons, lung tumor induction by, 26–27

I

Immune response
  histocompatibility-linked genes for, 121–173
  tumor growth and, 82–90
Immunoglobulin
  antigens to cell variants with, 358–364
  structural genes for, H-linked Ir genes and, 133–135
Influenza virus, lung tumors and, 24–25
Intestinal epithelial cells, division potential of, 267–268
5-Iodo-2'-deoxyuridine, variant-cell selection by, 329–330
Ionizing radiation, lung-tumor induction by, 35–36
β-Irradiation, variant cell resistance to, 377–378
γ-Irradiation, variant cell resistance to, 378

L

Leukemia
  feline
    horizontal transmission, 208–216
    pathology, 205–208
    virus induction of, 194–197
  human, viremic cats and, 233–235
Leukemia virus, lung tumors and, 25
Lung tumors
  in carcinogenesis assay, 1–58
  in mice
    age effects, 17–18
    bioassay, 38–44
    biochemical aspects, 13–15

environmental factors, 20–23
explants and embryos, 44–46
frequency and distribution, 3–5
growth and transplantation, 11–13
hereditary factors, 15–17
histogenesis, 7–11
host factors, 15–20
immunologic factors, 18–20
induction, 25–38
morphology, 5–7
virus aspects, 23–25
Lymphoid cells, culture of, 255–256

M

Malignant tissue, cell death in, 59–120
Mammalian cells, variant and mutant, in culture, 273–390
Mammary tumor virus, lung tumors and, 25
6-Mercaptopurine, variant-cell selection by, 308–309
Metals, lung-tumor induction by, 38
6-Methylthiopurine ribonucleoside variant-cell selection by, 316–317
Mice
histocompatibility-linked immune response genes in, 124–129
mapping, 130–133
lung tumors in, use in bioassay, 1–58
Microcinematography, of cell death, 68–71
Microcytotoxicity tests, of tumor-cell death, 84–88
Moloney sarcoma virus, lung tumors and, 25
Mutagenesis
genetic basic for, 399–400
molecular basis for, 395–400
Mutant cells, mammalian, in culture, 273–390
Myxoviruses, lung tumors and, 24

N

β-Naphthoflavone, effect on mouse lung tumors, 22–23
4-Nitroquinoline-1-oxide, lung tumor induction by, 34
Nitrosamines, lung tumor induction by, 28–32

O

Oncogenic viruses, feline oncornaviruses compared to, 230–233
Oncornaviruses
feline, see Feline oncornaviruses
in lung tumors, 24
Ouabain, variant cell resistance to, 357

P

Phagocytosis, tumor cell death and, 90–93
Phenobarbital, effect on mouse lung tumors, 22
Photoreactivating repair enzymes, in DNA repair, 402–403
Pollutants, of air, lung-tumor induction by, 37–38
Polycyclic hydrocarbons, lung tumor induction by, 26–27
Purine base analogs, variant-cell selection by, 289–314
Purine nucleoside analogs, variant-cell selection by, 314–318
Puromycin, variant-cell selection by, 343–345

R

Rat, histocompatibility-linked immune response genes in, 129–130

S

Scanning electron microscopy, of cell death, 71–73
Senescence
cell type and, 253–261
cellular, theory of, 252–253
Smoking, lung-tumor induction and, 36–37
Somatic mutation
in carcinogenesis, 391–425
evolutionary aspects of, 417–419
Squamous epithelial cells, division potential of, 263–267
Steroids, variant-cell resistance to, 349–350
Streptomycin, variant cell resistance to, 357–358
Stromal cells, in culture, 254–255
Suppressor T cells, for GAT, 140–143

SUBJECT INDEX

T

T cells, suppressor type, 140–143
T-B cell interactions
  genetic requirements, 157–159
  histocompatibility gene products in, 143–159
6-Thioguanine, variant-cell selection by, 304–308
6-Thioguanosine, variant-cell selection by, 316
Thymidine and analogs, variant-cell selection by, 318
Tobacco, lung-tumor induction by, 36–37
Transmission electron microscopy, of cell death, 65–68
Tubercidin, variant-cell selection by, 317
Tumors
  blood supply of, 80–82
  cell cycle parameters within, 111–112
  cell death in, 78–79, 80–82
  cell loss in
    mathematical studies, 108–114
    modes, 113–114
  experimental, cell loss in, 96–100
  feline oncornavirus induction of, 194–199
  human
    cell loss in, 100–106
    lymphoid infiltration in, 88–90

U

Ultraviolet irradiation, variant cell resistance to, 377
Uracil analogs, variant-cell selection by, 334–335
Uridine analogs, variant-cell selection by, 334–335

V

Variant cells, mammalian, in culture, 273–390
Vinblastine, variant cell resistance to, 358
Virus, effect on mouse lung tumors, 23–25

X

X-rays, variant cell resistance to, 378

CONTENTS OF PREVIOUS VOLUMES

Volume 1

Electronic Configuration and Carcinogenesis
 C. A. Coulson
Epidermal Carcinogenesis
 E. V. Cowdry
The Milk Agent in the Origin of Mammary Tumors in Mice
 L. Dmochowski
Hormonal Aspects of Experimental Tumorigenesis
 T. U. Gardner
Properties of the Agent of Rous No. 1 Sarcoma
 R. J. C. Harris
Applications of Radioisotopes to Studies of Carcinogenesis and Tumor Metabolism
 Charles Heidelberger
The Carcinogenic Aminoazo Dyes
 James A. Miller and Elizabeth C. Miller
The Chemistry of Cytotoxic Alkylating Agents
 M. C. J. Ross
Nutrition in Relation to Cancer
 Albert Tannenbaum and Herbert Silverstone
Plasma Proteins in Cancer
 Richard J. Winzler
AUTHOR INDEX–SUBJECT INDEX

Volume 2

The Reactions of Carcinogens with Macromolecules
 Peter Alexander
Chemical Constitution and Carcinogenic Activity
 G. M. Badger

Carcinogenesis and Tumor Pathogenesis
 I. Berenblum
Ionizing Radiations and Cancer
 Austin M. Brues
Survival and Preservation of Tumors in the Frozen State
 James Craigie
Energy and Nitrogen Metabolism in Cancer
 Leonard D. Fenninger and G. Burroughs Mider
Some Aspects of the Clinical Use of Nitrogen Mustards
 Calvin T. Klopp and Jeanne C. Bateman
Genetic Studies in Experimental Cancer
 L. W. Law
The Role of Viruses in the Production of Cancer
 C. Oberling and M. Guerin
Experimental Cancer Chemotherapy
 C. Chester Stock
AUTHOR INDEX–SUBJECT INDEX

Volume 3

Etiology of Lung Cancer
 Richard Doll
The Experimental Development and Metabolism of Thyroid Gland Tumors
 Harold P. Morris
Electronic Structure and Carcinogenic Activity and Aromatic Molecules: New Developments
 A. Pullman and B. Pullman
Some Aspects of Carcinogenesis
 P. Rondoni
Pulmonary Tumors in Experimental Animals
 Michael B. Shimkin

Oxidative Metabolism of Neoplastic
    Tissues
    Sidney Weinhouse
AUTHOR INDEX–SUBJECT INDEX

Volume 4

Advances in Chemotherapy of Cancer in
    Man
    Sidney Farber, Rudolf Toch, Edward
      Manning Sears, and Donald Pinkel
The Use of Myleran and Similar Agents
    in Chronic Leukemias
    D. A. G. Galton
The Employment of Methods of Inhibition Analysis in the Normal and Tumor-Bearing Mammalian Organism
    Abraham Goldin
Some Recent Work on Tumor Immunity
    P. A. Gorer
Inductive Tissue Interaction in Development
    Clifford Grobstein
Lipids in Cancer
    Frances L. Haven and W. R. Bloor
The Relation between Carcinogenic
    Activity and the Physical and
    Chemical Properties of Angular
    Benzacridines
    A. Lacassagne, N. P. Buu-Hoï, R.
      Daudel, and F. Zajdela
The Hormonal Genesis of Mammary
    Cancer
    O. Mühlbock
AUTHOR INDEX–SUBJECT INDEX

Volume 5

Tumor-Host Relations
    R. W. Begg
Primary Carcinoma of the Liver
    Charles Berman
Protein Synthesis with Special Reference
    to Growth Processes both Normal
    and Abnormal
    P. N. Campbell
The Newer Concept of Cancer Toxin
    Waro Nakahara and Fumiko Fukuoka

Chemically Induced Tumors of Fowls
    P. R. Peacock
Anemia in Cancer
    Vincent E. Price and Robert E.
      Greenfield
Specific Tumor Antigens
    L. A. Zilber
Chemistry, Carcinogenicity, and Metabolism of 2-Fluorenamine and Related
    Compounds
    Elizabeth K. Weisburger and John H.
      Weisburger
AUTHOR INDEX–SUBJECT INDEX

Volume 6

Blood Enzymes in Cancer and Other
    Diseases
    Oscar Bodansky
The Plant Tumor Problem
    Armin C. Braun and Henry N. Wood
Cancer Chemotherapy by Perfusion
    Oscar Creech, Jr. and Edward T.
      Krementz
Viral Etiology of Mouse Leukemia
    Ludwik Gross
Radiation Chimeras
    P. C. Koller, A. J. S. Davies, and Sheila
      M. A. Doak
Etiology and Pathogenesis of Mouse
    Leukemia
    J. F. A. P. Miller
Antagonists of Purine and Pyrimidine
    Metabolites and of Folic Acid
    G. M. Timmis
Behavior of Liver Enzymes in Hepatocarcinogenesis
    George Weber
AUTHOR INDEX–SUBJECT INDEX

Volume 7

Avian Virus Growths and Their Etiologic
    Agents
    J. W. Beard
Mechanisms of Resistance to Anticancer
    Agents
    R. W. Brockman

Cross Resistance and Collateral Sensitivity Studies in Cancer Chemotherapy
Dorris J. Hutchison

Cytogenic Studies in Chronic Myeloid Leukemia
W. M. Court Brown and Ishbel M. Tough

Ethionine Carcinogenesis
Emmanuel Farber

Atmospheric Factors in Pathogenesis of Lung Cancer
Paul Kotin and Hans L. Falk

Progress with Some Tumor Viruses of Chickens and Mammals: The Problem of Passenger Viruses
G. Negroni

AUTHOR INDEX–SUBJECT INDEX

Volume 8

The Structure of Tumor Viruses and Its Bearing on Their Relation to Viruses in General
A. F. Howatson

Nuclear Proteins of Neoplastic Cells
Harris Busch and William J. Steele

Nucleolar Chromosomes: Structures, Interactions, and Perspectives
M. J. Kopac and Gladys M. Mateyko

Carcinogenesis Related to Foods Contaminated by Processing and Fungal Metabolites
H. F. Kraybill and M. B. Shimkin

Experimental Tobacco Carcinogenesis
Ernest L. Wynder and Dietrich Hoffman

AUTHOR INDEX–SUBJECT INDEX

Volume 9

Urinary Enzymes and Their Diagnostic Value in Human Cancer
Richard Stambaugh and Sidney Weinhouse

The Relation of the Immune Reaction to Cancer
Louis V. Caso

Amino Acid Transport in Tumor Cells
R. M. Johnstone and P. G. Scholefield

Studies on the Development, Biochemistry, and Biology of Experimental Hepatomas
Harold P. Morris

Biochemistry of Normal and Leukemic Leucocytes, Thrombocytes, and Bone Marrow Cells
I. F. Seitz

AUTHOR INDEX–SUBJECT INDEX

Volume 10

Carcinogens, Enzyme Induction, and Gene Action
H. V. Gelboin

In Vitro Studies on Protein Synthesis by Malignant Cells
A. Clark Griffin

The Enzymatic Pattern of Neoplastic Tissue
W. Eugene Knox

Carcinogenic Nitroso Compounds
P. N. Magee and J. M. Barnes

The Sulfhydryl Group and Carcinogenesis
J. S. Harington

The Treatment of Plasma Cell Myeloma
Daniel E. Bergsagel, K. M. Griffith, A. Haut, and W. J. Stuckley, Jr.

AUTHOR INDEX–SUBJECT INDEX

Volume 11

The Carcinogenic Action and Metabolism of Urethan and N-Hydroxyurethan
Sidney S. Mirvish

Runting Syndromes, Autoimmunity, and Neoplasia
D. Keast

Viral-Induced Enzymes and the Problem of Viral Oncogenesis
Saul Kit

CONTENTS OF PREVIOUS VOLUMES

The Growth-Regulating Activity of Polyanions: A Theoretical Discussion of Their Place in the Intercellular Environment and Their Role in Cell Physiology
William Regelson

Molecular Geometry and Carcinogenic Activity of Aromatic Compounds. New Perspectives
Joseph C. Arcos and Mary F. Argus

AUTHOR INDEX–SUBJECT INDEX
CUMULATIVE INDEX

Volume 12

Antigens Induced by the Mouse Leukemia Viruses
G. Pasternak

Immunological Aspects of Carcinogenesis by Deoxyribonucleic Acid Tumor Viruses
G. I. Deichman

Replication of Oncogenic Viruses in Virus-Induced Tumor Cells—Their Persistence and Interaction with Other Viruses
H. Hanafusa

Cellular Immunity against Tumor Antigens
Karl Erik Hellström and Ingegerd Hellstrom

Perspectives in the Epidemiology of Leukemia
Irving L. Kessler and Abraham M. Lilienfeld

AUTHOR INDEX–SUBJECT INDEX

Volume 13

The Role of Immunoblasts in Host Resistance and Immunotherapy of Primary Sarcomata
P. Alexander and J. G. Hall

Evidence for the Viral Etiology of Leukemia in the Domestic Mammals
Oswald Jarrett

The Function of the Delayed Sensitivity Reaction as Revealed in the Graft Reaction Culture
Haim Ginsburg

Epigenetic Processes and Their Relevance to the Study of Neoplasia
Gajanan V. Sherbet

The Characteristics of Animal Cells Transformed in Vitro
Ian Macpherson

Role of Cell Association in Virus Infection and Virus Rescue
J. Svoboda and I. Hloźánek

Cancer of the Urinary Tract
D. B. Clayson and E. H. Cooper

Aspects of the EB Virus
M. A. Epstein

AUTHOR INDEX–SUBJECT INDEX

Volume 14

Active Immunotherapy
Georges Mathé

The Investigation of Oncogenic Viral Genomes in Transformed Cells by Nucleic Acid Hybridization
Ernest Winocour

Viral Genome and Oncogenic Transformation: Nuclear and Plasma Membrane Events
Georges Meyer

Passive Immunotherapy of Leukemia and Other Cancer
Roland Motta

Humoral Regulators in the Development and Progression of Leukemia
Donald Metcalf

Complement and Tumor Immunology
Kusuya Nishioka

Alpha-Fetoprotein in Ontogenesis and Its Association with Malignant Tumors
G. I. Abeler

Low Dose Radiation Cancers in Man
Alice Stewart

AUTHOR INDEX–SUBJECT INDEX

Volume 15

Oncogenicity and Cell Transformation by Papovavirus SV40: The Role of the Viral Genome
J. S. Butel, S. S. Tevethia, and J. L. Melnick

Nasopharyngeal Carcinoma (NPC)
J. H. C. Ho

Transcriptional Regulation in Eukaryotic Cells
A. J. MacGillivray, J. Paul, and G. Threlfall

Atypical Transfer RNA's and Their Origin in Neoplastic Cells
Ernest Borek and Sylvia J. Kerr

Use of Genetic Markers to Study Cellular Origin and Development of Tumors in Human Females
Philip J. Fialkow

Electron Spin Resonance Studies of Carcinogenesis
Harold M. Swartz

Some Biochemical Aspects of the Relationship between the Tumor and the Host
V. S. Shapot

Nuclear Proteins and the Cell Cycle
Gary Stein and Renato Baserga

AUTHOR INDEX–SUBJECT INDEX

Volume 16

Polysaccharides in Cancer
Vijai N. Nigam and Antonio Cantero

Antitumor Effects of Interferon
Ion Gresser

Transformation by Polyoma Virus and Simian Virus 40
Joe Sambrook

Molecular Repair, Wound Healing, and Carcinogenesis: Tumor Production a Possible Overhealing?
Sir Alexander Haddow

The Expression of Normal Histocompatibility Antigens in Tumor Cells
Alena Lengerová

1,3-Bis(2-chloroethyl)-1-nitrosourea (BCNU) and Other Nitrosoureas in Cancer Treatment: A Review
Stephen K. Carter, Frank M. Schabel, Jr., Lawrence E. Broder, and Thomas P. Johnston

AUTHOR INDEX–SUBJECT INDEX

Volume 17

Polysaccharides in Cancer: Glycoproteins and Glycolipids
Vijai N. Nigam and Antonio Cantero

Some Aspects of the Epidemiology and Etiology of Esophageal Cancer with Particular Emphasis on the Transkei, South Africa
Gerald P. Warwick and John S. Harington

Genetic Control of Murine Viral Leukemogenesis
Frank Lilly and Theodore Pincus

Marek's Disease: A Neoplastic Disease of Chickens Caused by a Herpesvirus
K. Nazerian

Mutation and Human Cancer
Alfred G. Knudson, Jr.

Mammary Neoplasia in Mice
S. Nandi and Charles M. McGrath

AUTHOR INDEX–SUBJECT INDEX

Volume 18

Immunological Aspects of Chemical Carcinogenesis
R. W. Baldwin

Isozymes and Cancer
Fanny Schapira

Physiological and Biochemical Reviews of Sex Differences and Carcinogenesis with Particular Reference to the Liver
Yee Chu Toh

Immunodeficiency and Cancer
John H. Kersey, Beatrice D. Spector, and Robert A. Good

Recent Observations Related to the

Chemotherapy and Immunology of Gestational Choriocarcinoma
K. D. Bagshawe

Glycolipids of Tumor Cell Membrane
Sen-itiroh Hakomori

Chemical Oncogenesis in Culture
Charles Heidelberger

AUTHOR INDEX–SUBJECT INDEX

Volume 19

Comparative Aspects of Mammary Tumors
J. M. Hamilton

The Cellular and Molecular Biology of RNA Tumor Viruses, Especially Avian Leukosis-Sarcoma Viruses, and Their Relatives
Howard M. Temin

Cancer, Differentiation, and Embryonic Antigens: Some Central Problems
J. H. Coggin, Jr. and N. G. Anderson

Simian Herpesviruses and Neoplasia
Fredrich W. Deinhardt, Lawrence A. Falk, and Lauren G. Wolfe

Cell Mediated Immunity to Tumor Cells
Ronald B. Herberman

Herpesviruses and Cancer
Fred Rapp

Cyclic AMP and the Transformation of Fibroblasts
Ira Pastan and George S. Johnson

Tumor Angiogenesis
Judah Folkman

SUBJECT INDEX

Volume 20

Tumor Cell Surfaces: General Alterations Detected by Agglutinins
Annette M. C. Rapin and Max M. Burger

Principles of Immunological Tolerance and Immunocyte Receptor Blockade
G. J. V. Nossal

The Role of Macrophages in Defense against Neoplastic Disease
Michael H. Levy and E. Frederick Wheelock

Epoxides in Polycyclic Aromatic Hydrocarbon Metabolism and Carcinogenesis
P. Sims and P. L. Grover

Virion and Tumor Cell Antigens of C-Type RNA Tumor Viruses
Heinz Bauer

Addendum to "Molecular Repair, Wound Healing, and Carcinogenesis: Tumor Production a Possible Overhealing?"
Sir Alexander Haddow

SUBJECT INDEX

RC
267
A45
v.21
1975

NOV 4 1975